Dermatomyositis

Lyubomir A. Dourmishev · Assen L. Dourmishev†

Dermatomyositis

Advances in Recognition, Understanding and Management

Foreword by Gerd Plewig

Springer

Lyubomir Dourmishev MD, PhD
Department of Dermatology
and Venereology
Medical University Sofia
1, St. Georgi Sofiiski Str.
1431 Sofia, Bulgaria

Assen L. Dourmishev MD, PhD, DSc †
Sofia, Bulgaria

ISBN: 978-3-540-79312-0 e-ISBN: 978-3-540-79313-7

DOI: 10.1007/978-3-540-79313-7

Library of Congress Control Number: 2008939991

Cover design: Frido Steinen-Broo, eStudio Calamar, Spain

Printed on acid-free paper

9 8 7 6 5 4 3 2 1

springer.com

Dedication

In memoriam of my father
Prof. Assen L. Dourmishev M.D., Ph.D., D.Sc.
who was so enthusiastic in initiating this book,
but was unable to see it published…

Two things are spent in different ways;
money diminishes, but knowledge increases.

Ch. Stambolsky
(1843–1932)

Foreword

Is there still a need for printed media, or are electronics the tool of the future? The answer is a clear yes for the former, but also for the latter. Books and other print forms have been with us for some 500 years since the revolutionary invention of the *Buchdruckerkunst* by Johannes Gutenberg from Mainz in Germany, movable type.

For us in medicine, be it investigative or clinical, books and journals are our daily instruments for the care of patients. One may say without exaggeration that printed pages, text and illustrations, are of eminent importance for learning and teaching alike.

Dermatomyositis. Advances in Understanding and Management is a monograph. I personally like monographs very much, as they cover a single subject in greater detail than available elsewhere, yet include differential aspects at the same time.

This new book is a welcome addition to the growing list of monographs dealing with individual diseases in dermatology, such as psoriasis, lupus erythematosus, photodermatoses and acne, just to name a few.

Dermatomyositis is not a problem of a single medical specialty; rather, it is dealt with in dermatology, neurology, internal medicine, family medicine, pathology, pediatrics, and oncology. Dermatomyositis is seen in the pediatric population but also as a paraneoplastic dermatomyositis in the elderly. Classic cases are no diagnostic problem, but the many faces of this awful disease challenge the best of clinicians.

Our colleagues and friends from Bulgaria, the late Assen L. Dourmishev, Professor and Chairman of Dermatology in Sofia, and his son Lyubomir A. Dourmishev, now in the same institution, have made a great effort to bring together the pertinent facts.

When I heard some time ago about the manuscript, I without hesitation encouraged Lyubomir A. Dourmishev to finish the work of his father. Our Bulgarian colleagues of dermatology can be proud of this contribution, which hopefully will find the wide international acceptance it deserves.

Finally, Springer-Verlag, Heidelberg, Germany, again shows courage in publishing monographs.

Prof. Dr. Dr. h.c. mult. Gerd Plewig, FRCP

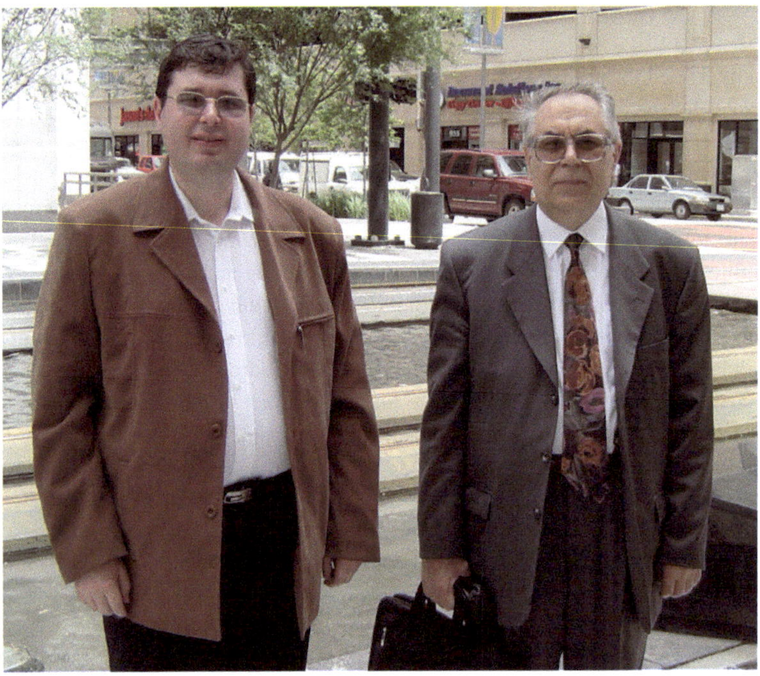

Lyubomir A. Dourmishev (left) Assen L. Dourmishev (right)

Preface

Although dermatomyositis is a rare disorder, it is of interest to different medical specialists such as rheumatologists, pediatricians, dermatologists, neurologists, and general practitioners, because of the diversity of clinical syndromes, the difficulties in diagnosis and therapeutic management, and the severe prognosis. The interdisciplinary disposition also complicates the diagnostic approach.

Sometimes the patient endures the long journey from one physician to another, and exact diagnosis takes a long period of time. The patient's saga becomes even more complicated following the definition of amyopathic dermatomyositis and drug-induced skin eruption resembling dermatomyositis. The author is one of the first clinicians who coined the possibility of the existence of "drug-induced dermatomyositis". It is true that dermatomyositis is difficult to diagnose if the physician does not expect it, or misdiagnoses it for another disease of connective tissue, for example lupus erythematosus, or even disregards its existence.

In my long practice, I have met many dermatomyositis patients, with unusual cases of disease, with different clinical manifestations and with variation in the diagnostic process. For example, a 46-year-old woman with breast cancer was removed from the operating table because the surgeon recognized a skin rash of face and extremities as "allergy" against anesthesia. In fact, the lady had paraneoplastic dermatomyositis.

This advanced monograph gives a description of the clinical symptoms of dermatomyositis and a methodology for diagnosis preparation, as well as new diagnostic immunological and photobiological methods and treatment modalities. The authors have personal experience with diagnoses, treatment, and management control of many dermatomyositis patients.

I hope that this book will be interesting and useful for many colleagues.

Sofia — Professor Dr. Assen L. Dourmishev PhD, DSc

Contents

Clinical Manifestations of Dermatomyositis

Complications of Dermatomyositis

List of Abbreviations

ADM	Amyopathic dermatomyositis
CK	Creatine kinase
CTD	Connective tissue disease
DM	Dermatomyositis
EP	Eosinophilic polymyositis
HLA	Human leukocyte antigen
IBM	Inclusion body myositis
IIM	Idiopathic inflammatory myopathies
ILD	Interstitial lung disease
IVIG	Intravenous immunoglobulin
JDM	Juvenile dermatomyositis
MAAs	Myosin-associated antibodies
MRI	Magnetic resonance imaging
MSAs	Myosin-specific antibodies
PDM	Paraneoplastic dermatomyositis
PM	Polymyositis
OS	Ovelap syndrome
SLE	Systemic lupus erythematosus
SSc	Systemic sclerosis (scleroderma)
TNF	Tissue necrosis factor
vWf	von Wilibrand factor
VCAM	Vascular cell adhesion molecule

1 Introduction

Dermatomyositis (DM) is a rare idiopathic inflammatory myopathy with muscle weakness and characteristic cutaneous manifestations. The disease is a rare assembly of systemic disorders in which idiopathic inflammatory myopathy (IIM) which does not affect neuromuscular transmission is associated with characteristic skin exanthema [1–3]. Today, several autoimmune disorders are subjoined to the group of DM and polymyositis, presented with cutaneous and muscle syndrome, with unclear etiology and probably different genesis. Clinical profile of DM is heterogeneous [4], and this heterogenous character of disease is supported by [5]:

(a) A strong association with malignancy [6, 7]
(b) A combination with features of other connective tissue diseases [6, 8], and a high level of autoantibodies [9]
(c) The existence of a separate cutaneous form without muscle damage [10]
(d) The absence of autoantibodies in two-thirds of patients [9]
(e) A different therapeutic response to immunosuppressive therapy depending upon the presence of high titers of antinuclear antibody (ANA) or myositis-specific autoantibody (MSAs) and malignancy [11, 12]
(f) Drug induction of clinical features of DM [13]

The investigation is hard to do because of the relatively seldom frequency of the disorder, the impossibility of carrying out simultaneous comparative surveillance, the atypical evolution and difficulties in differentiation from other disorders of connective tissue diseases, the presence of diverse clinical variants, and the availability sometimes of artifacts in implementing muscle biopsy [14]. Because the pathology in myositis is sometimes segmental [15] and the reading of biopsies is subjective, some patients with myositis will inevitably undergo non-diagnostic muscle biopsies [16]. This is the reason why patients with classic DM, especially children, with acute onset of symmetrical proximal weakness, raised levels of muscle enzymes in serum, MSAs, and pathognomonic rashes often do not undergo biopsy [16]. In one survey, a large percentage of pediatric rheumatologists indicated that they found electromyography (EMG) and muscle biopsy to have low incremental value when the hallmark cutaneous manifestations of DM present along with a typical pattern of muscle weakness [17, 18]. Moreover, the activities of muscle enzymes in serum are sometimes normal in patients with myositis [15].

L.A. Dourmishev and A.L. Dourmishev, *Dermatomyositis: Advances in Recognition, Understanding and Management*,

1

Dermatologists play a primary role in diagnosis and control of DM. In one retrospective study of juvenile DM, 25% of patients complained only of a rash on initial presentation, and 38% of patients presented to a dermatologist first, regardless of other symptoms [19]. Cutaneous manifestations of DM usually precede the onset of myositis by several months and for up to 2 years or more. In addition, skin involvement can be the most active or severe component of DM, failing to respond to therapeutic interventions that are adequate for myositis and other systemic involvement [20].

Most of the available information about DM is not of practical relevance to practicing dermatologists, for several reasons [21]:

(i) Dermatologists in Bulgaria as in other countries (e.g., USA) are involved only in the management of patients having cutaneous manifestations of DM.
(ii) Rheumatologists are primarily involved with the management of systemic manifestations of DM and other diseases involving IIM.
(iii) General discussions of the IIM often underemphasize the importance of:

  (a) Hallmark cutaneous manifestations of DM in the diagnosis of major disease subsets of IIM
  (b) The profound clinical impact which cutaneous inflammation can have on the quality of life of DM patients, whether or not they have myositis or other systemic disease manifestations
  (c) The existence of DM subsets that have clinical expression only or predominantly in the skin. The information related to the incidence of amyopathic DM in the USA derives predominantly from the outpatient practices of academic dermatologists.

The importance of investigations in this area is determined by the fact that, regardless of the restricted number of DM patients, the disorder may have acute evolution and may finish with fatal outcome, or in another cases, with a chronic, protracted march that leads to serious invalidity and in the final stage needs special care. Serious prognosis and high mortality rate of the disease ranges between 3% in juvenile DM in the USA [22] and 13% in adults [23] to 57.5% in patients with *Pneumocystis carinii* pneumonia [24] requiring the elaboration of new contemporary approaches for diagnostic and treatment. Cutaneous symptoms frequently precede by months or years the evolution of myositis, and early diagnosing, monitoring of clinical and laboratory indicators, as well as the implementation of an adequate therapy can dramatically improve the quality of patients' life and prolong its continuation.

In addition to the medical aspect, the disease requires the resolution of important social-economic problems and the consequence of affecting the working capacity of such patients.

References

1. Dalakas M. Polymyositis, dermatomyositis and inclusion body myositis. *N Engl J Med* 1991; 325(21): 1487–1498.
2. Drake L, Dinehart SM, Farmer ER, et al. Guidelines of care for dermatomyositis. *J Am Acad Dermatol* 1996; 34: 824–829.
3. Callen JP. Dermatomyositis. *Lancet* 2000; 355: 53–57.

4. Rybojad M, Ducloy G, Pricent F, et al. La dermatomyositis amyopathique de l'énfant: 5 cas. *Ann Dermatol Venereol* 2001; 128: 813–814.
5. Dourmishev LA, Dourmishev AL, Schwartz RA. Dermatomyositis: cutaneous manifestations of its variants. *Int J Dermatol* 2002; 41: 625–630.
6. Bohan A, Peter JB, Bowman RL, Pearson CM. A computer-assisted analysis of 153 patients with polymyositis and dermatomyositis. *Medicine* 1977; 56: 255–286.
7. Manchul LA, Jin A, Pritchard K, et al. The frequency of malignant neoplasms in patients with polymyositis-dermatomyositis. *Arch Int Med* 1985; 145: 1835–1839.
8. Jablonska S, Chorselski TP, Blaszczyk M, et al. Scleroderma/polymyositis overlap syndromes and their immunologic markers. *Clin Dermatol* 1992; 10: 457–472.
9. Targoff IN. Humoral immunity in polymyositis/dermatomyositis. *J Invest Dermatol* 1993; 100: 116S–125S.
10. Euwer RL, Sontheimer RD. Amyopathic dermatomyositis (dermatomyositis sine myositis). Presentation of six new cases and review of the literature. *J Am Acad Dermatol* 1991; 24: 959–966.
11. Love LA, Leff RL, Fraser DD, et al. A new approach to the classification of idiopathic inflammatory myopathy: myositis-specific autoantibodies define useful homogeneous patient groups. *Medicine* 1991; 70: 360–374.
12. Gottfried I, Seeber A, Anegg B, et al. High dose intravenous immunoglobulin (IVIG) in dermatomyositis: clinical responses and effect on sIL-2R levels. *Eur J Dermatol* 2000; 10: 29–35.
13. Dourmishev AL, Dourmishev LA. Dermatomyositis and drugs. *Adv Exp Med Biol* 1999; 455: 187–191.
14. Grau JM, Perea M. Dermatomyositis with features of inclusion body myositis associated with carcinoma of the bladder: a true association? *Br J Dermatol* 2001; 143: 645–690.
15. Bohan A, Peter JB. Polymyositis and dermatomyositis. *N Engl J Med* 1975; 292 (part I): 344–347.
16. Miller FW, Rider LG, Plotz PH, Isenberg DA, Oddis CV. Diagnostic criteria for polymyositis and dermatomyositis. *Lancet* 2003; 362: 1762–1763.
17. Moenkemoeller K, Petty RE, Malleson PN, et al. What criteria do pediatric rheumatologists use to make the diagnosis of juvenile dermatomyositis? *Arthritis Rheum* 2001; 44: S293.
18. Murray KJ. Juvenile dermatomyositis: advances in understanding and management. *APLAR J Rheumatol* 2003; 6: 50–63.
19. Peloro TM, Miller OF, Hahn TF, et al. Juvenile dermatomyositis: a retrospective review of a 30-year experience. *J Am Acad Dermatol* 2001; 45: 28–34.
20. Santmyire-Rosenberger B, Dugan EM. Skin involvement in dermatomyositis. *Curr Opin Rheumatol* 2003; 15(6): 714–722
21. Sontheimer RD. Dermatomyositis: an overview of recent progress with emphasasis on dermatologic aspects. *Dermatol Clin* 2002; 20: 387–408.
22. Pachman LM. Juvenile dermatomyositis. *Pediatr Clin North Am* 1995; 42: 1071–1098.
23. Clarke AE, Bloch DA, Medsger TA, et al. A longitudinal study of functional disability in a national cohort of patients with polymyositis/dermatomyositis. *Arthritis Rheum* 1995; 38: 1218–1224.
24. Ward MM, Donald F. *Pneumocystis carinii* pneumonia in patients with connective tissue diseases. *Arth Rheum* 1999; 42(4): 780–789.

History of Dermatomyositis

2

The first detailed descriptions of patients with rare muscle disease (acute form of myositis) with cutaneous lesions were reported by E. Wagner [1] in 1863 and P. Potain (1875) [2]. These authors introduced to the medical community a new group of IIMs, characterized by the damage of many skeletal muscles and by skin manifestations. These disorders are rare, but increasingly recognized. They have avariety of clinical manifestations, immunological abnormalities and courses, and form a diverse group of diseases with unclear causes. The most common forms of these disorders are dermatomyositis (DM) and polymyositis (PM) [3].

In 1887, Professor Hans Unvericht published a description of a peculiar muscle disease with fatigue and malaise, muscle pain and weakness, swelling of face, and bluish lesions over eyelids [4]. He reported a 27-year-old stonemason, who developed acute onset of weakness, stiffness, and pain in the proximal arm, leg, and back muscles. A week later, diffuse swelling of face and extremities, accompanied by a low-grade evening fevers and a bluish rash over his eyelids, had developed. Over the next few days the patient noticed shortness of breath, thickening of the voice, and dysphagia. After several weeks, the patient died with cyanosis and clinical manifestation of a pulmonary arrest. Autopsy showed fluid-filled lungs and swollen proximal muscles. Histopathological examination showed various stages of degeneration of muscle fibers, and focal round-cell interstitial infiltration of the affected muscles. In 1891, Unvericht reported a second case and gave a name to this disorder — **dermatomyositis** [5].

Up to the end of the nineteenth century, several authors published independently clinical descriptions of these disorders. Twenty-eight cases had been reported, and the name of the disease was coined variously as myositis universalis acuta, polymyositis, pseudotrichinosis, or DM [6–10].

In the first decade of the twentieth century, Jacoby observed a patient with skin atrophy, edema of the face and eyelids, arthralgias, and weakness of muscles, and reported the case as poikiloderma vascularis atrophicans [11].

In 1916 the first two cases of DM with association of malignancy (i.e., paraneoplastic DM) [12, 13] were published. Stertz [12] reported a patient of DM associated with gastric cancer, and Krenkeleit reported DM associated with breast cancer [13].

Petges and Clejat (1926) reported a case with idiopathic atrophic sclerosis of the skin, subcutaneous calcinosis, and myositis [14]. Gottron [15] in 1930 provided an extensive

L.A. Dourmishev and A.L. Dourmishev, *Dermatomyositis: Advances in Recognition, Understanding and Management,* © Springer-Verlag Berlin Heidelberg 2009

2

description of cutaneous manifestations of DM, and introduced erythematous papules and macular lesions covering bony prominences as a specific hallmark of the disease. Mills in 1993 [16] noted that no extensive clinical experience was reported in English literature until that of O'Leary and Waismann (1940) from the Mayo Clinic, who analyzed 40 cases.

The first cases of DM in children were reported by Hecht in 1940 [17]. The vascular pathology of juvenile DM was initially recognized by Wedgewood et al. [18] in 1953. Later on, Everett and Curtis (1957) [19] and Banker and Victor (1966) [20], emphasized the differences between juvenile and adult DM.

Keil (1942) [21] was among in the first who differentiated DM from systemic lupus erythematosus (SLE) and accepted the idea that cutaneous manifestations of DM may precedes the muscle disease.

The first cases of DM in Bulgaria were described in 1941 and 1943 by V. Ganev [22] and L. Popov [23].

Two periods are recognized in the development of the concept of DM in the twentieth century: the first is up to the mid-1970s, when the main parameters of the diseases were identified and the criteria for diagnosis of myopathy were formulated [24]. In 1977 Bohan and Peter defined five diagnostic criteria for the idiopathic nonsuppurative inflammatory disorders of striated muscles, which became useful for accurate diagnosis in clinical practice [24]. Although empirically derived, these criteria are useful to include cases within a well-defined range and to exclude patients in which the diagnosis may be in doubt in prospective and retrospective studies [25].

DM sine myositis was first described in six patients by Krain in 1975 [26], but the term amyopathic DM was introduced by Pearson in 1979 [27] for the patients who had typical cutaneous findings of DM but did not have any clinical or laboratory signs of muscle disease for at least 2 years after the onset of the skin pathology.

The second period in the development of the concept of DM in the twentieth century started with the determination of cutaneous signs and formulation of new clinical forms [28–32]. At the same time, some MSAs were identified [32–35], and new therapeutic modalities were introduced.

Serologic studies during the past 25 years have demonstrated the presence of autoantibodies in DM/PM patients, and have helped to classify some of these patients into specific subsets (i.e., the antisynthetase syndrome) [36]. Between 1976 and 1985 Reichlin, in collaboration with Nishikai, Arnett, and Targoff, detailed the multiplicity of autoantibodies in DM and PM, including recognition of anti-Mi-2 and anti-Jo-1 antibodies, in a series of articles [33–38].

References

1. Wagner E. Fall einer seltnen Muskelkrankheit. *Dtsch Arch Heilk* 1863; 4: 282–283.
2. Poten PC. Morve chronique de forme anormal. *Bull et Mem Hop Paris* 1875; 12: 314–318.
3. Bohan A, Peter JB. Polymyositis and dermatomyositis (part 1). *N Engl J Med* 1975; 292: 344–347.
4. Unverricht H. Polymyositis acuta progressive. *Z Klin Med* 1887; 12: 553.
5. Unverricht H. Dermatomyositis acuta. *Dtsch Med Wochenschr* 1891; 17: 41–44.

6. Unverricht H. Über eine eigenthümliche Form von akuter Muskelentzündung mit einem der Trichinose-ähnelnden Krankheitsbilde. *Müncher Med Wochnschrf* 1887; 34: 488–492.
7. Hepp P. Über einen Fall von acuter parenhymatoser Myositis, welche Geschwulste bildete und Fluctuation vortauschte. *Berlin Klin Wochenschr* 1887; 24: 389.
8. Jackson H. A case of acute, infectious universal myositis. *Boston Med Surg J* 1887; 116: 498.
9. Wagner E. Fall einer seltenen Muskelkrankheit. *Arch Heikd* 1886; 4: 242.
10. Wagner E. Ein Fall von acuter Polymyositis. *Dtsch Arch Klin Med* 1886–1887; 11: 241.
11. Jacobi E. Fall für Diagnose (Poikilodermia vascularis atrophicans). *Verh Dtsch Dermatol Ges* 1907; 9: 321–323.
12. Stertz G. Polymyositis. *Berl Klin Wochenshr* 1916; 53: 489.
13. Kankeleit H. Über primaire nichteitrige Polymyositis. *Dtsch Arch Klin Med.* 1916; 120: 335–339.
14. Patjes G, Clejat C. Sclerose atrophic de la peau et myosite. *Ann Derm et Syphil Paris* 1926; 550–568.
15. Gottron H. Hautveränderungen bei Dermatomyositis. VIII Congres Intern. Dermatol. et Syphilogr., Copenhagen, 5–8 Agout, 1930, *Compt rend Seancy*, Ed. S.Lomholt, Copenhagen 1931; 826–830.
16. Mills JA. Dermatomyositis. In: *Dermatology in General Medicine*, Fitzpatrick TB, Eisen AZ, Wolff K, et al. (eds), McGraw-Hill, New York, 1993; 2148–2155.
17. Hecht MS. Dermatomyositis in children. *J Pediatr* 1940; 17: 791.
18. Wedgwood RJ, Cook CD, Cohen J. Dermatomyositis: report of 26 cases in children with a discussion of endocrine therapy in 13. *Pediatrics* 1953; 12: 447–466.
19. Everett MA, Curtis AC. Dermatomyositis: a review of 19 cases in adolescents and children. *Arch Intern Med* 1957; 100: 70–76.
20. Banker B, Viktor M. Dermatomyositis (systemic angiopathy) of childhood. *Medicine* 1966; 45: 261–289.
21. Keil H. The manifestations in the skin and mucus membranes in dermatomyositis with special reference to the differential diagnosis from systemic lupus erythematosus. *Ann Intern Med* 1942; 16: 827.
22. Ganev V. Dermatomyositis. *Bulg Clin* 1941; 13(1): 1–15 [Bulgarian].
23. Popov L. Dermatomyositis (Morbus Wagner-Potain). *Bulg Clin* 1943; 15(3): 117–139 [Bulgarian].
24. Bohan A, Peter JB, Bowman RL, Pearson CM. A computer-assisted analysis of 153 patients with polymyositis and dermatomyositis. *Medicine* 1977; 56: 255–286.
25. Caro I. Dermatomyositis as a systemic disease. *Med Clin North Am* 1989; 73: 1181–1192.
26. Krain LS. Dermatomyositis in six patients without initial muscle involvement. *Arch Dermatol* 1975; 111: 241–246.
27. Pearson CM. Polymyositis and dermatomyositis. In: *Arthritis (and Allied Conditions)*, Mc Carty DJ (ed.), 9th ed. Lea & Febiger, Philadelphia, 1979; 742.
28. Euwer RL, Sontheimer RD. Amyopathic dermatomyositis (dermatomyositis sine myositis). Presentation of six new cases and review of the literature. *J Am Acad Dermatol* 1991; 24: 959–966
29. Blaszczyk M, Jablonska S, Szymanska-Jagiello W, et al. Childhood sclero-myositis: an overlap syndrome associated with PM-Scl antibody. *Pediatr Dermatol* 1991; 8: 1–8.
30. Basset-Seguin N, Roujeau JC, Gherardi R, et al. Prognostic factors and predictive signs of malignancy in adult dermatomyositis. A study of 32 cases. *Arch Dermatol* 1990; 126: 633–637.
31. Chapurlat R, Tebib JG, Noel E, et al. Dermatomyosite induite par la d-penicillamine au cours d'une polyarthrite rheumatoide. *Rheumatologie* 1995; 47: 203–207.
32. Love LA, Feff RL, Fraser DD, et al. A new approach to the classification of idiopathic inflammatory myopathy: myositis-specific autoantibodies define useful homogeneous patient group. *Medicine* 1991; 70: 360–374.

33. Nishikai M, Reichlin M. Heterogeneity of precipitating antibodies in polymyositis and dermatomyositis. Characterization of the Jo-1 antibody system. *Arthritis Rheum* 1980; 23: 881–888.
34. Targoff IN, Reichlin M. The association between Mi-2 antibodies and dermatomyositis. *Arthritis Rheum* 1985; 28: 796–803.
35. Targoff IN, Johnson AE, Miller FW. Antibody to signal recognition particle in polymyositis. *Arthritis Rheum* 1990; 33: 1361–1370.
36. Targoff IN. Humoral immunity in polymyositis/dermatomyositis. *J Invest Dermatol* 1993; 100: 116s–123s.
37. Arnett FC, Hirsch TJ, Bias WB, Nishikai M, Reichlin M. The Jo-1 antibody system in myositis. Relationships to clinical features and HLA. *J Rheumatol* 1981; 8: 925–930.
38. Nilasena DS, Trieu EP, Targoff IN. Analysis of the MI-2 autoantigen of dermatomyositis. *Arthritis Rheum* 1995; 38: 123–128.

Classification of Dermatomyositis 3

Idiopathic inflammatory myopathies (IIMs) or myositis are a heterogeneous group of acquired systemic diseases that are characterized by weakness and chronic inflammation in skeletal muscles and other target organs, with variability in their clinical and laboratory parameters, prognosis, and response to therapy [1, 2]. In 1975, Bohan and Peter [3, 4] wrote a classic article that suggested five subsets of myositis and PM and DM classified according to subtypes and prevalence (Table 3.1). A combined sensitivity for defined and probable PM or DM was determined to range from 74% to 100% in several studies that included a total of 885 patients [5–7].

One of the limitations of Bohan and Peter's [3–5] classification is that inclusion body myositis (IBM) was not recognized as a subset of myositis. Dalakas [1] suggested a new classification of acquired inflammatory myopathies which included PM, DM, and IBM. Based on well-defined clinical, demographic, histologic, and immunopathologic criteria, a new subset known as IBM has been identified as a distinct variety of IIM [1, 8, 9].

In 1991 Euwer and Sontheimer [10], based on the cases previously reported in literature [4, 11, 12] and their own observations, proposed a revision of Bohan and Peter's original classification system of DM/PM, and included "amyopathic DM" or "DM sine myositis"as the sixth type of the disease. Amyopathic DM refers to a condition in which the typical cutaneous eruption of DM is present but muscle disease is lacking [10]. This clinical variant of DM is the opposite of polymyositis, in which muscle disease is present but cutaneous disease is lacking. In fact, the category of amyopathic DM is controversial according to the strict Bohan and Peter criteria, since patients with such clinical presentation fulfill only one criterion and may have "suspected DM" [13]. However, the Bohan and Peter definition has no criteria for "possible DM" without muscle affection, and because of the low specificity of skin lesions it may be difficult to distinguish cases of amyopathic DM from other early connective tissue diseases — for example, lupus erythematosus (LE) [14, 15].

The clinical entity amyopathic DM included patients with either cutaneous disease alone [16], or patients with cutaneous disease and minimal muscle involvement [10, 12]. A classification scheme for patients having cutaneous manifestation of DM with three groups was proposed [16, 17]: (i) patients with skin changes only (amyopathic DM), (ii) patients with cutaneous manifestations at baseline and subsequent evolution to myositis

3

Table 3.1 Classification of dermatomyositis (DM) and polymyositis (PM) [3, 4]

I.	Polymyositis	30–40%
II.	Dermatomyositis	20–30%
III.	Dermatomyositis and polymyositis with malignancy	10–15%
IV.	Juvenile dermatomyositis	10%
V.	Overlap syndrome (DM/PM with another connective tissue disease)	20%

Table 3.2 Comprehensive classification of cutaneous manifestations of the idiopathic inflammatory myopathies (IIMs) (Adapted from an earlier published version [21])

Type of myositis	Distinguishing features	Cutaneous lesions	Reference
1. Polymyositis	Myositis with proximal weakness	None of the features below	[5]
2. Classic DM	Muscle involvement and characteristic skin lesions	Heliotrope eruption and Gottron's papules and signs	[5]
3. Paraneoplastic DM	Cancer diagnosed within 1–2 years after the onset of myositis	Epidermal necrosis	[22]
4. Juvenile DM	Onset before the age of 18, frequent gastrointestinal vasculitis	Typical rash, vasculopathic/ulcerative lesions	[23]
5. Overlap syndrome/DM	Association with another connective tissue disease	Gottron's papules, mechanic's hands	[24]
6. Amyopathic DM	Characteristic skin lesions without muscle involvement	Gottron's papules and signs, heliotrope rash	[20]
7. Drug-induced DM/PM	Onset associated with intake of medicine	Heliotrope eruption and Gottron's papules	[18]
8. Inclusion body myositis	Distal involvement; ringlet vacuoles in myofibers; intracellular tubofibrillar inclusion bodies; deposits of ectopic beta-amyloid, ubiquitin	Heliotrope eruption, erythema, and periorbital edema	[25]
9. Granulomatous myositis	Chronic inflammation with prominent granulomas in the muscle biopsy		[19]
10. Eosinophilic myositis/ perimyositis	Chronic inflammation with prominent eosinophils on biopsy	Cellulitis-like subcutaneous induration, erythema, angioedema, urticarial, and papular lesions	[26]

(continued)

Table 3.2 (continued)

Type of myositis	Distinguishing features	Cutaneous lesions	Reference
11. Focal nodular myositis	Focal involvement of one or more extremities with pain, swelling, and inflammatory nodules		[19]
12. Orbital myositis	Cellular infiltration of lymphocytes, macrophages, and giant cells in the endomyocardial biopsy	Periorbital edema and erythema of the eyelids	[27]

(classic DM), and (iii) cases with skin lesions and normal muscle enzymes in whom diagnostic evaluations revealed subclinical myositis (hypomyopathic DM).

Various medications have been reported that may cause myopathy and cutaneous lesions, so an eighth subset known as "drug-induced DM/PM" has been recognized [18].

Based on the clinical and pathological features, several subgroups of myositis syndromes such as focal myositis, orbital myositis, eosinophilic myositis, granulomatous myositis, etc. are differentiated [19, 20]. The distinction between DM and PM is perhaps more academic than practical, since the presence of any cutaneous findings precludes the disgnosis of PM. Recently, cutaneous findings have been reported in patients with IBM, eosinophilic perimyositis (EP), and ocular myositis with giant cell myocarditis [21] (Table 3.2).

Within these IIM categories, the different clinical syndromes are recognized. Distinct clinical phenotypes have been reported to be associated with certain myositis-specific autoantibodies (MSAs), which could be useful for subclassification of myositis and have prognostic implications [19, 28]. The comparison of clinical and laboratory studies of MSAs to the standard myositis subsets (DM, PM, IBM) suggests that each group of these autoantibodies defines an IIM syndrome that is different from others in immunogenetics, clinical manifestations, severity of disease and prognosis and can be considered as a distinct disorder [19, 28, 29]. Three subsets of IIM have been reported: (i) "antisynthetase syndrome" [28], (ii) anti-signal recognition particle syndrome [29], and (iii) anti-Mi-2 autoantibody syndrome [28] (see also Chapter 31).

References

1. Dalakas M. Polymyositis, dermatomyositis and inclusion body myositis. *N Engl J Med* 1991; 325(21): 1487–1498.
2. Plotz PH, Rider LG, Targoff, et al. NIH conference. Myositis: immunologic contributions to understanding cause, pathogenesis, and therapy. *Ann Intern Med* 1995; 122: 715–724.
3. Bohan A, Peter JB. Polymyositis and dermatomyositis (part 1). *N Engl J Med.* 1975; 292: 344–347.
4. Bohan A, Peter JB. Polymyositis and dermatomyositis (part 2). *N Engl J Med.* 1975; 292: 403–407.
5. Bohan A, Peter JB, Bowman RL, Pearson CM. A computer-assisted analysis of 153 patients with polymyositis and dermatomyositis. *Medicine* 1977; 6: 55–286.

6. Medsger TA, Oddis CV. Classification and diagnostic criteria for polymyositis and dermatomyositis. *Medicine* 1997; 56: 255–286.
7. Targoff IN, Miller FW, Medsger TA Jr, et al. Classification criteria for the idiopathic inflammatory myopathies. *Curr Opin Rheum* 1997; 9: 527–535.
8. Carpenter S, Karpati G, Heller I, et al. Inclusion body myositis: a distinct variety of idiopathic inflammatory myopathy. *Neurology* 1978; 28: 8–17.
9. Sayers ME, Chou SM, Calabrese LH. Inclusion body myositis: analysis of 32 cases. *J Rheumatol* 1992; 19(9): 1385–1389.
10. Euwer RL, Sontheimer RD. Amyopathic dermatomyositis (dermatomyositis sine myositis). Presentation of six new cases and review of the literature. *J Am Acad Dermatol* 1991; 24: 959–966.
11. Krain LS. Dermatomyositis in six patients without initial muscle involvement. *Arch Dermatol* 1975; 111: 241–246.
12. Pearson CM. Polymyositis and dermatomyositis. In: *Arthritis (and Allied Conditions)*. Mc Carty DJ (ed.), 9th ed. Lea & Febiger, Philadelphia, 1979; 742.
13. Kovacs SO, Kovacs SC. Dermatomyositis. *J Am Acad Dermatol* 1998; 39: 899–920.
14. Whitmore SE, Watson R, Rosenshein NB, Provost TT. Dermatomyositis sine myositis: association with malignancy. *J Rheumatol* 1996; 23(1): 101–105.
15. Smith CA, Pinals RS. Periorbital edema in systemic lupus erythematosus. *Arch Intern Med* 1982; 142(9): 1711–1712.
16. Stonecipher MR, Jorizzo JL, White WL, et al. Cutaneous changes of dermatomyositis in patients with normal muscle enzymes: dermatomyositis sine myositis. *J Am Acad Dermatol* 1993; 28(6): 951–956.
17. Park JH, Olsen NJ. Utility of magnetic resonance imaging in the evolution of patients with inflammatory myopathies. *Curr Rheumatol Rep* 2001; 3: 334–345.
18. Dourmishev AL, Dourmishev LA. Dermatomyositis and drugs. *Adv Exp Med Biol* 1999; 455: 187–191.
19. Miller FW. Myositis-specific autoantibodies: Touchstones for understanding the inflammatory myopathies. *JAMA* 1993; 270: 1846–1849.
20. Sontheimer RD. Dermatomyositis: an overview of recent progress with emphasis on dermatologic aspects. *Dermatol Clin* 2002; 20: 387–408.
21. Dourmishev, LA, Dourmishev AL Schwartz, RA. Dermatomyositis: cutaneous manifestations of its variants. *Int J Dermatol* 2002; 41: 625–630.
22. Mautner GH, Grossman ME, Silvers DN, et al. Epidermal necrosis as a predictive sign of malignancy in adult dermatomyositis. *Cutis* 1998; 61(4): 190–194.
23. Murray KJ. Juvenile dermatomyositis: advances in understanding and management. *APLAR J Rheumatol* 2003; 6: 50–63.
24. Jablonska S, Blaszcyk M. Scleromyositis: a scleroderma/polymyositis overlap syndrome. *Clin Rheumatol* 1998; 17: 465–467.
25. Talanin NY, Bushore D, Rasberry R, et al. Dermatomyositis with the features of inclusion body myositis associated with carcinoma of the bladder. *Br J Dermatol* 1999; 141: 926–930.
26. Trüeb RM, Pericin M, Winzeler B, et al. Eosinophilic myositis/ perimyositis: frequency and spectrum of cutaneous manifestations. *J Am Acad Dermatol* 1997; 37: 385–391.
27. Stevens AW, Grossman ME, Barr ML. Orbital myositis, vitiligo and giant cell myocarditis. *J Am Acad Dermatol* 1996; 35: 310–312.
28. Love LA, Feff RL, Fraser DD, et al. A new approach to the classification of idiopathic inflammatory myopathy: myositis-specific autoantibodies define useful homogeneous patient group. *Medicine* 1991; 70: 360–374.
29. Targoff IN, Johnson AE, Miller FW. Antibody to signal recognition particle in polymyositis. *Arthritis Rheum* 1990; 33: 1361–1370.

Diagnostic Criteria 4

4.1 Helpful Hints

The purpose of classification criteria for idiopathic inflammatory myopathies is to define homogenous groups of patients [1]. These criteria can be used in studies that aim to increase the knowledge about disease mechanisms and to improve the treatment in disorders in which etiology is unknown. Great progress has been made during the past 30 years in characterizing the clinical features of IIMs. In 1975 Bohan and Peter, focusing upon non-neurogenic muscle involvement, suggested five diagnostic criteria for the diagnosis of PM/DM, which today are an accepted standard [2, 3] (Table 4.1). The presence of distinguishing skin features, including heliotrope rash, Gottron's papules, and characteristically distributed macular erythemas, is the fifth criterion. Although these are the most typical cutaneous manifestations, skin findings of DM can be heterogeneous, and these hallmark cutaneous lesions may not be evident at the time of presentation [4].

The presence of three or four criteria for myositis plus the cutaneous rash in a patient defines a definitive diagnosis for DM, and the availability of four criteria without the skin rash provides the same for PM. Bohan and Peter outlined a systemic way to describe the probability of having the diseases as definite, probable, and possible. The patients who fulfill four criteria have definite PM/DM, those who cover three criteria have probable PM/DM, and patients with two criteria — possible PM/DM. Cutaneous eruption must be one of the stated number of criteria in patients with definite, probable, or possible DM.

One of the limitations of the criteria proposed by Bohan and Peter is the imprecise definition of the individual criterion [1]. The degree of abnormality for the serum levels of muscle enzymes, EMG, or histopathological changes in muscle biopsies was not defined [1]. A wide variety of skin lesions were included in the original criteria for DM.

The Japanese research committees for Autoimmune Diseases, Scleroderma, and Neuro-Immunological Diseases outlined new criteria for DM and added them to those of Bohan and Peter, showing high sensitivity and specificity [5] (Table 4.2).

Patients presenting at least one finding from item 1 and four findings from items 2 to 9 have DM with 94.1% sensitivity and 90.3% specificity of skin lesions against LE and systemic sclerosis (SSc). Patients presenting at least four findings have PM (98.9% sensitivity,

4

Table 4.1 Diagnostic criteria for polymyositis/dermatomyositis [2, 3]

1. Symmetrical proximal muscle weakness of the limb girdle muscles and anterior neck flexors, with or without dysphagia or respiratory muscle involvement; progressing weeks to months
2. Elevation of serum levels of skeletal-muscle enzymes
3. Evidence of an inflammatory myopathy on muscle biopsy
4. Electromyographic features of a myopathy
5. Characteristic cutaneous eruption present in DM, but not in PM

Table 4.2 Classification criteria for dermatomyositis [5]

1. Skin lesions
– Heliotrope rash (red purple edematous erythema on the upper eyelids)
– Gottron's papules and sign
– Shawl sign/V-sign
2. Proximal muscle weakness
3. Elevated muscle enzymes (CK and aldolase)
4. Muscle pain on grasping or spontaneous pain
5. Myogenic changes on EMG
6. Positive anti-Jo-1 antibody test
7. Nondestructive arthritis or arthralgias
8. Systemic inflammatory signs
Temperature ≥37°C (98.6°F) at axilla
Accelerated ESR ≥20 mm/h by Westergren, or
Elevated serum C-reactive protein level
9. Pathologic findings compatible with inflammatory myositis

and 95.2% specificity of PM and DM against all control diseases). Cutaneous lesions shown to have a high specificity compared with SLE and SSc were the heliotope rash, Gottron's sign, and erythema on extensor surface of joints (98.7%, 99.6%, and 90.7% specificity, respectively) [5]. The Gottron's papules and sign were considered to be diagnostic for DM [6], whereas the heliotrope rash and erythema over extensor surfaces of extremities were found to be less specific by a committee from the American Academy of Dermatology [7]. Three of the four additional new criteria (spontaneous muscle pain or pain on grasping, arthritis or arthralgias, and systemic inflammatory signs such as fever, elevated C-reactive protein, or erythrocyte sedimentation rate (ESR) are uncommon in non-inflammatory neuromuscular disease but are common in other connective tissue diseases, and thus not particularly helpful in establishing diagnosis in individual patients from a rheumatology perspective [1]. The fourth proposed criterion, the presence of anti-Jo-1 antibodies, is a more specific feature of myositis, and has been suggested for inclusion in classification criteria for IIM [5].

It has been recognized, however, that there is a subset of patients with skin lesions typical for DM who never developed clinical evidence of muscle disease, and this group is termed "amyopatic DM" or "DM sine myositis" [6]. These patients have only skin lesions as their

Table 4.3 Revised criteria for diagnosis of IIM [10]

1. Symmetric proximal muscle weakness[a]
2. Elevation of serum levels of skeletal-muscle enzymes[a]
3. Abnormal EMG
4. Features of inflammatory infiltration, degeneration, or perifascicular atrophy in muscle biopsy
5. One of the MSAs (antisynthetase, anti-Mi2, or anti-SRP)
6. Typical skin rash of DM: Gottron's sign, Gottron's papules, or heliotrope rash

Definite IIM = any four criteria; Probable IIM = any three criteria; Possible IIM = any two criteria
[a]Results of MRI that are consistent with muscle inflammation may be substituted for either criterion 1 or 2.

primary manifestation of DM. Amyopathic DM is accepted by dermatologists, but has not been widely recognized outside the field of dermatology. This can be partially accounted for by the fact that the accepted criteria for PM/DM require myositis. This category is controversial in that, by strict Bohan and Peter criteria, patients with this presentation only fulfill one criteria and may have suspected DM [6]. Tanimoto's classification and diagnostic criteria for PM and DM also do not recognize the amyopathic DM variant [8].

Recent data on myositis-specific antibodies (MSA) provide a better categorization for the evaluation of patients [9]. The possibility of determining MSA, as well as the feasibility of using MRI as a diagnostic tool in IIMs, led to a proposal for revised classification criteria for these diseases, with the aim of increasing the sensitivity without reducing specificity. The addition of MSA and the use of MRI to identify muscle inflammation in order to improve the sensitivity of criteria for the diagnosis of DM have been proposed [10] (Table 4.3).

For diagnostic purposes, both testing for Jo-1, Mi-2, and MRI of the muscles and musculoskeletal ultrasound could be helpful, as well as previously suggested clinical symptoms, muscle enzymes, EMG, and muscle biopsy [1, 10–12].

The subject of diagnostic criteria remains unsettled, because the various proposed criteria [13] have not been properly validated. The criteria of Bohan and Peter cannot distinguish PM from IBM or from certain dystrophies [14]. Muscle biopsy is needed for the confirmation of an inflammatory myopathy and for the exclusion of other muscle disorders as well as for subclassification of the IIMs. Because the immunopathological characteristics confer specificity for each subset, the diagnostic criteria should rely on histopathology and immunopathology as the best means of separating PM from other myopathies [14].

4.2 Myositis Diagnostic Tests

4.2.1 Confirmatory Tests

The conventional procedures for diagnosis and therapeutic evaluations of DM include: (i) physical examination for muscle strength and endurance, (ii) measurement of serum levels of muscle enzymes, (iii) detection of MSA, (iv) electromyography, and (v) the presence of active muscle inflammation in muscle biopsy MRI or ultrasound investigations. These procedures are limited by subjectivity, low specificity, and invasiveness.

(i) **Physical examination for muscle strength and endurance**

The diagnosis of muscle involvement can be determined by physical examination demonstrating muscle weakness or loss of power. The strength of muscles may be graded according to their ability to act against pressure and resistance offered by an examiner, as proposed by the well-known MRC grading system. This can be done with formal quantitative muscle testing as well as by assessing the ability of patients to perform their daily activities. For this purpose the following functional tests are used:

(a) **Functional tests** based on questionnaires [15].
(b) **Manual Muscle Test (MMT)** with the **Medical Research Council (MRC) scale** is the the most commonly used technique for assessing the muscle function [16, 17].
(c) **Functional Index of Myositis** is a reliable functional test for clinical practice [18], which measures muscle strength and endurance. It is feasible for a follow-up study of exercise [19].

(ii) **Measurement of serum levels of muscle enzymes**

The most frequently elevated serum muscle enzymes in DM/PM [20] are present in Table 4.4.

Creatine kinase (CK), is the most sensitive and the most specific (MM subtype) for skeletal-muscle damage.

(iii) **Determination of serum levels of myositis-specific autoantibodies (MSA)**

A positive MSAs has a highly predictive value for myositis [10, 21]. MSAs determined in patients with DM are presented in Table 4.5. The fact that none of the MSAs has prevalence greater than 20% of IIM patients' sera makes routine clinical testing for these autoantibodies clinically significant (see Chapter 31)

(iv) **Abnormal electromyogram**

EMG is helpful in distinguishing myopathy from neuropathy [22]. An abnormal EMG (short-duration, polyphasic motor unit potentials with spontaneous fibrillation potentials) has been recorded in 90% of patients with DM/PM [23, 24].

(v) **Presence of active inflammation in muscle biopsy, MRI, or ultrasound**

(a) **Muscle biopsy.** A definitive diagnosis of DM/PM is established by muscle biopsy, since other clinical conditions can produce muscle weakness and mimic an

Table 4.4 Sarcoplasmatic muscle enzymes elevated in DM/PM

1. Creatine kinase (CK)
2. Aspartate aminotransferase (AST)
3. Alanine aminotransferase (ALT)
4. Lactate dehydrogenase (LDH, isoenzymes 4 and 5)
5. Aldolase (subtype A)
6. Carbonic anhydrase (isoenzyme III)

Table 4.5 MSAs determined in DM

	Antibody	Target	Frequency (%)
Anti-Mi-2			~20
		Antisynthetase	
	Anti-Jo-1	Histidyl-tRNA synthetase	~20
	Anti-PL-7	Threonyl-tRNA synthetase	~3
	Anti-PL-12	Alanyl-tRNA synthetase	~3
	Anti-OJ	Isoleucyl-tRNA synthetase	~1
	Anti-EJ	Glycyl-tRNA synthetase	~1
	Anti-KS	Asparginyl-tRNA synthetase	<1
Anti-SRP			3

inflammatory muscle disease. Muscle biopsy is the most sensitive way to assess muscle changes, but it may not be an ideal way to monitor the efficacy of therapy, due to the inconvenience for the patient and costs [25]. This problem could be overcome by performing percutaneous conchotome muscle biopsies which can be performed in an out-patient clinic, with little discomfort for the patient, and with a very low complication rate [26, 27]. The preferred site for muscle biopsy is the quadriceps or biceps muscles. EMG or MRI can assist in selecting the site for muscle biopsy [28]. Biopsies of muscle identified by EMG must be interpreted with caution, since the inserting of needles for EMG may induce nonspecific inflammation and necrosis [29].

(b) **Magnetic resonance imaging (MRI)**. T2-weighted images of the thigh muscles have shown increased signal intensity, with focal and inhomogeous involvement predominantly in the vastus lateralis; T1 and T2 values of the vastus lateralis were significantly higher than those of the control subjects [30].

(c) **High-frequency muscle ultrasound** (20 MHz) has also been used to show active muscle inflammation and fascial involvement [11, 31]. Ultrasound may also reveal the earliest indications of calcinosis before obvious X-ray changes, with characteristic signal dropout.

However, the use of any of these methods alone yields either low sensitivity or low specificity for the evaluation of disease activity [32], particularly in those patients with amyopatic DM with normal enzyme levels and free from myositis.

4.3 Cutaneous Diagnostic Criteria

The skin lesions are essentially pathognomonic for DM, and are unique distinguishing clinical features from PM [9] without which the diagnosis of DM cannot be made with confidence [33]. Cutaneous rash is almost always present at the time when muscle weakness presents, but it may precede the myositis, or in a few cases to be a unique clinical manifestation of the disease [6]. Most studies suggest that the diagnosis of DM is often missed, even by dermatologists. This can lead to a delay in diagnosing the muscle disease and in investigation for occult malignancy.

According to American Academy of Dermatology Guidelines, the diagnosis of DM is confirmed by the presence of diagnostic skin lesions (1–2) or by characteristic muscle findings and less specific cutaneous changes (3–7) [7]:

1. Gottron's sign
2. Gottron's papules
3. Periorbital heliotrope erythema often associated with edema
4. Photosensitive poikiloderma
5. Violaceous erythema over the extensor aspects of the arms and hands
6. Telangiectasias and erythema of the proximal nailfold, erythema of the nail bed, cuticle abnormalities, and nail plate
7. Scalp disease

The primary, classic cutaneous feature of DM is a violaceous macular erythema distributed symmetrically [9]. As the disease progresses, the erythema becomes poikilodermatous or indurated, as a result of the mucin deposit.

4.3.1 Diagnostic Cutaneous Lesions for Dermatomyositis

Cutaneous manifestations of DM are generally grouped as pathognomonic, characteristic, compatible [6], and less common and rare [4, 34] (Table 4.6).

(i) **Pathognomonic cutaneous manifestations of DM**

The more **specific** or pathognomic manifestations of DM are the "classic" periorbital heliotrope rash and erythematous maculo-papular lesions covering bony prominences, which were described by Gottron (1931) and are named after him, and they constitute the primary cutaneous findings [35].

(a) **"Heliotrope" rash** (Gr *helios* sun; Gr *trope* a turn, turning; a heliotrope being a red/purple-colored flower that tracks the course of the sun during the day) [36].

Table 4.6 Cutaneous manifestations of dermatomyositis

Pathognomonic	Characteristic	Compatible	Less common manifestations	Rare manifestations
Heliotrope rash	Shawl sign/V-sign	Periorbital edema/facial swelling	Cutaneous vasculitis	Mechanic's hands
Gottron's papules	Nailfold changes	Photosensitive poikiloderma	Panniculitis	Follicular hyperkeratosis
Gottron's sign	Scalp scaly dermatosis	Prurutus	Calcinosis	Zebra-like erythema
				Erythroderma
				Vesiculo-bullous lesions
				Epidermal necrosis

Confluent, palpebral, or periorbital (facial) dusky macular erythema (violaceous/lilac/cyanotic/purplish-red exanthema) that involves symmetrically the eyelids, the upper cheeks, the forehead, and the temples is often associated with edema of the eyelids and periorbital tissues. A distinctive, but often more subtle, sign is an erythematous blush on the margin of the eyelids (particularly the upper eyelids) and around the eyes. It has a lavender shade similar to the flower of the valerian, from which the term heliotrope erythema comes [33]. The intensity of the blush may vary considerably from hour to hour. This heliotrope erythema may be the only cutaneous symptom in children and some adults.

(b) **Gottron's papules** are bluish-red, slightly elevated, violaceous papules, or dusky erythematous scaly plaques overlying around the base of the nails, that occur over bony prominences, particularly over the proximal or distal dorsal interphalangeal or metacarpophalangeal joints, elbow, or knee joints, feet, or a combination of those [35]. The characteristic violaceous to erythematous hues of Gottron's papules often extend from metacarpophalangeal joints onto dorsal hands and fingers as linear streaking over the distribution of extensor tendon sheaths [37]. When fully formed, these papules become slightly depressed at the center, which can assume a white, atrophic appearance [36]. Associated telangiectasia can be present. In contrast to subacute lupus erythematosus, the rash does not involve the phalanges [38].

(c) **Gottron's sign** consists of symmetrical, polymorphic, non-scaling, violaceous erythemas, with or without edema, or depigmented porcelain-white atrophic spots localized overlying the dorsal aspect of the interphalangeal/metacarpophalangeal joints, olecranon processes, patellae, and medial malleoli [7].

(ii) **Characteristic cutaneous manifestations of DM**

The **characteristic cutaneous features of DM**, in spite of not being pathognomic, are the following [6, 39, 40]:

(a) **Shawl sign** — violaceous erythema disposed in a "shawl" distribution over the neck, upper back, shoulders, and extensor parts of arms, hands, and fingers, with predominance over the extensor tendon sheaths [5]. Confluent, macular, violaceous erythema might be "V"- shaped on the anterior neck and upper chest (**V-sign**), or with central aspect over the face and forehead, and scalp [41]. Photosensitivity, and erythema on sun-exposed skin or a flare of cutaneous lesions after sunlight exposure may also occur [42, 43].

(b) **Nailfold changes** is a grossly visible syndrome consisting of: (i) **periungual erythema** (diffuse redness and shininess of the nailfolds), (ii) **telangiectases** (dilated, irregular, and tortous capillary loops) at the mago ocultus of nail margin, (iii) **cuticular hypertophy**, a characteristic cuticular change known as **Keining sign** (irregular, thickened, rough, and distorted cuticles with minimal or no redness or inflammation) [44–46], which are associated with (iv) small, punctate, **hemorrhagic infarcts** in a few thrombosed vessels [47, 48]. Cutaneous nailfold telangiectasias are an important diagnostic marker of DM in elderly patients with a chronic course of the disease [45].

4

(c) **Scalp scaly dermatosis** – is pruritic, diffuse, erythematous to violaceous scaly dermatosis resembling a psoriasiform dermatitis, with or without diffuse noncicatricial alopecia which is frequent, and often misdiagnosed [49].

(iii) **Compatible cutaneous manifestations of DM**

Compatible cutaneous manifestations of DM have also been observed in other skin diseases, and include:

(a) **Periorbital edema** (facial swelling) can be a dominant physical sign of DM [50]. The heliotrope macular rash and periorbital edema create a "tearful appearance" on the patient's face. Some authors described edematous eyelids as "driver's spectacles" [51, 52]. Sometimes DM patients have only periorbital edema [50, 53–55], and this could be the only visible finding of the disease in patients with VI type pigmentation (African-American patients) [56]. Edema of the hands and arms and sometimes of the body may also be found.
(b) **Poikilodermia vascularis atrophicans** (photosensitive poikiloderma) consists of a circumscribed violaceous erythema with associated reticulate telangiectasia, dyschromias (hypo- and hyperpigmentation), and superficial atrophy, scarring, and scales, in sun-exposed areas over the posterior shoulders, back, buttocks, and V-shaped area of the anterior neck and chest (mostly in chronic forms) [39, 57, 58]. The pigmentary changes, telangiectasia, and atrophy are a postinflammatory reaction.
(c) **Pruritus** is a condition commonly evident in DM patients. Intractable itch can produce great discomfort or even complete disabling in some patients [7, 59].

(iv) **Less common manifestations of DM** are the following:

(a) **Cutaneous vasculitis** manifests as (i) palpable purpura [60], (ii) periungual infarcts, (iii) eschares, (iv) urticaria-like lesions, (v) livedo reticularis, and (vi) digital or oral **ulcerations** [37, 60], and may occur particularly in severe, acute childhood form, but also in adult DM patients [12, 60].
(b) **Panniculitis** is a characteristic component of DM in children and adults [61–65], and in 10% of skin biopsies from cutaneous lesions of DM, patients have histological data for panniculitis [66].
(c) **Calcinosis cutis** is manifested by firm, yellow, or flesh-colored nodules, commonly over bony prominences [40], or in traumatized areas. Calcification is frequent in children or adolescents with DM [67] and rare in adults [68], and is associated with the activity of the disease. Skin calcification associated with DM presents as two different subtypes: (i) the presence of superficial calcifications as small and hard plaques or nodules that can be felt just below the skin surface; and (ii) subcutaneous calcifications — large tumorous deposits of calcium, which often appear "popcorn-like" on X-ray examination. Subcutaneous calcifications occur only in DM; in some cases, nodules can extrude through the surface of the skin and cause ulcerations, infections, and pain, especially at sites of compression (elbows, buttocks, back) [69]. Skin calcinosis over the extensor surfaces of extremities frequently leads to chronic ulcers which heal with difficulty [68].

(v) **Rare cutaneous manifestations of DM**

(a) **"Mechanic's hands"**—presents with confluent, nonpruritic, bilateral, symmetric, rough and cracked, hyperkeratotic, scaly, fissured patches and hyperpigmentation with irregular "dirty" horizontal lines, having the appearance of that produced by manual labor, distributed on the ulnar aspect of the thumb and radial aspect of the fingers with occasional extension to the palmar surfaces [70, 71].

(b) **Follicular hyperkeratosis (type Wong)** — patients with DM on rare occasions develop cutaneous hyperkeratotic lesions (orange-red scaling plaques with follicular plugging and follicular papules) over the extensor aspects of the upper extremities, and histologically show follicular hyperkeratosis, follicular destruction and degenerative findings and arrector pilorum myositis [72–75].

(c) **Centripetal linear or flagellate erythema** (zebra-like DM)—isolated persistent, asymptomatic, erythematous, violaceous macular lesions in linear streaks or centripetal flagellate erythema, extremely rarely found over various areas of the body (suggesting that the trauma or scratching may have played a role in the pathogenesis (Koebner's phenomenon) [76]. This rare clinical manifestation of DM is not associated with dermographism [77–79].

(d) **Erythroderma (erythrodermic dermatomyositis)** — widespread erythema of the face, trunk, and extremities, or diffuse rash (exfoliative dermatitis-like exanthema) in patients with DM is a rare clinical manifestation [80, 81]. In 75% of cases, erythroderma has preceded the signs of DM by several weeks [82].

(e) **Vesicular** and subepidermal **bullous lesions** are rare manifestations of DM, and frequently lead to erosions and scar formation [83–86]. They are accompanied by dyschromia, telangiectasias, and atrophy. A specimen from the lesion has demonstrated a subepidermal blister with the features of toxic epidermal necrolysis, including full-thickness epidermal necrosis [86]. Vesiculo-bullous lesions are frequently associated with malignancies (gynecologic or gastric) [85, 86].

(f) **Epidermal necrosis** – The term "cutaneous necrosis" regroups a fairly wide range of symptoms: small digital necroses, superficial epidermal necroses and also large necrotic plaques with loss of substance [87–90]. It has been suggested as a predictive sign of concomitant neoplasia in adult DM [89–91]. Cutaneous necrosis in patients with DM associated with malignancy has low sensitivity (63%), and 89% specificity; in the study by Burnouf et al., its positive predictive value was of 71% and its negative predictive value was of 84% [92].

(vi) **Oral mucosal lesions characteristic of DM**

The typical lesions of oral mucosa in DM are: (i) erythema and edema, (ii) hemorrhage, (iii) vesicles, (iv) erosions or ulcers, (v) leukoplakia-like plaques, and (vi) a net of dilated superficial vessels [93–96].

(a) **Gingival telangiectases** at the mucosal gingiva are proposed as an important diagnostic marker of juvenile DM [94], but have also been observed in adults [95, 96].

(b) **Dysphasia (changes of voice)**: (i) "hoarse voice" resulting from the laryngeal swelling is a frequent feature of the disease [97], and (ii) "nasal speech" is due to the involvement of the cricopharyngeal and other muscles in the hypopharynx.

4

4.4 Cutaneous Disease Indexes

Recently, new scoring methods for cutaneous disease measurement have been proposed [98].

The **Cutaneous Dermatomyositis Disease Area and Severity Index (CDASI)** assesses four activity measures (erythema, scale, excoriation, ulceration) with subscore ranging from 0 to 116, and two damage measures (poikiloderma, calcinosis) with subscore from 0 to 32 for 15 anatomical locations. The total score ranges from 0 to 148 points, and describes the extent of disease in terms of the severity of involvement; the higher the score, the worse the disease.

The **Dermatomyositis Skin Severity Index (DSSI)** measures disease activity based on the percentage involvement of four body surface areas (head, trunk, upper extremity, lower extremity), and estimates the severity by three symptom scores (redness, induration, scaliness). DSSI ranges from 0 to 72, and higher scores represent advanced disease.

The **Cutaneous Assessment Tool (CAT)** is an extended instrument that uses 21 items, divided into ten activity, four damage and seven combined lesions. The characteristic DM lesions are divided by subclass (pathognomonic lesions, erythematous lesions, vasculopathic lesions, characteristic acral lesions, etc.) Activity is assessed with a specific set of criteria for each lesion, including the intensity of erythema or hyperpigmentation, and damage is assessed by presence or absence of atrophy, hypopigmentation, calcinosis, lipodystrophy, atrophy, scar, and poikiloderma. CAT activity ranges from 0 to 175 and damage subscales from 0 to 33, with higher scores indicating worse disease [99].

4.5 Cutaneous Laboratory Tests

(a) **Skin biopsy**. The histopathologic examination of DM skin lesions demonstrates an interface dermatitis and a patchy mononuclear inflammatory infiltrate high in the reticular and papillary dermis. Blood vessel dilatation may be prominent. The histopathological alternations found in DM skin lesions are nonspecific, but histology may exlude other dermatoses that could be confused with DM cutaneous lesions [7, 100].

(b) Immunohistochemistry form skin lesions present **deposits of membrane attack complex** of C5b-9 complement (MAC) along the dermoepidermal junction (in 86% of DM cases) and into the walls of papillar dermis vessels (in 77% of biopsy specimens) and lack of MAC in uninvolved skin [101].

(c) **Nailfold capillary microscopy** is a useful method for monitoring the overall disease activity and predicting the severity and clinical course in classical adult and juvenile DM [102].

(d) **Cutaneous photosensitivity to ultraviolet B (UVB) light** may be useful for the diagnosis of disease [103].

4.6 Markers for Inflammatory Disease

(a) **Erythrocyte sedimentation rate (ESR)** is elevated in 50% of DM patients in active phase [5, 104]; high levels are seen in patients with a severe ulcerative/vasculopathic juvenile DM or with associated infection [12]. ESR does not correlate well with disease activity, and might be a potential marker of malignancy in association with cutaneous necrosis [88].
(b) **Neopterin** and **factor VIII-related antigen (von Willebrand factor)** are serological indicators of disease activity in childhood DM. Neopterin is found elevated in about 60 % of juvenile DM, and its levels correlate with disease activity [105]; however, as factor VIII-related antigen they are not specific to juvenile DM. It may indicate ongoing inflammation when muscle enzymes may have returned to normal [106], and thus are useful for monitoring the disease activity in some patients.
(c) **Rheumatoid factor** is found elevated in 20% of DM patients, often in those with overlap syndrome [107].
(d) Increased level of **C-reactive protein** — often modestly elevated in juvenile DM [12]; may be a predictive sign of malignancy in adult DM [108].
(e) **Urinary creatine** estimations of the 24-h urinary creatine level provide useful information of disease activity [109, 110].

For other markers of inflammatory disease, see Chapter 32.

References

1. Dorph C, Lundberg IE. Idiopathic inflammatory myopathies – myositis. *Best Pract Res Clin Rheumatol* 2002; 16(5): 817–832.
2. Bohan A, Peter JB. Polymyositis and dermatomyositis (part I). *N Engl J Med* 1975; 292: 344–347.
3. Bohan A, Peter JB. Polymyositis and dermatomyositis (part II). *N Engl J Med* 1975; 292: 403–407.
4. Santmyire-Rosenberger B, Dugan EM. Skin involvement in dermatomyositis. *Curr Opin Rheumatol* 2003; 15(6): 714–722.
5. Tanimoto K, Nakano K, Kano S, et al. Classification criteria for polymyositis and dermatomyositis. *J Rheumatol* 1995; 22: 668–674.
6. Euwer RL, Sontheimer RD. Amyopathic dermatomyositis (dermatomyositis sine myositis). Presentation of six new cases and review of the literature. *J Am Acad Dermatol* 1991; 24: 959–966.
7. Drake L, Dinehart SM, Farmer ER, et al. Guidelines of care for dermatomyositis. *J Am Acad Dermatol* 1996; 34: 824–829.
8. Zuber M. Taninato's classification and diagnostic criteria for polymyositis and dermatomyositis do not recognize the variant of amyopathic dermatomyositis. *J Rheumatol* 1996; 23: 191.
9. Kovacs SO, Kovacs SC. Dermatomyositis. *J Am Acad Dermatol* 1998; 39: 899–920.
10. Targoff IN, Miller FW, Medsger TA Jr, et al. Classification criteria for the idiopathic inflammatory myopathies. *Curr Opin Rheum* 1997; 9: 527–535.
11. Owen NJ, Owens CM, Bose S, et al. The role of musculoskeletal ultrasound at diagnosis and follow-up in patients with juvenile dermatomyositis. *Radiology* 2002; 217: S495.

4

12. Murray KJ. Juvenile dermatomyositis: Advances in understanding and management. *APLAR J Rheumatol* 2003; 6: 50–63.
13. Mastaglia FL, Phillips BA. Idiopathic inflammatory myopathies: epidemiology, classification, and diagnostic criteria. *Rheum Dis Clin North Am* 2002; 28(4): 723–741.
14. Dalakas MC, Hohfeld R. Polymyositis and dermatomyositis. *Lancet* 2003; 362: 971–982.
15. Feldman BM, Ayling-Campos A, Luy L, et al. Measuring disability in juvenile dermatomyositis: validity of the childhood health assessement questionnaire. *J Rheumatol* 1995; 22: 326–331.
16. Daniels L, Worthingham C. *Muscle Testing*, 4th ed. WB Saunders, Philadelphia, 1972.
17. Florence JM, Pandya S, King WM, et al. Intrarater reliability of manual muscle test (Medical Research Council scale) grades in Duchenne's muscular dystrophy. *Phys Ther* 1992; 72: 115–122.
18. Josefson A, Romanus E, Carlson J. A functional index in myositis. *J Rheumatol* 1996; 23: 1380–1384.
19. Alexanderson H, Stenström C, Lundberg I. Safety of a home exercise programme in patients with polymyositis and dermatomyositis: a pilot study. *Rheumatology* 1999; 38: 608–611.
20. Bohlmeyer TJ, Wu AH, Perryman MB. Evaluation of laboratory tests as a guide to diagnosis and therapy of myositis. *Rheum Dis Clin North Am* 1994; 20: 845–856.
21. Love LA, Leff RL, Fraser DD, et al. A new approach to the classification of idiopathic inflammatory myopathy: myositis-specific autoantibodies define useful homogeneous patient groups. *Medicine* 1991; 70: 360–374.
22. Oester YT, Rodriguez AA, Fudema JJ. Electromyographic findings in dermatomyositis. *Arch Dermatol* 1957; 76: 91–95.
23. Rider LG, Miller FW. Laboratory evaluation of the inflammatory myopathies. *Clin Diagn Lab Immunol* 1995; 2: 1–9.
24. Sultan SM, Ioannou Y, Moss K, et al. Outcome in patients with idiopathic inflammatory myositis: morbidity and mortality. *Rheumatology* 2002; 41: 22–26.
25. Lundberg I, Chung Y-L. Treatment and investigation of idiopathic inflammatory myopathies. *Rheumatology* 2000; 39: 7–17.
26. Henriksson KG. "Semi-open" muscle biopsy technique. *Acta Neurol Scand* 1979; 59: 317–323.
27. Lundberg IE, Dorph C, Nennesmo I. Percutaneous conchotome technique – a valuable and safe procedure for muscle biopsies. *Arthritis Rheum* 1998; 1024: S203.
28. Pitt AM, Fleckenstein JL, Greenlee RG, et al. MRI-guided biopsy in inflammatory myopathy: initial results. *Magn Reson Imaging* 1993; 11: 1093–1099.
29. Strauss KW, Herman G-B, Khamasha MA, et al. Polymyositis-dermatomyositis: a clinical review. *Postgrad Med J* 1989; 65: 437–443.
30. Park SK, Cho KH, Kang SK. Acute renal failure associated with dermatomyositis and colon cancer. *Nephron* 1990; 55: 225–226.
31. Stonecipher MR, Jorizzo JR, Monu J, et al. Dermatomyositis with normal muscle enzyme concentration. A single-blind study of the diagnostic value of magnetic resonance imaging and ultrasound. *Arch Dermatol* 1994; 130: 1294–1299.
32. Kroll M, Otis J, Kagen L. Serum enzyme, myoglobin and muscle strength relationships in polymyositis and dermatomyositis. *J Rheumatol* 1986; 13: 349–355.
33. Mills JA. Dermatomyositis. In: *Dermatology in General Medicine*, Fitzpatrick TB, Eisen AZ, Wolff K, et al. (eds), McGraw-Hill, New York, 1993; 2148–2155.
34. Koler RA, Montemarano A. Dermatomyositis. *Am Fam Physician* 2001; 64: 1564–1572.
35. Gottron H. Hautveränderungen bei Dermatomyositis. VIII Congres Intern. Dermatol. et Syphilogr., Copenhagen, 5–8 Agout 1930, *Compt rend Sieancy* Ed. S. Lomholt, Copenhagen 1931; 826–830.
36. Sontheimer RD. Dermatomyositis: an overview of recent progress with emphasasis on dermatologic aspects. *Dermatol Clin* 2002; 20: 387–408.
37. Caro I. Dermatomyositis as a systemic disease. *Med Clin North Am* 1989; 73: 1181–1192.

38. Plotz PH, Dalakas M, Leff RL, et al. Current concepts in the idiopathic inflammatory myopathies: polymyositis, dermatomyositis and related disorders. *Ann Intern Med* 1989; 111: 143–157.
39. Stonecipher MR, Callen JP, Jorizzo JL. The red face: dermatomyositis. *Clin Dermatol* 1993; 11: 261–273.
40. Callen JP. Dermatomyositis. *Lancet* 2000; 355: 53–57.
41. Sontheimer RD. Skin manifestations of systemic autoimmune connective tissue disease: diagnostics and therapeutics. *Best Pract Res Clin Rheumatol* 2004; 18(3): 429–462.
42. Woo TR, Rasmunsen J, Callen JP. Recurrent photosensitive dermatitis preceding juvenile dermatomyositis. *Pediatr Dematol* 1985; 3: 207–212.
43. Badawy Abdel-Nasser M, Chun SC, Gollnick H, Orfanos CE. Amyopathic dermatomyositis (dermatomyositis sine myositis) in a male patient and possible induction by UV light. *Eur J Dermatol* 1993; 3: 367–370.
44. Keining E. Versammlungen Casus 3 und 4. *Dermatol Wochenschr* 1939; 109: 1198–1199.
45. Samitz MH. Cuticular changes in dermatomyositis: a clinical sign. *Arch Dermatol* 1974; 110: 866.
46. Franks AG. Important cutaneous markers of dermatomyositis. *J Musculoskeletal Med* 1988; 5: 39–63.
47. Maricq HR, Spencer-Green G, LeRoy EC. Skin capillary abnormalities as indicators of organ involvement in scleroderma (systemic sclerosis), Raynaud's syndrome and dermatomyositis. *Am J Med* 1976; 61(6): 862–870.
48. Maricq HR, Maize JC. Nailfold capillary abnormalities. *Clin Rheum Dis* 1982; 8: 455–478.
49. Kasteler JS, Callen JP. Scalp involvement in dermatomyositis: often overlooked or misdiagnosed. *JAMA* 1994; 272: 1939–1941.
50. Dicken CH. Periorbital edema: an important physical finding in dermatomyositis. *Cutis* 1991; 48: 116–117.
51. Iotzov M. Contribution to clinic, histopathology, and pathogenesis of dermatomyositis. *Ann Med Acad (bulg)* 1950; 29: 267–315 [Bulgarian].
52. Zografsky B, Balabanov G. A case report of polymyositis. *Savr Med (bulg)* 1951; 1: 66–73 [Bulgarian].
53. Cunningham JD, Lowry LD. Head and neck manifestations of dermatomyositis-polymyositis. *Otolaryngol Head Neck Surg* 1985; 93: 673–677.
54. Sevigny GM, Mathes BM. Periorbital edema as the presenting sign of juvenile dermatomyositis. *Pediatr Dermatol* 1999; 16: 43–45.
55. Hall VC, Keeling JH, Davis MD. Periorbital edema as the presenting sign of dermatomyositis. *Int J Dermatol* 2003; 42: 466–467.
56. Bridges BF. The rashes of dermatomyositis in a black patient. *Am J Med* 1991; 91: 661–662.
57. Jacobi E. Fall für Diagnose (Poikilodermia vascularis atrophicans). *Verh Dtsch Dermatol Ges* 1907; 9: 321–323.
58. Popov L. Dermatomyositis. Morbus Wagner-Potain. *Bulg Clinica* 1943; 15(3): 117–139 [Bulgarian].
59. Shirani MZ, Kucenic J, Carroll CL, et al. Pruritus in adult dermatomyositis. *Clin Exp Dermatol* 2004; 29: 273–276.
60. Feldman D, Hochberg MC, Zizic TM, et al. Cutaneous vasculitis in adult polymyositis/dermatomyositis. *J Rheumatol* 1983; 10: 85–89.
61. Winkelmann WJ, Billick RC, Srolowitz H. Dermatomyositis presenting as panniculitis. *J Am Acad Dermatol* 1990; 23: 127–128.
62. Fusade T, Belanyi P, Joly P, et al. Subcutaneous changes in dermatomyositis. *Br J Dermatol* 1993; 128: 451–453.
63. Naidenbach PJ, Sahn EE, Helton J. Panniculitis in juvenile dermatomyositis. *J Am Acad Dermatol* 1995; 33: 305–307.

4

64. Molnar K, Kemeny L, Korom, et al. Panniculitis in dermatomyositis: report of two cases. *Br J Dermatol* 1998; 139: 152–169.
65. Chao YY, Yang LJ. Dermatomyositis presenting as panniculitis. *Int J Dermatol* 2000; 39: 141–144.
66. Janis FJ, Winkelmann RK. Histopathology of the skin in dermatomyositis. *Arch Dermatol* 1968; 97: 640–650.
67. Ichiki Y, Akiyama T, Shimozawa N, et al. An extremely severe case of cutaneous calcinosis with juvenile dermatomyositis, and successful treatment with diltiazem. *Br J Dermatol* 2001; 144: 894–897.
68. Dasgeb B, Phillips TJ. Adult-onset dermatomyositis complicated by calcinosis cutis. *Wounds* 2004; 16(12): 364–370.
69. Dalakas MC. Calcifications in dermatomyositis. *N Engl J Med* 1995; 333: 978.
70. Sthal NI, Klippel JH, Decker JL. A cutaneous lesion associated with myositis. *Ann J Med* 1979; 91: 577–579.
71. Mitra D, Loevell CL, Macleod TI, et al. Clinical and histological features of "mechanic's hands" in a patient with antibodies to Jo-1 — a case report. *Clin Exp Dermatol* 1994; 19: 146–148.
72. Wong KO. Dermatomyositis: a clinical investigation of 23 cases in Hong Kong. *Br J Dermatol* 1969; 81: 544–547.
73. Dupre A, Floutard X, Christol B, et al. Dermatomyositis avec spinulosisme (dermatomyositis type Wong). Etude histologique: essai d'interpretation pathogénique. *Ann Dermatol Syphiligr* (Paris) 1976; 103: 141–149.
74. Tribonniere X, Delaporte E, Alfandari S, et al. Dermatomyositis with follicular hypekeratosis. *Dermatology* 1995; 191: 242–244.
75. Lupton JR, Figueroa P, Berberian BJ, Sulica VI. An unusual presentation of dermatomyositis: the type Wong variant revised. *J Am Acad Dermatol* 2000; 43: 908–912.
76. Provost TT, Flyn JA. Dermatomyositis. In: *Cutaneous Medicine, Cutaneous Manifestations of Systemic Diseases*, BC Decker, Hamilton/London, 2001; 82–103.
77. Dupre A, Viraben R, Bonafe JL, et al. Zebra-like dermatomyositis. *Arch Dermatol* 1981; 117: 63–64.
78. Bachmeyer C, Blum L, Danne O, et al. Isolated flagellate eruptions in dermatomyositis. *Dermatology* 1998; 197: 92–93.
79. Kimyai-Asadi A, Tausk FA, Nousari HC. A patient with dermatomyositis and linear streaks on the back. *Arch Dermatol* 2000; 136(5): 667–670.
80. Miyagawa S, Okazaki A, Minowa R, et al. Dermatomyositis presenting as erythroderma. *J Am Acad Dermatol* 1992; 26: 489–490.
81. Pierson JC, Taylor JS. Erythrodermic dermatomyositis. *J Am Acad Dermatol* 1993; 28: 136.
82. Maruani A, Armingaud P, Nseir A, et al. Erythroderma and cutaneous necrosis in patient with dermatomyositis. *Ann Dermatol Venereol* 2003; 150: 353–356.
83. Glover M, Leigh I. Dermatomyositis pemphigoides: a case with coexistent dermatomyositis and bullous pemphigoid. *J Am Acad Dermatol* 1992; 27: 849–852.
84. Barrows-Wade L, Jordon RE, Axnett FC. Linear IgA bullous dermatosis associated with dermatomyositis (letter). *Arch Dermatol* 1992; 128: 413.
85. Kubo M, Sato S, Kitahara H, et al. Vesicle formattion in dermatomyositis associated with gynecologic malignancies. *J Am Acad Dermatol* 1996; 34: 391–394.
86. Fujimoto M, Murakami T, Murata S, et al. Acute onset vesiculo-bullous dermatomyositis associated with massive mucosal necrosis of the intestines. *Clin Exp Dermatol* 2002; 27: 714–722.
87. Bonafé JL, Touron P, Viraben R, et al. Dermatomyositis associated with lethal pulmonary fibrosis and cutaneous necrosis. *Ann Dermatol Venereol* 1981; 108(4): 363–368 [French].

88. Basset-Seguin N, Roujeau J, Gherardi R, et al. Prognostic factors and predicative signs of malignancy in adult dermatomyositis. *Arch Dermatol* 1990; 126: 633–637.
89. Gallais V, Crickx B, Belaïch S. Facteurs pronostiques et signes prédictifs de cancer au cours de la dermatomyosite de l'adulte. *Ann Dermatol Venereol* 1996; 123: 722–726.
90. Mautner G, Grossman M, Silvers D, et al. Epidermal necrosis as a predicative sign of malignancy in adult dermatomyositis. *Cutis* 1998; 61: 190–194.
91. Chen YJ, Wu CY, Shen JL. Predicting factors of malignancy in dermatomyositis and polymyositis: a case-control study. *Br J Dermatol* 2001; 144: 825–831.
92. Burnouf M, Mahe E, Verpillat P, et al. Cutaneous necrosis is predictive of cancer in adult dermatomyositis. *Ann Dermatol Venereol* 2003; 130: 313–316.
93. Keil H. The manifestations in the skin and mucus membranes in dermatomyositis with special reference to the differential diagnosis from systemic lupus erythematosus. *Ann Intern Med* 1942; 16: 827.
94. Ghali FE, Stein LD, Fine JD, et al. Gingival telangiectases: an underappreciated physical sign of juvenile dermatomyositis. *Arch Dermatol* 1999; 135: 1370–1374.
95. Márton K, Hermann P, Dankó K, et al. Evaluation of oral manifestations and masticatory force in patients with polymyositis and dermatomyositis. *J Oral Pathol Med* 2005; 34(3): 164–169.
96. Dourmishev LA, Dourmishev AL, Schwartz RA. Dermatomyositis: an association of gingival telangiectases and anti Jo-1 antibody in the adult. *Acta Dermatoven APA* 2007; 16(2): 67–72.
97. Metheny JA. Dermatomyositis: a vocal and swallowing disease entity. *Laryngoscope* 1978; 88: 147–161.
98. Klein RQ, Bangert CA, Costner M, et al. Comparison of the reliability and validity of outcome instruments for cutaneous dermatomyositis. *Br J Dermatol* 2008; 159(4): 887–894.
99. Huber AM, Dugan EM, Lachenbruch PA, et al. Preliminary validation and clinical meaning of the cutaneous assessment tool in juvenile dermatomyositis. *Arthritis Rheum* 2008; 59: 214–221.
100. Dourmishev L, Obreshkova E. Histological changes in skin of dermatomyositis patiesnts. *Dermatol i Venereol* 2001; 40(1): 18–22 [Bulgarian].
101. Mascaro JM, Hausmann G, Herrero C, et al. Membrane attack complex deposits in cutaneous lesions of dermatomyositis. *Arch Dermatol* 1995; 131: 1386–1392.
102. Dolezalova P, Young SP, Bacon PA, Southwood TR. Nailfold capillary microscopy in healthy children and in childhood rheumatic diseases: a prospective single blind observational study. *Ann Rheum Dis* 2003; 62(5): 444–449.
103. Dourmishev L, Meffert H, Piazena H. Dermatomyositis: comparative studies of cutaneous photosensitivity in lupus erythematosus and normal subjects. *Photoderm Photoimmun Photomed* 2004; 20(5): 230–234.
104. Scola RH, Werneck LC, Prevedello DMS, et al. Diagnosis of dermatomyositis and polymyositis: a study of 102 cases. *Arq Neuropsoquiatr* 2000; 58: 789–799.
105. Pachman LM. An update on juvenile dermatomyositis. *Curr Opin Rheumatol* 1995; 7(5): 437–441.
106. Bloom BJ, Tucker LB, Miller LC, et al. von Willebrand factor in juvenile dermatomyositis. *J Rheumatol* 1995; 22: 320–325.
107. van Paassen P, Damoiseaux J, Tervaert J. Laboratory assessment in musculoskeletal disorders. *Best Pract Res Clin Rheumatol* 2003; 17: 475–494.
108. Rose C, Hatron PY, Brouillard M, et al. Signes prédicatifs de cancers au cours de la dermatomyosite. Etude de 29 observations. *Rev Med Int* 1994; 15(1): 19–24.
109. Rowell NR. Urinary creatine excretion and the management of dermatomyositis. *Dermatol Monatsschr* 1984; 170: 34.
110. Rowell NR, Fairris GM. Biochemical markers of myositis in dermatomyositis. *Clin Exp Dermatol* 1986; 11: 69–72.

Epidemiology of Dermatomyositis

5

The idiopathic inflammatory myopathies are relatively rare diseases that occur throughout the world. The occurrence of DM/PM is uncommon. The absence of reliable epidemiologic data for DM is rather surprising and may relate to several reasons: (i) the rarity of disease, (ii) the lack of consistent use of diagnostic criteria, (iii) the indolent clinical course, (iv) the fact that the numbers result from studies on hospitalized patients, (v) the management of outpatients by physicians from many different specialties (including pediatric and adult rheumatologists, neurologists, dermatologists, other specialists, and general practitioners), and (vi) the lack of prospective studies of associated myositis in connective tissue disease [1].

Dermatomyositis affects both children and adults. The incidence of DM is approximately 10–20 times lower than the incidence of lupus erythematosus, or other connective tissue diseases — systemic sclerosis or rheumatoid polyarthritis [2, 3]. The relative prevalence of DM in relation to PM varies between different studies.

The prevalence of the disease in the USA is about 5 cases/million population [4]. It seems to be increasing, although this may simply be a result of increased detection, as well as better diagnosis and reporting [5]. The incidence of hospital-diagnosed PM and DM in the population from Allegheny County, Pennsylvania, USA between 1963 and 1982 was determined to be 5.5 cases/million population [6]. A similar incidence rate of 5 cases/million population was reported in an earlier hospital-based study from the USA [7], as well as a rate of 6 cases/million population from a population-based study in Olmsted County, Minnesota, between 1951 and 1970 [8]. According to other studies, the incidence of DM ranges from 7 to 10 cases/million adults in various populations [6, 9, 10] or even more, between 10 and 60 cases/million population/year [11]. This figure includes patients with PM/DM, and most likely does not include patients with amyopathic DM. An annual incidence of 7.6 cases/million population was estimated in a country-based Swedish study [12]. A similar incidence rate of 7.4 cases/million person-years was reported from the state of Victoria, Australia [13]. The estimated annual incidence of PM/DM in the northern Stockholm County between March 1998 and September 2000, was approximately 8.5 cases/million population [14]. In one Israeli study, a slightly lower incidence of 2.2 cases/million population was reported [15]. Prevalence data for PM and DM vary from 5/100,000 population in Japan and 11/100,000 in a county-based survey in Sweden [16]. The prevalence of DM in Sofia is about 1.1 cases/100,000 population [17].

5

In children, PM is a very rare disease, and as has recently been confirmed, DM is the most frequent IIM [18]. According to the pediatric inflammatory myopathy group, the juvenile DM accounting about 85% of IIMs in children [18]. Demographic data show that juvenile DM affects children with an incidence between 1 and 3.3 cases per million children, and morbidity is 5% of all connective tissue diseases [18–21]. The results from the Canadian Pediatric Rheumatology Association Disease Registry show that juvenile DM is a relatively uncommon connective tissue disease, with an estimated annual incidence of 2 cases/million children [22]. An estimated incidence rate for juvenile IIM of 1.9 cases/million children aged under 16 years was reported in a nation-wide study in the UK and Ireland [23]. Only three out of 51 cases were classified as PM. In one population-based study of juvenile IIM from Shelby County, USA, the combined incidence of PM and DM was 3.2 cases/million population aged under 20 years [19]. DM was more common than PM. The incidence in the USA has been documented at a rate of 3.1 cases/million children/year by a NIH-sponsored registry of new-onset juvenile DM, using capture–recapture methodology [24]. In one region of the UK determined to be ethnically diverse, the West Midlands, the incidence and ethnic distribution of juvenile DM among other rheumatic diseases was evaluated as high as 4 cases/million children/year [25]. The differences in risk depend on age, race, gender, and seasons (Table 5.1).

5.1 Age

Although DM/PM have been observed at any age, a bimodal pattern is established; with an initial peak at 10–15 years in adolescent age, and a second larger peak in adulthood between 40 and 60 years of age [6, 26]. A mean onset age of 55.1 years was reported in a

Table 5.1 DM: distribution by age, sex, and clinical variants [95]

Clinical variant	Sex	*N*	Age range (years)	Average age (years)
"Classic" DM in adults:	Male	10	21–70	42.9 ± 15.6
M/F = 1/2.4	Female	24	25–74	54 ± 13
Paraneoplastic DM:	Male	4	62–81	70.8 ± 8.8
M/F = 1/3	Female	12	41–80	56.1 ± 13.3
Overlap syndrome:	Male	1	61	–
M/F = 1/11	Female	11	34–65	55.8 ± 9.3
Amyopathic DM:	Male	1	67	–
M/F = 1/2	Female	2	67–76	71.5 ± 6.4
Juvenile DM:	Male	2	13–16	14.5 ± 2.1
M/F = 2/0	Female	0	–	–
Total = 67:	Male	18	13–81	48 ± 21
M/F = 1/2.7	Female	49	25–80	55.6 ± 12.3

population-based study in Australia including juvenile cases [13]. In Bulgaria, 73% of DM patients are between 40 and 70 years, and the ratio of female to male is 2.7:1 [17].

Juvenile DM has also a bimodal age distribution with peaks at 5 and 9 and 10–14 years of age [6, 11]. In two studies, the mean onset age of juvenile DM was 6.8 and 7.8 years for the USA and Europe respectively [23, 27]. The average age at the onset is estimated between 8 and 9 years, although there is not a great difference in prevalence with children between 2 and 3 years [28]. The mean age of disease onset also varies worldwide. In the USA, the mean age of disease onset is 6.9 years [23, 24]. In one Indian study, the median age at diagnosis was 12 years, with a range of 2.5–16 years, and the median duration of the disease prior to diagnosis was 12 months [29]. Among the children studied in the West Midlands, juvenile DM showed a bimodal age distribution, with the highest annual incidence rates in children under the age of 5 years and in children of 12–13 years, with a mean age of onset of 7.1 years [25]. This bimodal incidence distribution around 2–6 years of age and during the teenage years is consistent with the incidence patterns reported previously [25]. Pachman et al. [30] reported that 18% of patients are diagnosed at 4 years of age or even younger.

5.2 Gender

With DM there is a female predominance in most epidemiological studies, although this was most pronounced during childbearing age. Both DM and PM in adults affect women twice as often as men, and female to male ratio is commonly 1.5–2:1, with an increase to 5:1 during childbearing years [6]. Females, especially African-Americans, are at increased risk. The onset is often later in men than in women [31] and, as expected, the elderly have an even higher incidence of malignancy [32]. A higher incidence was reported in black women compared with white women in two studies from the USA, with a ratio of 2.8:1, and with an incident rate of 17.1cases/million population for black women [6, 7].

The gender ratio varies somewhat among children with juvenile DM throughout the world. In the USA, girls are affected twice as often as boys, whereas in the UK and in Ireland the female to male ratio is reported as being 5:1 [23, 27]. Data from the West Midlands study noted a female to male ratio of 1.75:1 [25]. In China, the data are similar to that reported for the UK [33]. In a series with juvenile DM in India, 12/19 (63%) of patients were boys (female:male ratio of 1:1.7) [29]. In Japan, boys were marginally more frequently affected than girls (female to male ratio 1:1.3) [33]. Other series suggest an equal incidence by sex in juvenile patients.

5.3 Race

Ethnic and racial factors may play an important role in epidemiology of DM. DM appears about ten times more common in Bantu than in the white population of Transvaal [34]. African-Americans are affected twice as often as Caucasians [35]. Blacks affected by

5

DM/PM outnumber whites by 4:1, and black women have the highest incidence, with 32.2 cases/million/year [6].

5.4 Ethnicity

Ethnicity of the affected child may vary by geographic location. In the USA, 71% of affected children are Caucasian, 12% Hispanic, and 9% African-Americans [33]. In the West Midlands study, similar results were reported, with most affected children being white (79%) [25]. Reports from Singapore, Hong Kong, and Taiwan indicate that DM patients of those ethnic backgrounds are more likely to be male than female, while females are affected more often in white populations [36]. DM-associated interstitial lung disease (ILD) seems to occur more commonly in Japanese DM patients than in other ethnic groups [36]. Emerging information on the genetic background of various ethnic groups may allow identification of immune-response genes that predispose certain populations to DM or PM [37, 38].

5.5 Familial DM

During recent years, data supporting the role of genetic influence on susceptibility to IIMs have been presented [39]. These data come from observational studies based on reports of occurrence of multiple cases in single families, as well as from studies of candidate genes in patients cohorts [40]. Several recent reports address the rare familial occurrence of adult and juvenile DM-IIM [41–43]. Familial occurence of juvenile DM is quite variable, and only 11 reported instances of two or more cases from one family have been published. Familial juvenile DM has been reported in monozygotic twins [44–46], in siblings (in two sisters [47] and in a family with two sisters, one with classical juvenile DM and the other with the amyopathic DM [48]), in cousins [49, 50], and in parental relationships [51–53]. The appearance of adult DM in a 29-year-old Caucasian female whose father had the disease for 17 years when he was 40 years old has been reported [43]. This is an interesting example of the differences in clinical presentation and the age of the onset between two successive generations with DM.

5.6 HLA

Genetic factors may play an important role, as was suggested by the rare familial occurrences and the association with certain HLA genes, such as DRB1*0301 alleles for PM [54] and IBM [55], HLA DQA1 0501 for juvenile DM [56], or TNF 308A polymorphism for photosensitivity in DM [57]. From these studies, it is evident that several genes could be important for the development of IIM, but also that genetic factors by themselves are not enough to develop myositis [54]. The association with certain HLA types has been demonstrated in several myositis populations. Only limited genetic studies have been done, with the strongest association in patient cohorts being with the HLA-DQA*0501 allele [58]. The HLA class II genes HLA DRB1*0301 and DQA1*0501 have been determined to be risk factors for all of the major clinical forms of sporadic and familial IIM in both adults and children in the USA and Europe [59–63]. Studies on multiplex families with one or more family members having adult and juvenile DM indicate the etiological role of multiple genetic risk factors; however, HLA-DRB1*0301 is a common genetic risk factor for familial and sporadic IIM [41]. In white juvenile DM cases, HLA class II alleles DMA*0103 and DMB*0102 were suggested as possible risk factors [64]. Other genetic risk factors have also been observed in diverse ethnic groups: in Caucasian IIM (PM and DM) patients, HLA-B8 and DR3 have been reported [61, 65]; African-American IIMs are associated with DR8 and DQA1*0501, and/or DQA1*0401 [61]; in Japanese patients HLA B7 and DR8 have been reported [66]. However, in Korean IIM patients no genetic risk factor has been determined so far; nevertheless, the HLA DRB1*14 genotype seems to be a protective factor for myositis [54, 63]. The frequency of the HLA-DRB1*1302-DQA1*0102-DQB1*0604 haplotype in Japanese DM patients was significantly higher than in healthy controls (42.1% vs 17.7%) and in PM patients (42.1% vs 9.4%) [67]. Furthermore, the frequency of the HLA-DRB1* 0405-DQA1*03-DQB1*0401 haplotype was higher in the PM patients with ILD than in controls (50.0% vs 17.7%), and than in PM without ILD (50.0% vs 5.5%) [67].

Juvenile DM has been associated with HLA-D3 in Caucasians and Hispanics, and with HLA-B8 in Caucasians only [59]. Recently, the association with DR3 was found to be due to linkage disequilibrium with HLA-DQA1*0501 in all ethnic groups [68, 69]. This has been confirmed in studies in different populations and ethnic groups [68]. Indirect evidence has suggested that amyopathic DM shares HLA associations similar to those found in classic DM [61]. Homozygosity of HLA-DQA1 is a distinct risk factor for familial IIM [41]. The C4 null allele is highly associated with Caucasian juvenile DM [70], but no link was found with Caucasian or African-American adult myositis [71]. Anti-PM-Scl autoantibodies are strongly associated with the HLA-DR3 haplotype, which is found in 75–100% of the patients with anti-PM-Scl and also in 30% of the normal, Caucasian population. In sclerodermatomyositis, all Polish patients associated with PM-Scl antibodies had HLA-DQA1*0501, and 94% of them also HLA-DRB1*0301 suballeles [62]. Whereas HLA-DR3 is found in less than 1% of the Japanese population, anti-PM-Scl antibodies are not detected among Japanese patients with myositis overlap syndrome. One of the reasons for this ethnic discrepancy of anti-PM-Scl appears to be attributed to the genetic background [72].

The linkage to certain HLA types is even stronger when patients are classified according to the presence of MSAs. Caucasian patients with "antisynthetase syndrome" are carriers of HLA-DR3 in 90% of cases [73]. Antisynthetase autoantibodies are associated with HLA-DRB1*0301 and HLA-DQA1*0501 allels in white patients, whereas HLA-DQA1*0501 and/or HLA-DQA1*0401, but no HLA-DRB1*0301, are associated with Jo-1 autoantibodies in black and Mexican-American patients [54]. Other genetic associations such as HLA-DR7, HLA-DRw53/, and HLA-DQA*0201 for patients with anti-Mi2

5

autoantibodies, and HLA-DR5, HLA-DRw52, and HLA-DQA1*0301 for patients with anti-SRP autoantibodies, have been determined [74–76]. Drug-induced DM is associated with HLA-B18, HLA-B35, and HLA-DR4 [77].

An association with non-HLA genes has recently been reported [39]. IL-1RN gene encoding IL-1 receptor antagonist did not correlate with circulating levels of IL-1Ra (IL-1 receptor antagonist) that were elevated in IIM patients compared with controls [78]. The IL-1RN A1 allele, associated with increased proinflammatory activity, was found to be a risk factor for Caucasians with juvenile IIMs but not for African-Americans, in whom such a possible risk factor is A3 allele [78].

Recently a group of interferon-inducible genes being overexpressed in DM and relative to IBM and PM has been determined [79]. Profound interferon-inducible genes dysregulation was found in muscle biopsies from DQA1*0501 allele positive children with juvenile DM [80–82]. An association has also been found of the overproducing TNF alpha-308A variant with adult DM and with subacute cutaneous LE [57]. The significantly increased incidence of specific genes that correlate with overproduction or decreased clearance of apototic cells, along with HLA genes involved with antigen presentation, supports the concept of the relationship between genetic and environmental influences that trigger cutaneous autoimmune disease [83].

5.7 Seasons and Climate

The role of the environment in the evolution of DM, whether in regard to climate or geographic location, has not been fully identified and may vary by years and locations. Epidemiological data encompassing the period from 1989 to 1992 in the USA revealed an increased frequency of juvenile DM onset in spring and summer months in all geographic regions of the country [26]. Some demographic studies have suggested that more cases with juvenile DM and patients with antisynthetase (Jo-1) syndrome in adults arise in spring than during other times of the year [84, 85]. A seasonal pattern in the onset of the adult IIM has been reported in the USA [86]. A peak of the onset of anti-Jo-1-synthetase syndrome has been determined between February and July, and in patients with anti-SRP positive myositis between September and February [86]. The seasonal onset of the disease for Japanese PM/DM patients with anti-SRP autoantibodies is between June and August [87]. Recently, in a study of 503 patients in the USA, no significant seasonal patterns of the disease onset were reported in myositis patients as a whole or in the total PM or DM populations [88]. Significant seasonal associations were present, however, in the serologically defined groups. In a group of 131 categorized as "nonblack" patients with "antisynthetase syndrome" myositis, the onset has a peak in March–April predominantly in men with PM [88]. In contrast to previous findings, patients with anti-SRP autoantibodies did not have significant seasonal alterations in the disease onset [88]. Women suffering from IIMs without MSA showed a significant peak of the disease onset in summer, in June–July, whereas in men there was no seasonal pattern [88].

A recent study, suggesting that seasonal early environmental exposures may influence later development of autoimmune disease, assessed birth patterns of patients with IIM [89]. Seasonal birth distributions appear rather in juvenile than in adult IIM subgroups, hypothesizing an influence of perinatal exposures on childhood-onset disease [89].

5.8 Latitude

An increasing relative prevalence of DM along the geographical latitude in Europe has been reported [46]. Patients with DM were more prevalent in the cohorts from the southern countries of Europe (Greece, Italy, Slovenia), while the prevalence of patients with PM was more pronounced in the northern countries (Finland, Iceland, Sweden). The relative prevalence of DM increases from 0.08 in Iceland (latitude 64) to 0.56 in Athens (latitude 38) [46]. It is suggested that both genetic and environmental factors could be involved.

A latitudinal gradient similar to the DM prevalence was found for the MSAs (antisynthetase, anti-M2, and anti-SPR autoantibodies), which occurs more commonly in the southern countries [90]. In contrast, the myositis-associated autoantibodies (MAAs), with the exception of anti-Ro52 and anti-U1snRNP autoantibodies, were more commonly detected in patients from northern countries than in those from southern ones [90].

A study aimed at determining whether climatic and geographical factors influence the distribution of DM, PM, and associated autoantibodies around the world found that surface ultraviolet radiation intensity most strongly contributed to the relative proportion of DM, and was strongly related to the proportion of anti-Mi-2 autoantibodies [91]. It was suggested that ultraviolet radiation may modulate the clinical and histopathological expression of autoimmune muscle disease in various populations.

5.9 Evolution

It has been estimated that approximately 34–40% of DM-affected children have an acute monocyclic disease course that resolves within a 2-year period and remains in remission indefinitely [92]. The remaining 60–66% have chronic disease, requiring immunosuppressive therapy for more than 2 years, and have either disease which remains continuously active or which is characterized by polycyclic course of remissions and exacerbations. Over the past 40 years, the percentage of children with juvenile DM who have a monocyclic course has not changed significantly with the advent of corticosteroid and other immunosuppressive therapies [21]. Before the steroid era, 33% of affected children completely recovered, 33% died, and the remainder had significant disability [93]. After the 1960s, those with a chronic disease have had significantly less morbidity, and the mortality rate has dropped from approximately 33% to less than 5% at present [33].

5

5.10 Clinical Variants

The incidence and sex prevalence of disease are different in diverse variants of DM [17, 94]. Every fourth DM patient has neoplasma, and every sixth has features of other connective tissue disease [17]. Many studies have found a preponderance of female over male with a higher ratio in overlap syndromes [17, 94]. DM associated with a connective tissue disease occurs in younger women with higher preponderance in African-American persons [7, 60].

Amyopathic DM is more common in adults. In the USA it has been estimated to occur with approximately 10% of the incidence of classic DM [36]. In Europe, a similar incidence has been observed [95], whereas in Asia it seems to be relatively more common and varies between 14% in Taiwan [96] and 46% in Singapore [97]. Among children with juvenile DM, 3–5% have the amyopathic subtype with no clinical evidence of muscle weakness, but with the pathognomonic cutaneous manifestations of the disease [33, 98]. In a retrospective analysis of juvenile DM in Pennsylvania, 12% of 16 patients were categorized as having amyopathic DM [27].

References

1. Urbano-Marquez A, Casademont J, Grau JM. Polymyositis–dermatomyositis: the current position. *Ann Rheum Dis* 1991; 50: 191–195.
2. Dalakas M. Polymyositis, dermatomyositis and inclusion body myositis. *N Engl J Med* 1991; 325(21): 1487–1498.
3. Koh ET, Seow A, Ong B, et al. Adult-onset PM/DM: clinical and laboratory features and treatment response in 75 patients. *Ann Rheum Dis* 1993; 52: 857–861.
4. Drake L, Dinehart SM, Farmer ER, et al. Guidelines of care for dermatomyositis. *J Am Acad Dermatol* 1996; 34: 824–829.
5. Dawkins MA, Jorizzo JL, Walker FO, et al. Dermatomyositis: a dermatology-based case series. *J Am Acad Dermatol* 1998; 38: 397–404.
6. Oddis CV, Conte CG, Steen VD, et al. Incidence of PM/DM: a 20-year study of hospital-diagnosed cases in Allegheny County PA, 1963–82. *J Rheumatol* 1990; 17: 1329–1334.
7. Medsger TA, Dawson WN, Masi AT. The epidemiology of polymyositis. *Am J Med* 1970; 48: 715–723.
8. Kurland LT, hauser WA, Ferguson RH, et al. Epidemiologic features of diffuse connective tissue disorders in Rochester, Minn., 1951 through 1967, with special reference to systemic lupus erythematosus. *Mayo Clin Proc* 1969; 44: 649–663.
9. Medsger TA, Jr. Polymyositis and dermatomyositis. In: *Epidemiology of the Rheumatic Diseases*, Lawrence RC, Shulman LE (eds), Gower, New York, 1984; 176–180.
10. Benbassat J, Gefel D, Larholt K, et al. Prognostic factors in polymyostis/dermatomyositis. A computer-assisted analysis of ninety-two cases. *Arthritis Rheum* 1985; 28: 249–255.
11. Kovacs SO, Kovacs SC. Dermatomyositis. *J Am Acad Dermatol* 1998; 39: 899–920.
12. Weitoft T. Occurrence of polymyositis in the county of Gävleborg, Sweden. *Scand J Rheumatol* 1997; 26(2): 104–106.
13. Patrick M, Buchbinder R, Jolly D, et al. Incidence of inflammatory myopathies in Victoria, Australia, and evidence of spatial clustering. *J Rheumatol* 1999; 26: 1094–1100.

14. Fathi M, Dastmalchi M, Rasmussen E, et al. Interstitial lung disease, a common manifestation of newly diagnosed polymyositis and dermatomyositis. *Ann Rheum Dis* 2004; 63: 297–301.
15. Benbassat J, Geffel D, Zlotnick A. Epidemiology of polymyositis-dermatomyositis in Israel, 1960–76. *Isr J Med Sci* 1980; 16(3): 197–200.
16. Ahlstrom G, Gunnarsson LG, Leissner P, et al. Epidemiology of neuromuscular diseases, including the postpolio squelae, in a Swedish county. *Neuroepidemiology* 1993; 12: 262–269.
17. Dourmishev LA. Dermatomyositis: current aspects. Ph.D. thesis, Sofia, 2002; 140.
18. Ramanan AV, Feldman BM. Clinical outcomes in juvenile dermatomyositis. *Curr Opin Rheumatol* 2002; 14: 658–662.
19. Hanissian AS, Masi AT, Pitrier SE, et al. Polymyositis and dermatomyositis in children: an epidemiologic and clinical comparative analysis. *J Rheumatol* 1982; 9: 390–394.
20. Paller AS. Juvenile dermatomyositis and overlap syndromes. *Adv Dermatol* 1995; 10: 309–326.
21. Wargula JC. Update on juvenile dermatomyositis: new advances in understanding its etiopathogenesis. *Curr Opin Rheumatol* 2003; 15(5): 595–601.
22. Melleson PN, Fung MY, Rosenberg AM. The incidence of pediatric rheumatic disease: results from the Canadian Pediatric Rheumatology Association Disease Registry. *J Rheumatol* 1996; 23: 1981–1987.
23. Symmons DPM, Sills JA, Davis SM. The incidence of juvenile dermatomyositis: results from a nation-wide study. *Br J Rheumatol* 1995; 34: 732–736.
24. Mendez EP, Lipton R, Ramsey-Goldman R, et al. NIAMS Juvenile DM Registry Physician Referral Group. US incidence of juvenile dermatomyositis, 1995–1998: results from the National Institute of Arthritis and Musculoskeletal and Skin Diseases Registry. *Arthritis Rheum* 2003; 49(3): 300–305.
25. Gardner-Medwin JM, Dolezalova P, Cummins C, et al. Incidence of Henoch-Schönlein purpura, Kawasaki disease, and rare vasculitides in children of different ethnic origins. *Lancet* 2002; 360: 1197–1202.
26. Pachman LM, Hayford JR, Chung A, et al. Juvenile dermatomyositis at diagnosis: clinical characteristics of 79 children. *J Rheumatol* 1998; 25(6): 1198–1204.
27. Peloro TM, Miller OF, Hahn TF, et al. Juvenile dermatomyositis: a retrospective review of a 30-year experience. *J Am Acad Dermatol* 2001; 45: 28–34.
28. Malleson P. Juvenile dermatomyositis: a review. *J Royal Soc Med* 1982; 75: 33–37.
29. Chowdhary V, Wakhlu A, Agarwal A, et al. Outcome in juvenile dermatomyositis. *Indian Pediatr* 2002; 39: 931–935.
30. Pachman LM, Mendez E, Lou H, et al. Parent report of antecedent illness and environmental factors before onset of juvenile dermatomyositis (JDM): NIAMS JDM registry data [abstract]. *Arthritis Rheum* 1999; 42: S136.
31. Degos R, Civatte J, Belaich S, et al. The prognosis of adult dermatomyositis. *Trans St John's Hosp Dermatol Soc* 1971; 37: 98–104.
32. Marie I, Hatron PY, Levesque H, et al. The influence of age on characteristics of polymyositis and dermatomyositis in adults. *Medicine* 1998; 78: 139–147
33. Pachman LM. Juvenile dermatomyositis: immunogenetics, pathophysiology, and disease expression. *Rheum Dis Clin North Am* 2002; 28: 579–602.
34. Findlay GH, Whiting DA, Sinson IW. Dermatomyositis in the Transvaal and its occurrence in the Bantu. *S Afr Med J* 1969; 43: 694–697.
35. Hochberg MC. Epidemiology of polymyositis/dermatomyositis. *Mt Sinai J Med* 1988; 55: 447–452.
36. Sontheimer RD. Dermatomyositis: an overview of recent progress with emphasasis on dermatologic aspects. *Dermatol Clin* 2002; 20: 387–408.

37. Reed AM. Myositis in children. *Curr Opin Rheumatol* 2001; 13: 428–433.
38. Shamin EA, Rider LG, Pandey JP, et al. Differences in idiopathic inflammatory myopathy phenotypes and genotypes between Mesoamerican Mestizos and North American Caucasians. *Arthritis Rheum* 2002; 46: 1885–1893.
39. Dorph C, Lundberg IE. Idiopathic inflammatory myopathies — myositis. *Best Pract Res Clin Rheumatol* 2002; 16(5): 817–832.
40. Ginn LR, Lin JP, Plotz PH, et al. Familial autoimmunity in pedigrees of idiopathic inflammatory myopathy patients suggests common genetic risk factors for many autoimmune diseases. *Arthritis Rheum* 1998; 41: 400–405.
41. Rider LG, Gurley RC, Pandey JP, et al. Clinical serologic and immunogenetic features of familial idiopathic inflammatory myopathy. *Arthritis Rheum* 1998; 41: 710–719.
42. Plamondon S, Dent PB, Reed AM. Familial dermatomyositis. *J Rheumatol* 1999; 26: 2691–2692.
43. Davies MG, Hickling P. Familial adult dermatomyositis. *Br J Dermatol* 2001; 144: 415–416.
44. Wedgwood RJ, Cook CD, Cohen J. Dermatomyositis: report of 26 cases in children with a discussion of endocrine therapy in 13. *Pediatrics* 1953; 12: 447–466.
45. Harati Y, Niakan E, Bergman EW. Childhood dermatomyositis in monozygotic twins. *Neurology* 1986; 36: 721–723.
46. Hengstman GJD, van Venrooij WJ, Venkovsky J, et al. The relative prevalence of dermatomyositis and polymyositis in Europe exihibits a latitudinal gradient. *Ann Rheum Dis* 2000; 59: 141–142.
47. Christianson HB, Brunsting LA, Perry HO. Dermatomyositis: unusual features, complications, and treatment. *Arch Dermatol* 1956; 74: 581–584.
48. Plamondon S, Dent PB, Reed AM. Familial dermatomyositis. *J Rheumatol* 1999; 26(12): 2691–2692.
49. Lambie JA, Duff LF. Familial occurrence of dermatomyositis. Case report and a family survey. *Ann Intern Med* 1963; 59: 839–847.
50. Henekam RC, Hemstra I, Jennekens FG et al. Juvenile dermatomyositis in first cosins (letter). *N Engl J Med* 1990; 323: 199.
51. Andews A, Hickling P, Hutton C. Familial dermatomyositis. *Br J Rheumatol* 1998; 37: 231–232.
52. Lewkonia RM, Buxton PH. Myositis in father and daughter. *J Neurol Neurosurg Psychiatry* 1973; 36: 820–825.
53. Cassidy JT, Petty R. Dermatomyositis. In: *Textbook of Pediatric Rheumatology*, Cassidy JT, Petty R (eds), Churchill Livingstone, Edinburgh, 1990; 331–375.
54. Shamim EA, Rider LG, Miller FW. Update on the genetics of the idiopathic inflammatory myopathies. *Curr Opin Rheumatol* 2000; 12: 482–491.
55. Koffman BM, Sivakumar K, Simonis T, et al. HLA allele distribution distinguishes sporadic inclusion body myositis from hereditary inclusion body myopathies. *J Neuroimmunol* 1998; 84: 139–142.
56. Reed AM, Ytterberg SR. Genetic and environmental risk factors for idiopathic inflammatory myopathies. *Rheum Dis Clin N Am* 2002; 28: 891–916.
57. Werth VP, Callen JP, Ang G, Sullivan KE. Associations of tumor necrosis factor □ and HLA polymorphisms with adult dermatomyositis: implications for a unique pathogenesis. *J Invest Dermatol* 2002; 119: 617–620.
58. Reed AM, Pachman L, Ober C. Molecular genetic studies of major histocompatibility complex genes in children with juvenile dermatomyositis: increased risk associated with the HLA-DQA1*0501. *Hum Immunol* 1991; 32: 235–240.

59. Friedeman JM, Pachman LM, Maryjowski ML, et al. Immunogenetic studies of juvenile dermatomyositis: HLA-DR antigen frequencies. *Arthritis Rheum* 1983; 26: 214–216.
60. Love LA, Leff RL, Fraser DD, et al. A new approach to the classification of idiopathic inflammatory myopathy: myositis-specific autoantibodies define useful homogeneous patient groups. *Medicine* 1991; 70: 360–374.
61. Arnett FC, Targoff IN, Mimori T, et al. Interrelationship of major histocompatibility complex class II alleles and autoantibodies in four groups with various forms of myositis. *Arthritis Rheum* 1996; 39: 1507–1518.
62. Hausmanowa-Petrusewicz I, Kowalska-Oledzka E, Miller FW, et al. Clinical, serological and immunogenetic features in Polish patients with idiopathic inflammatory myopathies. *Arthritis Rheum* 1997; 40: 1257–1266.
63. Rider LG, Shamim E, Okada S et al. Genetic risk and protective factors for idiopathic inflammatory myopathy in Koreans and American whites: a tale of two loci. *Arthritis Rheum* 1999; 42: 1285–1290.
64. West JE, Reed AM. Analysis of HLA-DM polymorphism in juvenile dermatomyositis(JDM) patients. *Hum Immunol* 1999; 60: 255–258.
65. Garlepp MJ. Immunogenetics of inflammatory myopathies. *Baillieres Clin Neurol* 1992; 2: 579–597.
66. Furuya T, Hakoda M, Higami K et al. Association of HLA class I and class II Alleles with Myositis Japanese Patients. *J Rheumatol* 1998; 25: 1109–1114.
67. Horiki T, Ichikawa Y, Hoshina Y, et al. HLA class II haplotypes associated with pulmonary interstitial lesions of polymyositis/dermatomyositis in Japanese patients. *Tissue Antigens* 2002; 59: 25–30.
68. Reed AM, Stirling JD. Association of the HLA-DQA*0501 allele in multiple racial groups with juvenile dermatomyositis. *Hum Immunol* 1995; 44: 131–135.
69. Reed AM, Pachman LM, Hayford J, et al. Immunogenetic studies in families of children with juvenile dermatomyositis. *J Rheumatol* 1998; 25: 1000–1002.
70. Robb SA, Fielder AH, Saunders CE, et al. C4 complement allotypes in juvenile dermatomyositis. *Hum Immunol* 1988; 22: 31–38.
71. Moulds JM, Rolih C, Goldstein R, et al. C4 null genes in American whites and blacks with myositis. *J Rheumatol* 1990; 17: 331–334.
72. Mimori T. Autoantibodies in connective tissue diseases: clinical significance and analysis of target autoantigens. *Intern Med* 1999; 38: 523–532.
73. Goldstein R, Duvic M, Targoff I, et al. HLA-D region genes associated with autoantibody responses to Jo-1 (histidil-tRNA synthetase) and other translation- related factors in myositis. *Arthritis Rheum* 1990; 33: 657–665.
74. Targoff IN, Johnson AE, Miller FW. Antibody to signal recognition particle in polymyositis. *Arthritis Rheum* 1990; 33: 1361–1370.
75. Gurely RC, Love LA, Targoff IN, et al. Associations among myositis-specific autoantibodies (MSA) and HLA-DQA1 aleles [abstract]. *Arthritis Rheum* 1991; 34: S137.
76. Miller OF, Newman ED. Dermatomyositis and polymyositis. In: *Cutaneous Medicine and Surgery*, Arndt KA, Leboit PC, Robinson JK, et al. (eds), W.B. Saunders, Philadelphia, 1996; 283–290.
77. Wilson CL, Bradlow A, Wonjarowska F. Cutaneous problems with drug therapy in rheumatoid arthritis. *Int J Dermatol* 1991; 30: 148–149.
78. Rider LG, Artlett CM, Foster CB, et al. Polymorphisms in the IL-receptor antagonist gene VNTR are possible risk factors for juvenile idiopathic inflammatory myopathies. *Clin Exp Immunol* 2000; 121: 47–51.

79. Greenberg SA, Sanoudou D, Haslett JN, et al. Molecular profiles of inflammatory myopathies. *Neurology* 2002; 59: 1170–1182.
80. Pachman LM, Tezak Z, Bakay M, et al. Differential gene expression profiles in DQA1*0501(+) untreated JDM muscle are associated with increased IFN response compared with DQA1*0501 negative JDM. *Arthritis Rheum* 2001; 44: S399.
81. Tezak Z, Hoffman EP, Lutz JL, et al. Gene expression profiling in DQA1*0501+ children with untreated dermatomyositis: a novel model of pathogenesis. *J Immunol* 2002; 168: 4154–4163.
82. Hoffman EP, Rao D, Pachman LM. Clarifying the boundaries between the inflammatory and dystrophic myopathies: insights from molecular diagnostics and microarrays. *Rheum Dis Clin N Am* 2002; 28: 743–757.
83. Werth VP, Bashir M, Zhang W. Photosensitivity in rheumatic diseases. *J Invest Dermatol Symp Proc* 2004; 9: 57–63.
84. Plotz PH. Current comcepts in the idiopathic inflammatory myopathies: polymyositis, dermatomyositis, and related disorders. *Ann Intern Med* 1989; 111: 143–157.
85. Targoff IN. Dermatomyositis and polymyositis. *Curr Probl Dermatol* 1991; 3: 5.
86. Leff RL, Burgess SH, Miller FW, et al. Distinct seasonal patterns in the onset of adult idiopathic inflammatory myopathy in patients with anti-Jo-1 and anti-signal recognition particle autoantibodies. *Arthritis Rheum* 1991; 34: 1391–1396.
87. Satoh T, Okano T, Matsui T, et al. Novel autoantibodies against 7SL RNA in patients with polymyositis/dermatomyositis. *J Rheumatol* 2005; 32: 1727–1733.
88. Sarkar K, Weinberg CR, Oddis CV, et al. Seasonal influence on the onset of idiopathic inflammatory myopathies in serologically defined groups. *Arthritis Rheum* 2005; 52: 2433–2438.
89. Vegosen LJ, Weinberg CR, O'Hanlon TP, et al. Seasonal birth patterns in myositis subgroups suggest an etiologic role of early environmental exposures. *Arthritis Rheum* 2007; 56(8): 2719–2728.
90. Brower R, Hengstman GJD, Egberts WV, et al. Autoantibody profiles in the sera of European patients with myositis. *Ann Rheum Dis* 2001; 60: 116–123.
91. Okada S, Weatherhead E, Targoff IN, et al. Global surface ultraviolet radiation intensity may modulate the clinical and immunologic expression of autoimmune muscle disease. *Arthritis Rheum* 2003; 48: 2285–2293.
92. Rennebohm R. Juvenile dermatomyositis. *Pediatr Ann* 2002; 31: 426–433.
93. Bitnum S, Daeschner CW, Travis LB, et al. Dermatomyositis. *J Pediatr* 1964; 64: 101–130.
94. Dourmishev LA, Dourmishev AL, Schwartz RA. Dermatomyositis: cutaneous manifestations of its variants. *Int J Dermatol* 2002; 41: 625–630.
95. Caproni M, Cardinali C, Parodi A, et al. Amyopathic dermatomyositis, a review by the Italian Group of Immunodermatology. *Arch Dermatol* 2002; 138: 23–27.
96. Chen YJ, Wu CY, Shen JL. Predicting factors of malignancy in dermatomyositis and polymyositis: a case control study. *Br J Dermatol* 2001; 144: 825–831.
97. Ang P, Sugeng MW, Chau SH. Classic and amyopathic dermatomyositis seen at the National Skin Centere of Singapore: a 3-year retrospective review of their clinical characteristics and association with malignancy. *Ann Acad Med Singapore* 2000; 20: 219–223.
98. el-Azhary RA, Pakzad SY. Amyopathic dermatomyositis: retrospective review of 37 cases. *J Am Acad Dermatol* 2002; 46: 560–565.

Clinical Manifestations of Dermatomyositis

Dermatomyositis can impact a number of organ systems beyond the skeletal muscles and skin, including lungs, heart, gastrointestinal tract, and eyes.

6 Cutaneous Manifestations of Dermatomyositis

The cutaneous manifestations of DM appear to bear no relationship to the presence or absence of myositis, and the severity of the cutaneous lesions does not appear to be related to the severity of the myositis. In general, the cutaneous manifestations of DM occur approximately 1–3 months or more before the onset of muscle weakness. Skin features may also occur simultaneously with the recognition of myositis. However, it is uncommon for the myositis to occur before the onset of the cutaneous manifestations.

The cutaneous lesions of DM have recently been reviewed [1–4]. The primary, classic skin lesion is a symmetrically distributed violaceous macular erythema [5]. Cutaneous manifestations of DM are generally grouped as pathognomonic, characteristic, compatible [6], less common, and rare [4, 7] (Tables 6.1 and 6.2).

Because the cutaneous manifestations of DM are multiple, with great variety in appearance and with different frequency of appearance, they might be classified in three groups, as photosensitive, hyperkeratotic (isomorphic), and vascular features [8] (see Table 4.6).

The cutaneous lesions of DM are probably photoaggravated [9], despite the lack of symptoms reported by patients suggestive of photosensitivity [10, 11]. Skin lesions can be precipitated by both UVA and UVB light, from natural and artificial sources. A history of a severe sunburn preceding the onset of DM has been noted [12]. Clinical observations suggest that not only the skin lesions are exacerbed by light, but that the muscle disease may worsen after sun exposure [11]. Cutaneous lesions of DM patients may flare up after sun exposure, but in only a few of the cases does their muscle involvement aggravate [11]. However, phototesting cannot reliably reproduce the skin lesions, and thus, the wavelengths of light that cause or provoke the clinical manifestation remain unknown [11].

Photosensitive features of DM are: (i) "heliotrope" (periorbital, facial, malare) rash, with or without edema, (ii) "shawl" or "V"- sign and other erythemas on the extensor aspects, and (iii) photosensitive poikiloderma.

The "heliotrope rash" is violaceous to dusky erythematous exantem, with or without edema, in a symmetrical distribution involving mostly periorbital area and eyelids (Fig. 6.1). This sign can be slight, and may appear only as a mild discoloration along the eyeld margin [11]. Because DM occurs with high frequency in both adults and children of African origin, as well as in other nonwhite groups, the various macular erythematous rashes can be observed, and the activity of the disease can be obscured by the presence of hyperpigmentation

Table 6.1 Cutaneous manifestations of DM in 67 patients [165]

	N = 67	Percentage
Pathognomonic manifestations		
Heliotrope rash	59	88.1
Gottron's papules	38	56.7
Gottron's sign	48	71.6
Characteristic manifestations		
Shawl sign/V-sign	45	67.2
Nailfold changes	25	37.3
Scalp scaly dermatosis	51	73.1
Compatible manifestations		
Periorbital edema/facial swelling	–	–
Photosensitive poikiloderma	28	38.8%
Pruritus	–	–
Less common manifestations		
Cutaneous vasculitis	12	17.9
Panniculitis	–	–
Calcinosis	9	13.4
Rare manifestations	**≤1%**	

Table 6.2 Cutaneous manifestations of DM [165]

Features	Frequency > 50%	<50–>1%	<1%
Photosensitive	"Heliotrope" rash	Other erythemas on the extensor aspects poikiloderma atrophicans	
	"Shawl" or "V"- sign		
Hyperkeratotic (trauma-induced)	Gottron's papules and scalp scaly disease	Keining sign (cuticular hypertrophy)	Follicular hyperkeratosis
			"Mechanic's hands"
			"Holster sign"
Vascular		Proximal nailfold erythema, telangiectasia, infarcts, cutaneous vasculitis	Cutaneous necrosis
			Ulcers
Others		Pruritus	Edema
		Calcinosis	Panniculitis
			Zebra-like erythema
			Erythroderma
			Vesiculo-bullous

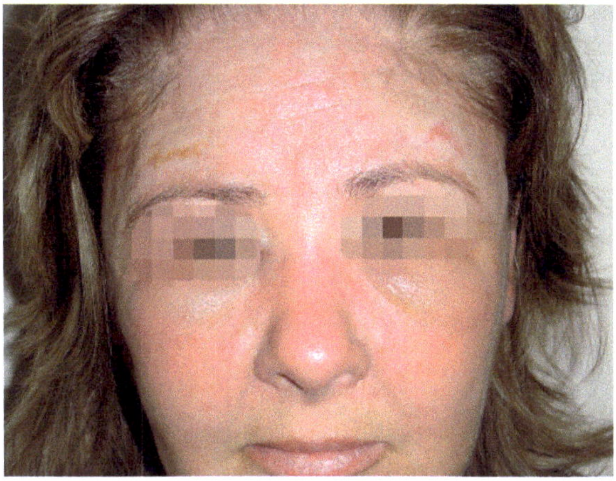

Fig. 6.1 Heliotrope erythema with symmetric periorbital edema in 58-year-old patient with "classic" DM in adults

in patients with darker complexions. The reliance on erythema can mask disease severity in black children compared with white. The presence of blanchable erythema can also be seen, even in areas of hyperpigmentation. Leading-edge erythema extending beyond hyperpigmented patches is also helpful in evaluating the presence of an active disease [4].

Facial-fold erythema, and seborrheic dermatitis-like pattern has been found relatively frequently in adult DM [13, 14]. This type of red, sharply erythema with absence of greasy scale is localized to nasal or periorbital facial folds. It usually precedes the other cutaneous manifestations. There were no significant differences between patients with and without facial fold erythema with regard to the development of complications such as lung fibrosis, internal malignancy, muscle involvement or abnormal laboratory data [14].

Sometimes DM in patients presents with only a periorbital edema [15–17], and this may be the only visible finding of the disease in patients with VI phototype skin (African-American patients) [18]. Depending on the stage of the disease, an initial presentation of intense red erythema, scaling, and edema of the face and upper trunk is followed by decreased edema and more violaceous skin color. As the disease becomes inactive, edema subsides and the color changes fade, leaving a "muddy" appearance of illdefined hypo- and hyperpigmentation. Facial swelling is a common observation in edema Quincke, urticaria, and other skin diseases, but persistent edema associated with violaceous erythema is highly suggestive of DM.

The characteristic lesions of the shawl sign and the V-sign appear as erythematous macules distributed in a "shawl" pattern over the shoulders, arms, and upper back and in a V-shaped distribution over the anterior neck and chest [3] (Fig. 6.2). The patients rarely complain of photosensity, despite the typical photodistribution of the rash. V-sign is difficult to recognize in dark-skinned people [19].

Photosensitive poikiloderma is a circumscribed reticulate telangiectatic erythema with dyschromias and superficial atrophy, resembling radiodermatitis [20–22]. It appears not only in the heliotrope and facial regions, but also over the the neck, upper chest, upper extremities, and back with a "shawl" or "V-shaped" pattern or even more widespread over extensor prominences, incuding knees and elbows [23]. It is most commonly found over the photoexposed

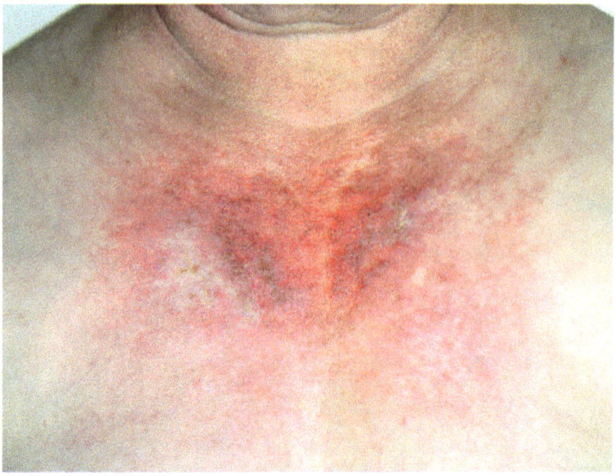

Fig. 6.2 V-shaped erythematous macules distributed over the anterior neck and chest in a "classic" DM in adults

areas, and is often a late finding [3]. The severe atrophy of the poikilodermatous skin can lead to fragility, superficial erosions, and even discrete, disproportionately painful, slow-healing ulceration, especially in the flexural areas of arms, legs, and neck [23]. Poikiloderma may become generalized, and then can resemble cutaneous T-cell lymphoma.

Dermatomyositis can present as generalized erythroderma distinct from both heliotrope rash and poikiloderma [24]. Erythroderma has been found to precede signs of DM by several weeks in 75% of cases [25]. In the classic review of Bohan et al. [26], a "diffuse rash" was described in 32 of 62 DM patients (51.8%). Since many of these patients are seen only by nondermatologists, the distinction between "erythroderma," and "diffuse rash," "widespread erythema" and "exfoliative dermatitis" is tenuous [27]. Ramirez et al. [28] have reported a patient with erythroderma in the UK. The presenting complaint in patients with erythroderma includes all typical clinical features: generalized, scaling, and edematous erythema, inability to maintain thermoregulation, and dermatopathic lymphadenitis [25]. Only six cases of erythrodermic DM have been published in the literature since 1970 [24, 25, 28–31]. No cutaneous necrosis was described in any cases, and only one of them was associated with a malignancy [30]. Moreover, only one report provided a complete description of the erythroderma, including the problem with thermoregulation [24]. Pierson and Taylor's report [27] should be noted, since it described a patient exhibiting extensive erythema, without any disorder in thermoregulation, preceding the onset of DM. Despite there being only a few clearly reported cases in the literature, it is possible that erythroderma might not be such an uncommon form of DM. Indeed, like Pierson and Taylor [27] who described an extensive erythema, Bohan et al. [26] reported diffuse cutaneous eruptions associated with hepatocellular carcinoma, myopathy, and dysphagia. Ramirez et al. described two cases of DM with "generalized eczema" [28]. It is impossible to estimate whether erythroderma is of prognostic value. Survival in three of the patients ranged from 7 [30] to 17 months [24], although it was not specified in other case reports [28, 29, 31]. On the other hand, erythroderma appeared to be an early manifestation of DM. In three of four cases, erythroderma preceded signs of DM, sometimes by several weeks [24, 28]. In the fourth case, the manifestations of erythroderma and DM occurred simultaneously [29]. It is difficult to assess the prevalence of erythrodermic DM and neoplasia in association, which according to all authors is a very poor prognostic sign, since few cases have been reported. An underlying malignancy was found in two out of six known cases of erythrodermic DM, hence the risk of malignancy is comparable with those of non-eythrodermic DM, which is reported to be 15–45%.

Centripetal linear or flagellate erythema is rarely observed in DM patients, and is not associated with photosensitivity. The presence of linear lesions in patients with DM was first described in Bohan's review [32]. Dupre et al. [33] reported a 14-year-old patient with "zebra-like" DM, with linear erythematous macules which gradually disappeared, responding to corticosteroid treatment. Similar cases have recently been reported [34–41]. This entity is observed more frequently in DM than is suggested by the review of the literature [38, 42] and and may correlate with the disease activity [42]. These peculiar cutaneous lesions of DM were located frequently on the back, and show similarity with cutaneous side-effects of patients treated with bleomycin [43]. Patients treated with bleomycin have shown an increased melanosome density in keratinocytes and a reduced epidermal turnover related with the onset of their flagellate erythema [44, 45]. Dupré et al. [46] observed that patients with DM show perinuclear vacuolisation of the arrector pili muscle, similar to those occurring in smooth muscle of cutaneous blood vessels in flagellate erythema [34]. A comparative study with prospective record analysis of patients with dermatomyositis suggested that flagellate erythema more frequent occurs in lupus erythematosus cases [47].

Another cutaneous feature of a DM is termed "holster sign" [3]. Patients with hallmark DM skin manifestations in typical locations have also bilaterally symmetric, patchy, macular violaceous erythema over the lateral aspects of upper thighs and hip. The lesions are extremely pruritic and located over the greater trochanter of the femur. "Holster sign" simulates the contact dermatitis of a leather pistol holster worn from a belt on the waist [3].

Hyperkeratic features of DM that resemble other skin diseases such as psoriasis, lupus erythematosus, lichen planus, pityriasis rubra pilaris are: (i) Gottron's papules, (ii) scalp scaly dermatosis, (iii) cuticular hypertophy, (iv) follicular hyperkeratosis, (v) "mechanic's hands", and (vi) "callosity feet".

Gottron's papular lesions covering bony prominences are pathognomonic cutaneous features of the disease. They are observed in more than 80% of DM patients, and are often distinctive and vary throughout the course of the illness. Gottron's papules might be slightly squamous, and rarely thick psoriasiform scales are observed [11]. The first lesions are small and discrete, then slightly raised, enlarge and coalesce, forming saturated wine-red plaques with scale and sometimes with telangiectasias, or small eschares (Fig. 6.3). If the evolution of the disease is chronic, the rash becomes scaly with a shiny appearance. There are commonly telangiectasias within the lesions. Later, they may become atrophic, or appear as hyperpigmented macules, and may extend as linear streaks over the dorsum of the hands (Gottron's sign).

Erythematous to violaceous scalp scaly dermatosis with atrophic plaques and diffuse noncicatricial alopecia is observed in more than 80% of adult DM patients, and is often misdiagnosed as psoriasis or seborrheic dermatitis [13, 48]. These features occur also in 25% of juvrenile DM patients [49]. Scalp involvement in DM has rarely been considered as a specific manifestation [13, 50] and is often overlooked (Fig. 6.4).

Cuticular changes can be prominent in DM patients. In 1939, Keining first described hyperkeratotic, thickened, rough, distorted cuticles in DM patients [51]. Gottron [52] noted that "Keining's sign" is "a specific symptom" of the disease [53]. The cuticles have

6

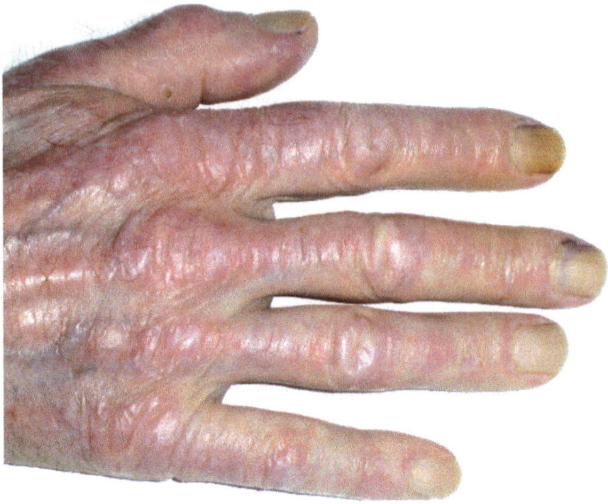

Fig. 6.3 Gottron papules over the dorsum of the hands in a patient with "classic" DM in adults

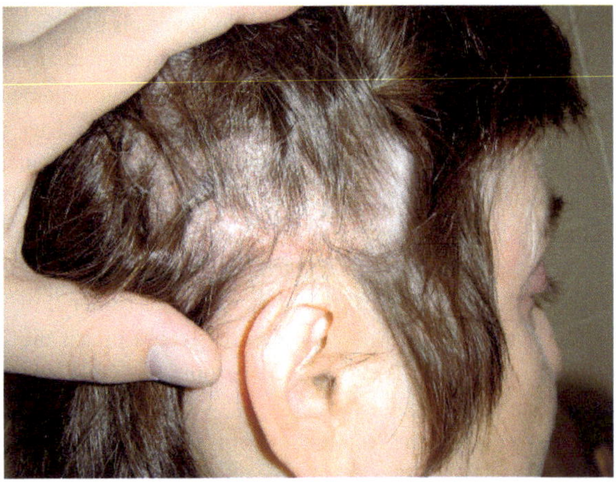

Fig. 6.4 Violaceous scalp erythema, descrete descamation and diffuse hair loss in a 64-year-old patient with "classic" DM in adults

an unkempt, picked appearance characterized by irregular overgrowth and thickening. Ragged cuticles are also found in other connective diseases such as SSc and SLE. A characteristic feature of DM is the association of cuticular changes with peringual erythema, telangiectasias, and hemorrhages. Cutaneous nailfold telangiectasias and cuticular changes are an important diagnostic marker of DM in elderly patients with a chronic course of the disease [54, 55].

Follicular hyperkeratosis (type Wong) is a rare subgroup of patients with DM in adults, who have follicular hyperkeratosis and erythematous papules occuring in a linear pattern [56–58]. To date, less than 20 similar cases have been reported in literature [59, 60]. This variant was named "Wong" since he reported the relatively large series of patients with these cutaneous features. In a series of 23 DM patients (12 of them with paraneoplastic DM) from South East Asia (Hong Kong), Wong announced 11 patients with generalized hyperkeratotic follicular erythematous and hyperkeratotic papules on the back of the hands, usually arranged in a linear array over the bony prominences, suggesting the influence of racial factors [56]. It was also suggested that this variant of DM is more common in Asian patients [61]. This entity was originally described by O'Leary in 1953 in a patient with erythroderma and a plantar keratoderma [62]. Later, Christianson et al. [63] reported 270 patients with DM who attended the Mayo Clinic, including O'Leary's patient and another patient with cutaneous lesions clinically resembling pityriasis rubra pilaris. A characteristic feature of the cutaneous involvement in this variant of DM is the occurrence of follicular hyperkeratosis with a perivascular lymphocytic infiltrate. Lesions involve at least the extremities, and the occurrence of diffuse erythema or spinulosis and palmoplantar keratoderma is possible [59]. The patients' condition clinically resembled pityriasis rubra pilaris, but they did not have characteristic findings such as yellow-orange, palmoplantar discoloration or desquamating hyperkeratosis, and could be distinguished on skin biopsy [64]. Eight additional patients have been reported since Wong's large series [57–60, 64–67]. Dupre et al. (1976) described generalized spinulosis and hyperkeratotic papules on the palms and soles in a 12-year-old child with DM, and found features of the erector pilli myositis in the cutaneous biopsy specimen [57]. Later, Ortonne et al. reported a 52-year-old patient with severe paraneoplastic DM, erythematous rash on the trunk, and erythematous papules on the back of the hands which was histologically confirmed as arrector pili myositis [67]. In 1997, Requena et al. [66] reported a 18-year-old woman with DM and generalized follicular hyperkeratosis and yellowish diffuse palmoplantar keratoderma. A biopsy specimen from the palm showed compact orthohyperkeratosis without evidence of epidermolytic hyperkeratosis. In a summarized review on DM with cutaneous eruptions resembling to pityriasis rubra pilaris, they indicated three other patients but without involvement of the palms and soles [65, 66, 68]. A 53-year-old woman with clinical findings of DM and pityriasis rubra pilaris-like lesions reported by Lupton et al. [64] also had no palmoplantar affection. The widespread patterns of involvement better simulated pityriasis rubra pilaris-like eruption [64, 66]; however, those patients did not have other classic features of pityriasis rubra pilaris such as desquamative palmar plantar hyperkeratosis [3]. Type Wong DM can simulate the appearance of florid keratosis pilaris, and some patients may have concomitant atopic dermatitis.

"Mechanic's hands" have been originally described in eight patients with connective tissue disease, all of whom have had an inflammatory myopathy [69]. Since then a very high incidence of mechanic's hands in patients with anti Jo-1 antibodies and other antisynthetases has been noted [70]. Later, it was suggested that the mechanic's hands skin lesion is associated with antisynthetase syndrome [70–72]. Mitra et al. [71] (1994) reported the clinical and histological features of mechanic's hands in a patient with PM characterized serologically by antibodies to histidyl tRNA synthetase (Jo-1). This feature is mentioned also in other case reports [72–74]. Further study of these cutaneous changes, however, fail to support such associations of mechanic's hands and antisynthetase syndrome [3, 75]. The mechanic's hands sign has been also observed in several patients with amyopathic DM without arthritis, Raynaud's phenomenon, interstitial pneumonia, or MSAs [3]. It has been found also in patients wth classic polymyositis [69, 76], systemic sclerosis [77], and in patients with anti PM-Scl antibody [77–79]. Only four of these patients were children with DM or sclerodermatomyositis [77, 80]. Recently, a 56-year-old woman presenting overlapping syndrome with scleromyositis and mechanic's hands, concomitant interstitial lung fibrosis and positive PM-Scl autoantibody has been reported [81].

Skin manifestations in DM patients consisting of plantar fissured, hyperkeratotic, and scaly eruption mimicking tinea pedis are referred as "callosity feet" [8]. This hyperkeratotic skin eruption, particularly localized on the soles is a rare manifestation of DM, and only a few cases have been reported in the literature. Usually they are associated incorrectly with pityriasis rubra pilaris. O'Leary [62] described a patient with DM with generalized erythema and thick keratinisation of soles, and "a biopsy confirmed clinical impression of pityriasis rubra pilaris." Yellowish diffuse palmoplantar keratoderma in DM patient was reported by Requena et al. [66].

The vascular features of DM included (i) proximal nailfold telangiectasias, (ii) hemorrhages or perungual infarcts, (iii) cutaneous vasculitis, (iv) livedo reticularis, and (v) scattered telangiectasias over the trunk. Histopathologic studies suggest that DM could be represented as a systemic angiopathy [82, 83]. It is suggested that microvascular injury plays an important role in the pathogenesis of cutaneous lesions of the disease [84]. Except for digital infarcts and ulcers, there are no reports specifically describing vascular damage in cutaneous lesions in DM [84]. Periungual areas are erythematous with telangiectases. The periungual telangiectases occur early in the course of the disease in 30–60% of the patients [5]. Capillary changes can parallel the clinical course, with reappearance of the normal cuticular vascular pattern during remission [50].

Cutaneous vasculitis may occur in severe, acute form in children and adults with DM as: (a) palpable purpura [85], (b) urticaria-like lesions [86], (c) livedo reticularis [87], (d) eschares, (e) periungual infarcts, and (f) digital or oral ulcerations [50, 87]. Leukocytoclastic vasculitis in adults suggests that it may be associated with underlying malignancy [85, 88]. However, necrotizing or leukocytoclastic vasculitis can occur also in children with juvenile DM [89]. Cutaneous vasculitis presenting as multiple digital infarcts in DM patients with ILD has been reported as a feature of severe pulmonary involvement [90]. DM with recurrent ulcers and vasculitis is supposed to have a poor prognosis [91].

In late stages of the disease in children, after the treatment discontinuation, scattered telangiectasias may develop over the trunk [92].

Raynaud's phenomenon occurs in approximately one quarter of DM patients. According to various clinical studies in a large group of patients with IIMs, Raynaud's phenomenon has been present in 7% of cases in Singapore [93], 15% in Brazil [94], 23% in Canada [95], 26% in the USA [96], 36% in the UK [28], 39% in Australia [97], and 59% in Sweden [98].

Dermatomyositis presenting as panniculitis is observed in children and adults [99–102]. It has been proposed that DM accompanied by panniculitis may comprise a distinct subset of DM [100]. Other authors have suggested that panniculitis is an inherent part of DM, and should be included as one of the diagnostic cutaneous features of the disease [99, 103]. Since 1924, when Weber and Gray [104] described the predominant involvement of subcutaneous fat in a patient with chronic relapsing DM, few cases with clinically manifested panniculitis have been published [105]. Although clinically manifestations of panniculitis are rarely found in DM, histologic data for panniculitis have frequently been observed and estimated to represent 10% of skin biopsy from cutaneous lesions of DM patients [106]. Common histopathological findings are the infiltration of lymphocytes, epithelioid cells, and plasma cells in the fat lobules, along with varying degrees of fat degeneration and fibrosis [107]. It has been interpreted that the discrepancy between the frequency of clinical manifestations and histologic changes supports the idea of the variable degrees of severity of the same process [103]. In contrast, although changes occurring in the adipose tissue are focal and infrequent, they are not characteristic enough to produce a clinical syndrome of panniculitis [108].

A 65-year-old woman with DM who developed panniculitis with a characteristic histological change known as a membranocystic lesion has been reported [107]. Only four cases of DM with a membranocystic lesion have been published in the literature [91, 107, 109]. Because all patients developed an acute interstitial pneumonia and three of them died from interstitial penumonia, an association of membranocystic lesion with interstitial pneumonia has been suggested in DM patients [91, 110].

Since the internal malignancy in DM patients is very rarely associated with panniculitis (one case with underlying rhabdomyosarcoma with good therapeutical response) [111], it has been suggested that panniculitis in DM could be a positive prognostic sign [100].

The cutaneous signs of DM include soft tissue calcifications. Calcinosis is more common in juvenile DM than in adult DM. Calcium deposition occurs in approximately 30% [112] to 70% [113] of cases of juvenile DM, and in only 10% of adult cases [114]. Calcium deposition occurs subcutaneously (tumor or popcorn-like form) or superficially. The calcinosis is most commonly present on the buttocks, elbows, knees, or areas of trauma, and is associated with increased disease activity and duration. Subcutaneous calcinosis over the extensor surfaces of extremities frequently leads to chronic and difficult healing ulcers [115].

Vesicle or bullae formation in DM was initially reported by Christian in 1903, with 33 subsequent cases being reported up to 2003 [116]. Bullous lesions are frequently observed in the classic form of DM in adults [117] or associated with significant edema [118], gynecologic [119], or gastric malignancies [120]. A specimen from a lesion has demonstrated a subepidermal blister with features of toxic epidermal necrolysis, including full-thickness epidermal necrosis [120]. These subepidermal blisters are not associated with immunoglobulin deposit [119]. Several case reports have described DM with vesicular and bullous lesions without immunofluorescence studies, and it is difficult to determine whether these patients had bullous pemphigoid or dermatitis herpetiformis. Moreover, the relationship between DM and bullous pemphigoid (BP) remains unclear. It has been proposed that the coexistence of the two diseases (DM + BP) may result from disruption of the basal membrane by the DM, which then exposes or realises the bullous pemphigoid antigen, the formation of antibodies, and the subsequent production of blisters in areas not clinically affected by DM [121]. However, in some cases the bullae often coincide with the onset of the DM [116]. Mechanical stress on edematous skin has been considered to be a major factor for the development of blisters in DM patients [120]. Moreover, epidermal necrosis may play a major role in the pathogenesis of bullous lesions [118].

A wide spectrum of nonspecific cutaneous features can frequently be observed in DM patients.

Pruritus, a common and underrecognized complaint of patients with DM, is often associated with secondary skin findings of excoriations and erosions [4]. A case review of 20 patients with juvenile DM revealed that 38% had complaints of pruritus [49]. Statistical analysis shows significant levels of itch sensation in a majority of DM patients [122]. From 26 DM respondents, only four (15%) had no associated pruritus. The pruritus is often refractory to standard therapy of antihistamines and topical corticosteroids.

The edema in DM is usually limited to periorbital and distal extremity areas [123]. Periorbital edema has been rarely reported as the dominant or sole physical sign of DM [15–17]. In four such cases, three were patients with adult DM [15,17], and in the fourth case periorbital edema was the presenting sign of juvenile DM [16]. Despite the female predominance in patients with inflammatory myopathies, most of the patients with associated edema were men. An equal number of patients with PM and DM were described, without significant difference in their clinical picture [124]. Affected patients usually have highly active disease, with pronounced muscle weakness and esophagic involvement. Edema usually begins early in the corse of the disease, ranging from 0.5 to 4 months in the reported cases [125]. Subcutaneous edema is a rare manifestation of inflammatory myopathies, which usually presents in patients with a very active disease [126]. Although few cases have been reported to date, the general prognosis seems good [124, 127–129]; nevetheless, some cases may have a fatal course [125, 131]. Edema is common in eyelids and other sites with loose, soft tissue, but generalized edema has rarely been observed. Generalized edema is an uncommon feature, and has been reported very rarely in an acute disease [126].

Anasarca due to inflammatory myopathies has been described in both male and female patients aged from 27 to 71 years [125]. About 12 cases of generalized edema secondary to inflammatory myopathies have been reported in literature [125], six of them in DM patients [124, 127–129, 130]. There have also been some case reports of generalized edema in juvenile DM [123, 132, 133]. Anasarca as the presenting feature of juvenile DM is suggested as an important prognostic sign [123]. Up to 2004, only 19 case reports of anasarca in juvenile DM have been observed in the literature [133] and the majority of them before 1965. Recently, two boys, 14 and 3.5 years old respectively, were reported with juvenile DM presenting with generalized edema [133, 134]. Magnetic resonance imaging (MRI) of the lower extremities and pelvis showed marked diffuse edema in the subcutaneous tissue, muscles, and myofascia. The mechanisms underlying the severe subcutaneous and diffuse edema in juvenile DM remain unclear. The inflammation of adjacent muscle tissue, coexistence of vasculitis, excessive vascular permeability in muscle, and subcutaneous tissue as a result of the deposition of immune complexes and vascular endothelial damage or even thrombosis of small vessels have been suggested [123, 124]. Zedan et al. even proposes juvenile DM (JDM) as a definite diagnosis in all patients presenting with anasarca in the absence of laboratory parameters of other causes of generalized edema and an appearance of heliotrope rash with muscle weakness [134].

Extremely rare associations with DM include localized lipoatrophy not clinically preceded by panniculitis [135]. Acquired lipodystrophy, increasingly recognized in juvenile DM, could be categorized as generalized, partial, or focal, based on the pattern of fat loss distribution [136]. It has been reported that lipodystrophy was associated with calcinosis [137] and metabolic abnormalities such as hypertriglyceridemia and diabetes [136, 138].

An unusual cutaneous finding in DM is the presence of mucinous papules and/or plaques over the creases of palms and fingers [3, 139], corrugated plaque on the abdominal wall [140], and reticular erythematous mucinosis [141]. Mucin deposits in the skin have been considered as a histological criterion in DM [106, 142]. Clinically evident mucin deposition is usually restricted to primary mucinosis. In secondary or catabolic mucinosis, the mucin deposits are usually microscopic, and associated with cutaneous lesions of associated diseases [139]. Other clinical forms of cutaneous mucinosis associated with DM include plaque-like mucinosis [143], scleromyxedema (lichen myxedematosus) [68, 144, 145] and cellulite-like massive mucinosis [117, 146]. The pathogenesis of mucinosis remains unclear; however, it probably involves fibroblast stimulation by cytokines such as interleukin-1 or interferon [146, 147]. In a review of eight cases of DM-associated macroscopic mucinosis, a pronounced female predominance was found, the age ranging between 21 and 67 years, and the onset of symptoms before diagnosis between 4 and 24 months [117]. Cutaneous lesions of mucinosis appear at the early stages of the disease, and seem to be associated with good response to the treatment [39].

Fasciitis and dermatosclerosis have also been observed in chronic DM [148].

Necrotic skin lesions are predictive of concomitant neoplasia [25, 149–151]. In a study including 32 patients with DM, eight of them had cutaneous necroses [149]. Dermatomyositis, erosions, and ulcers seem to be linked, and are thought to portend a poor prognosis in paraneoplastic dermatomyositis [149].

Rarely, localized or generalized acquired hypertrichosis has been reported in children with juvenile DM [152–156].

Dermatomyositis and acquired ichthyosis are both considered as paraneoplastic dermatoses [157].

Sarcoidosis is rarely associated with DM [158]. Only seven cases with clinically manifest sarcoidosis associated with DM have been described [158–164]. In 1976 Ogawa et al. reported the first case of sarcoidosis with DM [159]. Later, Itoh et al. reported a case of a sarcoid myopathy with a DM rash [160]. The skin biopsy showed the histological changes compatible with DM, and muscle biopsy showed sarcoidal granuloma. In a review of six cases of DM associated with sarcoidosis, the possibility of genetic predisposition of this association has been hypothesized, since two of the cases are Japanese patients; in one of them angiotensin-converting enzyme level was mildly increased [164].

The cutaneous involvement in DM patients sometimes waxes and wanes with the treatment, but no way reflects the severity of the associated myositis [5].

References

1. Euwer R, Sontheimer R. Amyopathic dermatomyositis: a review. *J Invest Dermatol* 1993; 100(1): 124S–128S.
2. Drake L, Dinehart SM, Farmer ER, et al. Guidelines of care for dermatomyositis. *J Am Acad Dermatol* 1996; 34: 824–829.
3. Sontheimer RD. Dermatomyositis: an overview of recent progress with emphasasis on dermatologic aspects. *Dermatol Clin* 2002; 20: 387–408.
4. Santmyire-Rosenberger B, Dugan EM. Skin involvement in dermatomyositis. *Curr Opin Rheumatol* 2003; 15(6): 714–722.
5. Kovacs SO, Kovacs SC. Dermatomyositis. *J Am Acad Dermatol* 1998; 39: 899–920.
6. Euwer R, Sontheimer R. Amyopathic dermatomyositis (dermatomyositis sine myositis). Presentation of six new cases and review of the literature. *J Am Acad Dermatol* 1991; 24: 959–966.

7. Koler RA, Montemarano A. Dermatomyositis. *Am Fam Physician* 2001; 64: 1565–1572.
8. Dourmishev LA, Dourmishev AL, Schwartz RA. Dermatomyositis: an association of gingival telangiectases and anti Jo-1 antibody in the adult. *Acta Dermatovenerol Alp Panonica Adriat* 2007; 16(2): 67–72.
9. Callen JP. Dermatomyositis. *Dis Mon* 1987; 323: 237–305.
10. Cheong WK, Hughes GR, Norris PG, et al. Cutaneous photosensitivity in dermatomyositis. *Br J Dermatol* 1994: 131: 205–208.
11. Callen JP. Dermatomyositis. *Lancet* 2000; 355: 53–57.
12. Rider LG, Okada S, Sherry DD, et al. Epidemiologic features and environmental exposures associated with illness onset in juvenile idiopathic inflammatory myopathy. *Arthritis Rheum* 1995; 38 (Suppl): 362.
13. Kasteler JS, Callen JP. Scalp involvement in dermatomyositis: often overlooked or misdiagnosed. *JAMA* 1994; 272: 1939–1941.
14. Katayama I, Sawada Y, Nishioka K. The seborrheic pattern of dermatomyositis. *Br J Dermatol* 1999; 140: 978–979.
15. Dicken CH. Periorbital edema: an important physical finding in dermatomyositis. *Cutis* 1991; 48: 116–117.
16. Sevigny GM, Mathes BM. Periorbital edema as the presenting sign of juvenile dermatomyositis. *Pediatr Dermatol* 1999;16:43–45.
17. Hall VC, Keeling JH, Davis MD. Periorbital edema as the presenting sign of dermatomyositis. *Int J Dermatol* 2003; 42: 466–467.
18. Bridges BF. The rashes of dermatomyositis in a black patient. *Am J Med* 1991; 91: 661–662.
19. Dalakas M. Polymyositis, dermatomyositis and inclusion body myositis. *N Engl J Med* 1991; 325(21): 1487–1498.
20. Popov L. Dermatomyositis (Morbus Wagner-Potain). *Bulg Clin* 1943; 15(3): 117–139 [Bulgarian].
21. Andreev V. Skin manifestations of cancer of internal organs. *Works of NIOI* 1952; 2(3): 175–258 [Bulgarian].
22. Stonecipher MR, Callen JP, Jorizzo JL. The red face: dermatomyositis. *Clin Dermatol* 1993; 11: 261–273.
23. Miller OF, Newman ED. Dermatomyositis and Polymyositis. In: *Cutaneous Medicine and Surgery*, Arndt KA, Leboit PC, Robinson JK, et al. (eds), W.B. Saunders, Philadelphia, 1996; 283–290.
24. Miyagawa S, Okazaki A, Minowa R, et al. Dermatomyositis presenting as erythroderma. *J Am Acad Dermatol* 1992; 26: 489–490.
25. Maruani A, Armingaud P, Nseir A, et al. Erythroderma and cutaneous necrosis in a patient with dermatomyositis. *Ann Dermatol Venereol* 2003; 150; 353–356.
26. Bohan A, Peter JB, Bowman RL, Pearson CM. A computer-assisted analysis of 153 patients with polymyositis and dermatomyositis. *Medicine* 1977; 56: 255–286.
27. Pierson JC, Taylor JS. Erythrodermic dermatomyositis. *J Am Acad Dermatol* 1993; 28: 136.
28. Ramirez G, Asherson RA, Khanashta MA, et al. Adult-onset polymyositis–dermatomyositis: description of 25 patients with emphasis on treatment. *Semin Arthritis Rheum* 1990; 20: 114–120.
29. Jove RP, Rey JP, Palou J. Modalidad eritrodérmica de dermatomiositis en tránsito a poiquilodermatomiositis. *Actas Dermosifiliogr* 1974; 65: 179–180.
30. Nousari HC, Kimyai-Asadi A, Spegman DJ. Paraneoplastic dermatomyositis presenting as erythroderma. *J Am Acad Dermatol* 1998; 39: 653–654.
31. Liu ZH, Wang XD. Acute-onset adult dermatomyositis presenting with erythroderma and diplopia. *Clin Exp Dermatol* 2007; 32(6): 751–752.
32. Bohan A, Peter JB. Polymyositis and dermatomyositis. *N Engl J Med* 1975; 292: 344–347.

33. Dupre A, Viraben R, Bonafe JL, et al. Zebra-like dermatomyositis. *Arch Dermatol* 1981; 117: 63–64.
34. Watanabe T, Tsuchida T. Flagellate erythema in dermatomyositis. *Dermatology* 1995; 190: 230–231.
35. Ferrer M, Herranz P, Manzano R, et al. Dermatomyositis with linear lesions. *Br J Dermatol* 1996;134:600–601.
36. Cordoliani F, Piette AM, Vignon-Pennamen MD, et al. Erytheme flagellate dorsal au cours de la dermatomyositis. *Ann Dermatol Venereol* 1996; 123: S203.
37. Jara M, Amerigo J, Duce S, Borbujo J. Dermatomyositis and flagellate erythema. *Clin Exp Dermatol* 1997; 21: 440–441.
38. Centeno PG, Sanchez-Aguilar D, Pereiro M, et al. Flagellate erythema and dermatomyositis. *Clin Exp Dermatol* 1998; 23, 239–240.
39. Bachmeyer C, Blum L, Danne O, et al. Isolated flagellate eruptions in dermatomyositis. *Dermatology* 1998; 197: 92–93.
40. Nousari HC, Ha VT, Laman SD, et al. "Centripetal flagellate erythema": a cutaneous manifestation associated with dermatomyositis. *J Rheumatol* 1999; 26: 692–695.
41. Kimyai-Asadi A, Tausk FA, Nousari HC. A patient with dermatomyositis and linear streaks on the back. *Arch Dermat* 2000; 136(5): 666A.
42. Parodi A, Caproni M, Marzano AV, et al. Dermatomyositis in 132 patients with different clinical subtypes: cutaneous signs, constitutional symptoms and circulating antibodies. *Acta Derm Venereol* 2002; 82: 48–51.
43. Mowad CM, Nguyen TV, Elenitsas R, et al. Bleomycin-induced flagellate dermatitis: A clinical and histopathological review. *Br J Dermatol* 1994; 131: 700–702.
44. Fernandez-Obregon AC, Hogan KP, Bibro MK. Flagellate pigmentation for intrapleural bleomycin. *J Am Acad Dermatol* 1985; 13: 464–468.
45. Zaki I, Haslam P, Scerri L. Flagellate erythema after intraperitoneal bleomycin. *Clin Exp Dermatol* 1994; 19: 366–367.
46. Dupré A, Bonafé JL, Delsol G, Oksman F. Dégénérescence des muscles arrecteurs dans une observation de dermatomyosite. *Dermatologica* 1976; 152: 33–39.
47. Magro CM, Crowson AN. The immunofluorescent profile of dermatomyositis: a comparative study with lupus erythematosus. *J Cutan Pathol* 1997; 24: 543–552.
48. Dourmishev A, Serafimova D, Dourmishev L, et al. Crusted scabies with scalp location in dermatomyositis patients. Three cases treated with oral ivermectin. *Int J Dermatol* 1998; 31: 231–234.
49. Peloro TM, Miller OF, Hahn TF, et al. Juvenile dermatomyositis: a retrospective review of a 30-year experience. *J Am Acad Dermatol* 2001; 45: 28–34.
50. Caro I. Dermatomyositis as a systemic disease. *Med Clin North Am* 1989; 73: 1181–1192.
51. Keining E. Versammlungen Casus 3 und 4. *Dermatol Wochenschr* 1939; 109: 1198–1199.
52. Gottron HA, Schönfeld W (eds). *Dermatologie und Venereologie*. Thieme, Stuttgart, 1958; Bd II, Teil 1: 548.
53. Kunte C, Plewig G. Das "Keining-Zeichen" bei Dermatomyositis. *Hautarzt* 1998; 49: 596–597.
54. Samitz MH. Cuticular changes in dermatomyositis: a clinical sign. *Arch Dermatol* 1974; 110: 866.
55. Franks AG. Important cutaneous markers of dermatomyositis. *J Musculoskeletal Med* 1988; 5: 39–63.
56. Wong KO. Dermatomyositis: a clinical investigation of 23 cases in Hong Kong. *Br J Dermatol* 1969; 81: 544–547.
57. Dupre A, Floutard X, Christol B, et al. Dermatomyositis avec spinulosisme (dermatomyositis type Wong). Etude histologique: essai d'interpretation pathogénique. *Ann Dermatol Syphiligr (Paris)* 1976; 103: 141–149.

58. Tribonniere X, Delaporte E, Alfandari S et al. Dermatomyositis with follicular hypekeratosis. *Dermatology* 1995; 191: 242–244.
59. Caporali R, Cavagna L, Bellosta M, et al. Inflammatory myopathy in a patient with cutaneous findings of pityriasis rubra pilaris: a case of Wong's dermatomyositis. *Clin Rheumatol* 2004; 23: 63–65.
60. Polat M, Lenk N, Ustün H, et al. Dermatomyositis with a pityriasis rubra pilaris-like eruption: an uncommon cutaneous manifestation in dermatomyositis. *Pediatr Dermatol* 2007; 24(2): 151–154.
61. Lister RK, Cooper ES, Paige DG. Papules and pustules of the elbows and knees: an uncommon clinical sign of dermatomyositis in oriental children. *Pediatr Dermatol* 1995; 191: 242–244.
62. O'Leary P. Dermatomyositis. *Arch Dermatol* 1953; 68: 101–102.
63. Christianson HB, Brunsting LA, Perry HO. Dermatomyositis: unusual features, complications and treatment. *Arch Dermatol* 1954; 74: 581–589.
64. Lupton JR, Figueroa P, Berberian BJ, et al. An unusual presentation of dermatomyositis: The type Wong variant revised. *J Am Acad Dermatol* 2000; 43:908–912.
65. Granier H, Bresollette L, Morand C, et al. Dermatomyositis de type Wong, chez une femme de 50 ans. *Ann Med Int (Paris)* 1991; 142: 389.
66. Requena L, Grilli R, Soriano L, et al. Dermatomyositis with a pityriasis rubra pilaris-like eruption: a little-known distinctive cutaneous manifestation of dermatomyositis. *Br J Dermatol* 1997; 136: 768–771.
67. Ortonne N, Viguier M, Vignon-Pennamen MD, et al. Arrector pili myositis in a patient with dermatomyositis: an unusual histological feature. *Ann Pathol* 2002; 22(1): 39–42 [French].
68. Von Nagy E, Szodoray L, Pongracz E. Gleichzeitiges Vorkommen von Hasimotos Struma, Dermatomyositis und Skleromyxedem. *Haut-Geschlkr* 1962; 33: 26–29.
69. Stahl NI, Klippel JH, Decker JK. A cutaneous lesion associated with myositis. *Ann Intern Med* 1979; 91: 577–579.
70. Love LA, Leff RL, Fraser DD, et al. A new approach to the classification of idiopathic inflammatory myopathy: myositis-specific autoantibodies define useful homogeneous patient groups. *Medicine (Baltimore)* 1991; 70(6): 360–374.
71. Mitra D, Lovell CL, Macleod TI, et al. Clinical and histological features of "mechanic's hands" in a patient with antibodies to Jo-1 — a case report. *Clin Exp Dermatol* 1994; 19(2): 146–148.
72. Moder KG, Gaffey TA, Matteson EL. Idiopathic inflammatory myopathy of the antisynthetase (Jo-1) type associated with noncaseating granulomas. *Arthritis Rheum* 1993; 36(12): 1743–1747.
73. Perret L, Salani I, Rivier G, et al. Le syndrome antisynthetase, un sous-groupe particulier des myopathies idiopathiques inflammatoires: à propos de trois observations. *Schweiz Rundsch Med Prax* 1996; 85: 508–512.
74. Mogulkoc N, Kabasakal Y, Ekren PK, Bishop PW. An unusual presentation of anti-Jo-1 syndrome, mimicking lung metastases, with massive pleural and pericardial effusions. *J Clin Rheumatol* 2006; 12(2): 90–92.
75. Watanabe C, Okubo Y, Ohi T, et al. A case of dermatomyositis associated with mechanic's hand. *J Dermatol* 2000; 27: 711–716.
76. Indard F, Espana A, Idoate MA, et al. A cutaneous lesion associated with primary polymyositis. *Arch Dermatol* 1993; 129: 1207–1208.
77. Oddis CV, Okano Y, Rudert WA, et al. Serum antibody to the nuclear antigen PM-Scl. *Arthritis Rheum* 1992; 35: 1211–1217.
78. Genth E, Mierau R, Genetzky P, et al. Immunogenetic associations of scleroderma-related antinuclear autoantibodies. *Arthritis Rheum* 1990; 33: 657–665.
79. Genth E, Mireau R. Diagnostische Bedeutung Sclerodermie- und Myositis-assozierter Autoantikörper. Z Rheumatol 1995; 1: 39–49.

80. Rider LG, Miller FW, Targoff IN, et al. A broadened spectrum of juvenile myositis. *Arthritis Rheum* 1994; 37: 1534–1538.
81. Török I, Dankó K, Cserni G, et al. PM-SCL autoantibody positive scleroderma with polymyositis (mechanic's hand: clinical aid in the diagnosis). *JEADV* 2004; 18: 356–359.
82. Wedgwood RJ, Cook CD, Cohen J. Dermatomyositis: report of 26 cases in children with a discussion of endocrine therapy in 13. *Pediatrics* 1953; 12: 447–466.
83. Banker BQ, Victor M. Dermatomyostis (systemic angiopathy) of childhood. *Medicine (Baltimore)* 1966; 45: 261–289.
84. Crowson AN, Margo CM. The role of microvascular injury in the pathogenesis of cutaneous lesions of dermatomyositis. *Hum Pathol* 1996; 27: 15–19.
85. Feldman D, Hochberg MC, Zizic TM, et al. Cutaneous vasculitis in adult polymyositis/ dermatmyositis. *J Rheumatol* 1983; 10: 85–89.
86. Payne CM, Thomas RH. Dermatomyositis with urticated lesions. *J R Soc Med* 1984; 77(2): 137–138.
87. Yosipovitch G, Feinmesser M, David M. Adult dermatomyositis with livedo reticularis and multiple skin ulcers. *J Eur Acad Dermatol Venereol* 1998; 11(1): 48–50.
88. Hunger RE, Durr C, Brands CU. Cutaneous vasculitis in dermatomyositis suggests malignancy. *Dermatology* 2001, 202: 123–126.
89. Jorizzo JL. Dermatomyositis. In: *Dermatology*. Bolognia JL, Jorizzo JL, Rapini RP (eds), Elsevier Science, Philadelphia, 2003; 155–163.
90. Tjiu JW, Lin SJ, Wang LF, et al. Digital infarcts showing microangiopathy in adult dermatomyositis suggest severe pulmonary involvement and poor prognosis. *Br J Dermatol* 2004; 150: 1214–1226.
91. Yamamoto T, Ohkubo H, Katayama I, et al. Dermatomyositis with multiple skin ulcers showing vasculitis and membrano-cystic lesion. *J Dermatol* 1994; 21: 687–689.
92. Norins AL. Juvenile dermatomyositis. *Med Clin North Am* 1989; 73: 1193–1209.
93. Koh ET, Seow A, Ong B, et al. Adult-onset polymyositis/dermatomyositis: clinical and laboratory features and treatment response in 75 patients. *Ann Rheum Dis* 1993; 52: 857–861.
94. Scola RH, Werneck LC, Prevedello DMS, et al. Diagnosis of dermatomyositis and polymyositis: a study of 102 cases. *Arq Neuropsiquiatr* 2000; 58: 789–799.
95. Uthman I, Vazquez-Abad D, Senexal JL. Distinctive features of idiopathic inflammatory myopathies in French Canadians. *Semin Arthritis Rheum* 1996; 26: 447–458.
96. Hochberg MC, Feldman D, Stevens MB. Adult-onset polymyositis/dermatomyositis: an analysis of clinical and laboratory features and survival in 76 patients with review of the literature. *Semin Arthritis Rheum* 1986; 15: 168–178.
97. Tymms KE, Webb J. Dermatopolymyositis and other connective tissue diseases: a review of 105 cases. *J Rheumatol* 1985; 12: 1140–1148.
98. Lundberg I, Nennesmo I, Hedfors E. A clinical, serological, and histopathological study of myositis patients with and without anti-RNP antibodies. *Semin Arthritis Rheum* 1992; 22: 127–138.
99. Neidenbach PJ, Sahn EE, Helton J. Panniculitis in juvenile dermatomyositis. *J Am Acad Dermatol* 1995; 33(2 Pt 1): 305–307.
100. Molnár K, Kemény L, Korom I, et al. Panniculitis in dermatomyositis: report of two cases. *Br J Dermatol* 1998; 139(1): 161–163.
101. Ghali FE, Reed AM, Groben PA, et al. Panniculitis in juvenile dermatomyositis. *Pediatr Dermatol* 1999; 16: 270–272.
102. Chao YY, Yang LJ. Dermatomyositis presenting as panniculitis. Int J Dermatol 2000; 39(2): 141–144.

6

103. Fusade T, Belanyi P, Joly P, et al. Subcutaneous changes in dermatomyositis. *Br J Dermatol* 1993; 128: 451–453.
104. Weber FP, Gray AM. Chronic relapsing polydermatomyositis with predominant involvement of subcutaneous fat. *Br J Dermatol* 1924; 36: 544–560.
105. Solans R, Cortés J, Selva A, et al. Panniculitis: a cutaneous manifestation of dermatomyositis. *J Am Acad Dermatol* 2002; 46(5 Suppl): S148–S150.
106. Janis FJ, Winkelmann RK. Histopathology of the skin in dermatomyositis. *Arch Dermatol* 1968; 97: 640–650.
107. Ishikawa O, Tamura A, Ryuzaki K, et al. Membranocystic changes in the panniculitis of dermatomyositis. *Br J Dermatol* 1996; 134: 773–776.
108. Winkelmann WJ, Billick RC, Srolovitz H. Dermatomyositis presenting as paniculitis. J Am Acad Dermatol 1990; 22: 966–969.
109. Nasu T, Fujiwara M, Suganuma T et al. An autopsy case of dermatomyositis accompanied by a membranocystic lesion (Nasu) in subcutaneous tissue. *Connective Tissue* 1976; 9: 25–31 [Japanese].
110. Tsuchida T, Tamaki K, Ando I, et al. Panniculitis and interstitial pneumonitis in dermatomyositis. Jpn J Dermatol 1987; 97: 1521–1530 [Japanese].
111. Kuyria N, Kninoshita N, Yokoyama N, et al. Dermatomyositis with rhabdomyosarcoma and panniculitis: report of an autopsy case. *Nippon Naika Gakai Zasshi* 1985; 74: 143–148 [Japanese].
112. Pachman LM, Friedman JM, Maryjowski-Sweeney ML, et al. Immunogenetic studies of juvenile dermatomyositis. III. Study of antibody to organ-specific and nuclear antigens. *Arthritis Rheum* 1985; 28(2): 151–157.
113. Bowyer SL, Blane CE, Sullivan DB, et al. Childhood dermatomyositis: factors predicting functional outcome and development of dystrophic calcification. *J Pediatr* 1983; 103: 882–888.
114. Orlow SJ, Watsky KL, Bolognia JL. Skin and bones II. *J Am Acad Dermatol* 1991; 25: 447–462.
115. Dasgeb B, Phillips TJ. Adult-onset dermatomyositis complicated by calcinosis cutis. *Wounds* 2004; 16(12): 364–370.
116. Tsukada Y, Kawase MK, Murashima A, et al. Bullous pemphigoid associated with dermatomyositis successfully controlled with minocycline. *Clin Exp Dermatol* 2003; 28: 554–564.
117. Chen GY, Liu MF, Lee J, et al. Combination of massive mucinosis, dermatomyositis, pyoderma gangrenosum-like ulcer, bullae and fatal intestinal vasculopathy in young female. *Eur J Dermatol* 2005; 15: 396–400.
118. McCollough ML, Cockerell CJ. Vesiculo-bullous dermatomyositis. *Am J Dermatopathol* 1998; 20: 170–174.
119. Kubo M, Sato S, Kitahara H, et al. Vesicle formation in dermatomyositis associated with gynecologic malignancies. *J Am Acad Dermatol* 1996; 34: 391–394.
120. Fujimoto M, Murakami T, Murata S, et al. Acute-onset vesiculo-bullous dermatomyositis associated with massive mucosal necrosis of the intestines. Clin Exp Dermatol 2002; 27(8): 718–720.
121. Glover M, Leigh I. Dermatomyositis pemphigoides: a case with coexistent dermatomyositis and bullous pemphigoid. J Am Acad Dermatol 1992; 27: 849–852.
122. Shirani Z, Kucenic MJ, Carroll CL, et al. Pruritus in adult dermatomyositis. *Clin Exp Dermatol* 2004; 29: 273–276.
123. Mitchell JP, Dennis GJ, Rider LG. Juvenile dermatomyositis presenting with anasarca: a possible indicator of severe disease activity. *J Pediatr* 2001; 138: 942–945.
124. Gorelik O, Almoznino-Sarafian D, Alon I, et al. Acute inflammatory myopathy with severe subcutaneous edema, a new variant? Report of two cases and review of the literature. *Rheumatol Int* 2001; 20: 163–166.

125. Werner de Castro GR, Appenzeller S, Bértolo MB, et al. Acute dermatomyositis with subcutaneous generalized edema. *Clin Rheumatol* 2006; 25(6): 898–900.
126. Andonopoulos AP, Gogos CA, Tzanakakis G. Subcutaneous oedema: an "unrecognized" feature of acute polymyositis. *Rheumatol Int* 1993; 13:159–161.
127. Smyth AE, Bell AL. Acute oedematous dermatomyositis. *Ann Rheum Dis* 2000; 59: 574–545.
128. Nitsche A. Edema de tronco y de pared abdominal en dermatomyositis. *Medicina (B Aires)* 2000; 48: 331–332.
129. Mroue KH, Sharana NH, Rbeiz JG, et al. A case of edematous dermatomyositis. *J Rheum* 2003; 30: 2722–2723.
130. Ito Y, Kawabata D, Yukawa N, et al. Severe subcutaneous generalized edema in a patient with dermatomyositis. *Mod Rheumatol* 2007; 17(2): 171–173.
131. Venables GS, Bates D, Cartlidge NE, et al. Acute polymyositis with subcutaneous oedema. *J Neurol Sci* 1982; 55(2): 161–164.
132. Mehndiratta S, Banerjee P. Juvenile dermatomyositis presenting with anasarca. *Indian Pediatr* 2004; 41: 752–753.
133. Karabiber H, Aslan M, Alkan A, et al. A rare complication of generalized edema in juvenile dermatomyositis: a report of one case. *Brain Dev* 2004; 26: 269–272.
134. Zedan M, El-Ayouty M, Abdel-Hady H, et al. Anasarca: not a nephrotic syndrome but dermatomyositis. *Eur J Pediatr* 2008; (Early online) doi: 10.1007/s00431-008-0716-z.
135. Commens C, O'Neill P, Walker G. Dermatomyositis associated with multifocal lipoatrophy. *J Am Acad Dermatol* 1990; 22: 966–969.
136. Bingham A, Mamyrova G, Rother KI, et al. Childhood Myositis Heterogeneity Study Group. Predictors of acquired lipodystrophy in juvenile-onset dermatomyositis and a gradient of severity. *Medicine (Baltimore)* 2008; 87(2): 70–86.
137. Rider L, Ruiz-Hidalgo M, Labora J, et al. Lipodystrophy in juvenile dermatomyositis is associated with calcinosis, but not with hepatocyte differentiation factor DLK levels. [Abstract]. *Arthritis Rheum* 2001; 44: S264.
138. Verma S, Singh S, Bhalla AK, et al. Study of subcutaneous fat in children with juvenile dermatomyositis. *Arthritis Rheum* 2006; 55(4): 564–568.
139. Del Pozo J, Almago M, Martinez W, et al. Dermatomyositis and mucinosis. *Int J Dermatol* 2001; 40: 120–124.
140. Requena L, Aguilar A, Yus ES. A corrugated plaque on the abdominal wall. *Arch Dermatol* 1990; 126: 1639–1644.
141. Kock JH, Heule, Vuzevski VD. Dermatomyositis en reticulaire erythemateuze mucinose. *Ned Tijdschr Geneeskd* 1994; 138: 1931.
142. Ackerman AB. Dermatomyositis. In: *Diagnosis of Inflammatory Skin Diseases. An Algorithmic Method Based on Pattern* Analysis. Williams & Wilkins, Baltimore, MD, 1997; 289–293.
143. Kaufmann R, Greiner D, Schmidt P, Wolter M. Dermatomyositis presenting as plaque-like mucinosis. *Br J Dermatol* 1998; 138: 889–892.
144. Johnson BL, Horowitz IR, Charles CR, et al. Dermatomyositis and lichen myxedematosus: a clinical, histopathological and electron microscopic study. *Dermatologica* 1973; 147: 109.
145. Launay D, Hatron PY, Delaporte E, et al. Scleromyxedema (lichen myxedematous) associated with dermatomyositis. *Br J Dermatol* 2001; 144: 359–362.
146. Igarashi M, Aizawa H, Tokudome Y, et al. Dermatomyositis with prominent mucinous skin change. Histochemical and biochemical aspects of glycosaminoglycans. Dermatologica 1985; 170(1): 6–11.
147. Caux F, Flageul F, Aractingi S, et al. Maladie de système et mucinose papulonodulaire. A propos de deux observations. *Ann Dermatol Venereol* 1993; 120: 737–739.

148. Dalakas MC, Hohlfeld R. Polymyositis and dermatomyositis. *Lancet* 2003; 362: 971–982.
149. Gallais V, Crickx B, Belaïch S. Facteurs pronostiques et signes prédictifs de cancer au cours de la dermatomyosite de l'adulte. *Ann Dermatol Venereol* 1996; 123: 722–726.
150. Mautner G, Grossman ME, Silvers DN, et al. Epidermal necrosis as a predictive sign of malignancy in adult dermatomyositis. *Cutis* 1998; 61: 190–194.
151. Chen YJ, Wu CY, Shen JL. Predicting factors of malignancy in dermatomyositis and polymyositis: a case-control study. *Br J Dermatol* 2001; 144: 825–831.
152. Turner JC. Dermatomyositis: a study of 3 cases. *N Engl J Med* 1937; 216: 158–161.
153. Reich NE, Reinchard JB. Dermatomyositis associated with hypertrichosis. *Arch Dermatol Syphilol* 1948; 57: 725–732.
154. Pope DN, Strimling RB, Mallory SB. Hypertrichosis in juvenile dermatomyositis. *J Am Acad Dermatol* 1994; 31: 383–387.
155. Faure Fontenla MA. Severe hypertrichosis as an uncommon feature of juvenile dermatomyositis. *J Am Acad Dermatol* 1995; 33(4): 691.
156. Piantanida NA, Person DA, Piantanida EW. Infrapatellar hypertrichosis: an unusual cutaneous manifestation of juvenile dermatomyositis. *Pediatr Dermatol* 2002; 19:135–137.
157. Inuzuka M, Tomita K, Tokura Y, et al. Acquired ichthyosis associated with dermatomyositis in a patient with hepatocellular carcinoma. *Br J Dermatol* 2001; 144(2): 416–417.
158. Ito A, Kazama T, Ito M. A unique case of sarcoidosis: coexistence of sarcoidal granuloma and histological changes consistent with dermatomyositis. *Br J Dermatol* 2003; 149: 430–432.
159. Ogawa K, Hongo O, Sekiguchi T. Dermatomyositis-like symptoms by muscle sarcoidosis. *Rinshyo Derm (Tokyo)* 1976; 18: 993–999.
160. Itoh J, Akiguchi I, Midorikawa R, et al. Sarcoid myopathy with typical rash of dermatomyositis. *Neurology* 1980; 30: 1118–1121.
161. Hart Y, Schwartz MS, Bruckner F, et al. Relapsing dermatomyositis associated with sarcoidosis. *J Neurol Neurosurg Psychiatry* 1988; 51: 311–313.
162. Lipton JH, McLeod BD, Brownell AK. Dermatomyositis and granulomatous myopathy associated with sarcoidosis. *Can J Neurol Sci* 1988; 15: 426–429.
163. Takano Y, Oida K, Kohri Y, et al. Dermatomyositis complicated by sarcoidosis. *Nippon Kyobu Shikkan Gakkai Zasshi* 1996; 34: 1255–1259 [Japanese].
164. Brateanu AC, Caracioni A, Smith HR. Sarcoidosis and dermatomyositis in a patient with hemoglobin SC. A case report and literature review. *Sarcoidosis Vasc Diffuse Lung Dis* 2000; 17: 190–193.
165. Dourmishev LA. Dermatomyositis: Current aspects. PhD Thesis, Sofia 2002; 140.

Oral Manifestations of Dermatomyositis

7

Oral lesions in DM have been only rarely described. This small number of reviews are limited only to mucosal symptoms [1–4], or are case reports [5, 6], mainly of juvenile DM patients [7, 8]. Mucous membrane involvement is reported in about 10–20% of cases [1, 4]. Mucosal edema, erythema, and telangiectasiae are the most common oral alterations [2, 4, 7, 8].

First, Oppenheimer in 1903 wrote the initial report describing mucous membrane involvement in DM patients [9]. Later, Schuerman [10] in a study of 263 DM patients reported that mucosal involvement of pharynx, larynx, and conujunctiva occurred in about 20% of DM patients. In 1942, Keil published details of mucous membrane involvement in DM. He described six main typical lesions of oral mucosa in DM patients, including: (i) erythema and edema, (ii) hemorrhage, (iii) vesicles, (iv) erosions or ulcers, (v) leukoplakia-like plaques, and (vi) a net of dilated superficial vessels [7]. Recently, several reports have been written on the oral manifestations of rheumatic disorders, and few are focused on DM [3, 4, 8, 11] (Table 7.1). Keil focused on the edema near the gingival margins and the prominent dusky red or bluish erythema on various portions of the oral mucous membrane, including gingiva, where closely set telangiectatic vessels could be observed [7]. The bluish red color was due to dilatation of the superficial capillaries. Marginal edematous gingivitis is believed to be a special sign of the capillary changes in PM and DM [2]. Edema of the mouth proper, near the gingival margins, is frequently observed with an increased tendency to bleed. Edema without erythema on the tongue, gingival, palate, and other intraoral sites is also noted.

Vesicules, erosions, and ulcerations can occasionally present on the oral mucosa. It has been suggested that leukoplakia-like lesions, which mainly affected the buccal mucosa, tongue, and palate, were one of the most important diagnostic features found in the oral cavity in DM [7]. Other authors confirmed these observations [8, 11]. Isolated reports of lip ulceration in paraneoplastic DM have been published in literature [12], as well as oral ulceration affecting the floor of the mouth in classic DM [13] and amyopathic DM [14]. In the latter case, biopsy of the oral ulcer showed necrotising vasculitis of a medium-sized artery in the floor of the ulcer. Recently, Healy et al. [6] reported a 65-year-old woman with amyopathic DM associated with non-Hodgkin's lymphoma and extremely painful extensive ulceration of the lips, the buccal mucosa, the lateral borders of the tongue, and

Table 7.1 Oral manifestations of DM

Features	References
Erythema	[2, 4, 7, 8]
Edema without an erythematous component	[2, 4, 7, 8]
Leukoplakia-like plaques	[2, 7, 8, 11]
Gingival telangiectases	[1, 2, 4, 7, 8, 15]
Vesicles	[7, 8, 11]
Erosions	[7, 8, 11]
Ulcers	[6, 12–14]
Hemorrhage	[2, 4, 7, 11]
Lip swelling	[12]
Intraoral pain	[6, 7, 11–14]
Hoarse voice	[17]
Nasal speech	[17]
Dysphagia	[5, 7, 16]

non-scarring alopecia. The oral ulceration and skin lesions resolved completely following the first course of CHOP (cyclophosphamide, doxorubicin, vincristine [oncovin], and prednisolone) combination chemotherapy.

Leukoplakia-like areas have been reported in the oral cavities of patients with lichen planus, or with other mixed connective tissue diseases. Whitish reticulated patches on the tongue, lichen-like lesions were also described, although authors declared that those are not specific characteristics of dermatomyositis [2, 7]. The presence of lip swelling and intraoral pain associated with DM has also been observed [7].

Gingival telangiectasia is mentioned as a symptom of childhood DM [8], but also in adult DM [1, 4, 7, 15]. Ghali et al. [8] reported five cases of juvenile DM with oral manifestations, primarily in the form of gingival telangiectases and proposed as an important diagnostic marker of juvenile DM, similar to the cutaneous nailfold telangiectasias in elderly patients with a chronic disease course. These mucosal changes have been observed in SLE and systemic sclerosis patients.

Recently, Marton et al. [4] evaluated the oral status of 34 patients with IIMs, 29 with PM and five with DM. Seven of them had telangiectasia (five on the lower lip, and one on the palatal mucosa); nine had subjective xerostomia, 11 had signs of salivary hypofunction, and 12 had fibrosis of the minor salivary glands. Masticatory force was significantly decreased in the first molar region in the patient group.

Marginal edematous gingivitis is believed to be a special sign of the capillary changes in PM and DM [2]. Increased gingival indices without severe periodontal disease can be seen as an unusual sign of IIM, which is probably caused by the edema and erythema secondary to the changes to the gingival capillaries [4].

Calcification is also a typical manifestation of the skin and the mucosa in DM but an unusual form, as a corollary sign of the generalized calcinosis, may result in the obliteration of the pulp chamber of the teeth [3].

Dysphagia affects 15–50% of the patients with IIM diseases [5, 7, 16], which is attributed to the esophagus dysmotility due to the striated muscles, and to the inflammatory macroglossia [5].

Voice change similar to "hoarse voice" resulting from swelling of the larynx is a frequent feature of the disease [17]. The involvement of cricopharyngeal muscle, and other muscles in the hypopharynx may produce nasal speech and hoarseness.

References

1. O'Leary PA, Waisman M. Dermatomyositis: a study of 40 cases. *Arch Dermatol Syphilol* 1940; 41: 1001.
2. Schuermann H, Greither A, Hornstein O (eds). Krankheiten der Mundschleimhaut und der Lippen, 3rd ed. Urban & Schwarzenberg, Munich, Germany, 1966; 28–32.
3. Sanger RG, Kirby JW. The oral and facial manifestations of dermatomyositis with calcinosis. *Oral Surg Oral Med Oral Pathol* 1973; 35: 476–488.
4. Marton K, Hermann P, Danko K, et al. Evaluation of oral manifestations and masticatory force in patients with polymyositis and dermatomyositis. *J Oral Pathol Med* 2005; 34: 164–169.
5. Chauvet E, Sailler L, Carreiro M, et al. Symptomatic macroglossia and tongue myositis in polymyositis. *Arthritis Rheum* 2002; 45: 2762–2764.
6. Healy CM, Tobin AM, Kirby B, et al. Oral lesions as an initial manifestation of dermatomyositis with occult malignancy. *Oral Surg Oral Med Oral Pathol Oral Radiol Endod* 2006; 101: 184–187.
7. Keil H. The manifestations in the skin and mucus membranes in dermatomyositis with special reference to the differential diagnosis from systemic lupus erythematosus. *Ann Intern Med* 1942; 16: 827.
8. Ghali FE, Stein LD, Fine JD, et al. Gingival telangiectases: an underappreciated physical sign of juvenile dermatomyositis. *Arch Dermatol* 1999; 135: 1370–1374.
9. Oppenheim H. Über die Polymyositis. *Berl Klin Wochenschr* 1903; 40: 381–385.
10. Schuerman H. Zür Klinik und Pathogenese der Dermatomyositis (Polymyositis). *Arch Dermatol Syph* 1939; 178: 414–468.
11. Callen JP. Oral manifestations of collagen vascular disease. *Sem Cut Med Surg* 1997; 16: 323–327.
12. Agbo-Godeau S, Bertrand J. Lip ulceration in paraneoplastic dermatomyositis. Case report. Review of the literature. *Rev Stomatol Chir Maxillofac* 1993; 94: 287–289.
13. Hall VC, Keeling JH, Davis MD. Periorbital edema as the presenting sign of dermatomyositis. *Int J Dermatol* 2003; 42: 466–467.
14. Seno A, Tokuda M, Yamasaki H, et al. A case of amyopathic dermatomyositis presenting blister and oral ulcer. *Ryumachi* 1999; 39: 836–840 [Japanese].
15. Dourmishev LA, Dourmishev AL, Schwartz RA. Dermatomyositis: an association of gingival telangiectases and anti Jo-1 antibody in the adult. *Acta Dermatoven APA* 2007; 16(2): 67–72.
16. Bohan A, Peter JB, Bowman RL, et al. Computer-assisted analysis of 153 patients with polymyositis and dermatomyositis. *Medicine* 1977; 56: 255–286.
17. Metheny JA. Dermatomyositis: a vocal and swallowing disease entity. *Laryngoscope* 1978; 88: 147–161.

8 Musculoskeletal Involvement in Dermatomyositis

The inflammatory myopathies are a heterogeneous group of chronic, subacute, or acute acquired diseases of skeletal muscle. Their common features are moderate to severe muscle weakness and inflammation in the skeletal muscles [1]. An analysis of 153 cases by Carl Pearson's group in 1977 forms the basis of current clinical knowledge of the musclar involvement in PM and DM [2].

Characteristically, DM patients develop progressive muscle weakness affecting the proximal muscles around the shoulders and hips (limb-girdle muscles), or neck muscles (ofthen in juvenile DM). The weakness is usually symmetric. In general, the onset is gradual and the disease develops relatively slowly, occurring over weeks to even months, and rarely appeares acute. In their series of 153 patients Bohan et al. (1977) reported that, on initial presentation, muscle strength was normal in 48 cases (31%) [2]. However, on occasions, the onset can be acute, with rapid development of weakness. The muscle involvement is the second most common presenting feature of DM, which varied between 53% and 96% of patients with skin rash [3–5] (Table 8.1). Almost all patients presented proximal muscle weakness in some studies [6, 7].

Often the initial complaint is fatigue rather than a specific weakness such as an inability to raise the arms for shaving or hair grooming. Patients have problems such as a difficulty in brushing the hair or reaching above the head, an inability to climb upstairs, a problem rising from a chair, getting out of bed, exiting a car, or even raising the head from the pillow, and may have difficulty with their gait. Patients may experience difficulty raising their arms and hands above their heads.

The more distal muscules are also involved, although their loss is not readily recognized [8]. Fine-motor movements that depend on the strength of distal muscles, such as buttoning a shirt, sewing, knitting, or writing, are affected only late in the course of DM [9].

The difficulties of chewing food due to masseter muscle involvement, and dysphagia (tongue and cricopharyngeal muscle involvement), although uncommon, can be potentially serious. Ocular muscles remain normal, except in advanced, nontreated cases, and if these muscles are affected, the diagnosis of orbital myositis should be suspected [10]. Rare involvement of the *orbicularis oculi* muscle may make the eyelids painful and tender [11]. The association of bilateral ocular myositis with primary inflammatory muscle disease is

L.A. Dourmishev and A.L. Dourmishev, *Dermatomyositis: Advances in Recognition, Understanding and Management,*

8

Table 8.1 Muscle involvement in 67 DM patients [5]

Muscle changes	DM patients	
	$n = 67$	%
1. Myalgia	30	44.8
2. Proximal muscle weakness of the upper limbs	54	80.6
3. Distal muscle weakness of the upper limbs	35	52.2
4. Proximal muscle weakness of the lower limbs	58	86.6
5. Distal muscle weakness of the lower limbs	28	41.8
6. Muscle weakness of the body	25	37.3
7. Asymmetry of the muscle power	10	14.9
8. Atrophy of the proximal muscles	19	28.4
9. Atrophy of the distal muscles	13	19.4
10. Myotonia	12	17.9
11. Dysphagia	31	47
12. Dysphonia	18	27.3
13. Febrility or subfebrility	16	24.2
14. Arthritis or arthralgias	31	47
15. Association with Sjögren syndrome	5	7.6
16. Loss of weight	24	35.8

rare [12]. The extraocular muscles are never affected, in contrast to myasthenia gravis in which they are affected early [9].

The facial muscles are usually spared. The neck-flexor muscles are often involved, causing fatigue and difficulty in holding up the head (head drop). In advanced and, rarely, in acute cases, dysphagia with choking episodes and respiratory muscle weakness occurs. Lumbar lordosis and Trendeleburg gait can also be seen [13]. In juvenile DM, children have difficulty rising to a standing position, using their hands to push off their bodies to get to a standing position (Gower's sign).

Aching, rather than pain, of the muscles might be mentioned. Muscle wasting is usually noted in long-standing cases. In general, muscle tenderness upon palpation, though present, is not a prominent feature in adult DM with a chronic course. However, muscle pain is common in the acute form of the disease [14]. Myalgia and muscle pain may occur usually early in the disease [15]. Because in some studies myalgia is a frequent symptom of DM/PM, it has already been proposed that it should be included in the diagnostic criteria [16]. In childhood DM, however, muscle pain on palpation may be prominent. Contrary to what was believed, myalgia is not as common, occurring in less than 30% of the patients with adult DM [1]. Fibromyalgia is a well-known symptomatic accompaniment of classic DM [17] and has also been reported in amyopathic DM [18]. However, the symptoms of fatigue, muscle pain, and muscle tenderness associated with fibromyalgia could falsely imply the development of myositis in patients with amyopathic DM [17].

Table 8.2 Comparison of the demographic data, clinical presentations, and laboratory features in DM/PM[a] (Adapted from [15])

	n	Female to male ratio	Proximal weak-ness (%)	Dys-phagia (%)	Arthral-gia (%)	Raynaud's phenom-enon (%)	CK (%)
Tymms 1985 Australia	105	2.4:1	85	29	65	39	68
Hochberg 1986 USA	76	3:1	93	45	29	26	96
Ramirez 1990 UK	37	2.5:1	100	–	28	36	84
Lundberg 1992 Sweden	49	3.8:1	100	52	45	59	–
Koh 1993 Singapore	75	1.9:1	87	11	35	7	90
Uthman 1996 Canada	30	2:1	90	43	47	23	90
Scola 2000 Brazil	59	1.5:1	95	30	27	15	71
Dourmishev 2002 Bulgaria[a]	67	2.7:1	83.6	47	47	21	68

[a]Only patients with DM.

Striated muscle involvement affects the ability of patients to swallow. The incidence of dysphagia varied in different studies from 12% [14] to 45% [4]. Esophageal manometry and cineradiography studies have shown abnormal proximal and distal esophageal motility and decreased amplitude of the lower esophageal contractions [19]. Nasal speech, nasal regurgitation of fluids, dysphagia, and palatal palsy can be rarely seen [20].

Sensation usually remains normal. The tendon reflexes are preserved, but may be absent in severely inflammatory affected or atrophied muscles [1].

In children, muscle involvement causes weakness but later leads to contractures [8]. Once a range of motion is lost to contracture, it is very difficult to restore. In the most severe cases, several years after the disease onset, untreated patients or those not responsive to the treatment developed great loss of muscle mass or muscle atrophy [8, 21].

The levels of muscle enzymes, mainly creatine kinase (CK), were increased in most patients with DM as also shown by some studies [15] (Table 8.2).

References

1. Dalakas MC, Hohlfeld R. Polymyositis and dermatomyositis. *Lancet* 2003; 362: 971–982.
2. Bohan A, Peter JB, Bowman RL,Pearson CM. A computer-assisted analysis of 153 patients with polymyositis and dermatomyositis. *Medicine* 1977; 56: 255–286.
3. Bohan A, Peter JB. Polymyositis and dermatomyositis. *N Engl J Med* 1975; 292: 344–347; 403–407.

8

4. Hochberg MC, Feldman D, Stevens MB. Adult-onset polymyositis/dermatomyositis: an analysis of clinical and laboratory features and survival in 76 patients with a review of the literature. *Sem Arthritis Rheum* 1986; 15: 168–178.
5. Dourmishev LA. Dermatomyositis: current aspects. PhD Thesis, Sofia 2002; 140.
6. Ramirez G, Asherson RA, Khamashta MA, et al. Adult onset polymyositis/dermatomyositis: description of 25 patients with emphasis of treatment. *Semin Arthritis Rheum* 1990; 20: 114–120.
7. Lundberg I, Nennesmo I, Hedfors E. A Clinical serological, and histopathological study of myositis patients with and without anti-RNP antibodies. *Semin Arthritis Rheum* 1992; 22: 127–138.
8. Norins AL. Juvenile dermatomyositis. *Med Clin North Am* 1989; 73(5): 1193–1209.
9. Dalakas M. Polymyositis, dermatomyositis and inclusion body myositis. *N Engl J Med* 1991; 325(21): 1487–1498.
10. Stevens AW, Grossman ME, Barr ML. Orbital myositis, vitiligo and giant cell myocarditis. *J Am Acad Dermatol* 1996; 35: 310–312.
11. Santmyire-Rosenberger B, Dugan EM. Skin involvement in dermatomyositis. *Curr Opin Rheumatol* 2003; 15(6): 714–722.
12. Kokotis P, Theodossiadis P, Bouros C, et al. Bilateral ocular myositis as a late complication of dermatomyositis. *J Rheumatol* 2005; 32(2): 379–381.
13. Adams-Gandhi LB, Boyd AS, King LE Jr. Diagnosis and management of dermatomyositis. *Compr Ther* 1996; 22(3): 156–164.
14. Mastaglia, FL, Ojeda VJ. Inflammatory myopathies: partes I and II. *Ann Neurol* 1985;17: 215–227; 317–323.
15. Scola RH, Werneck LC, Prevedello DM, et al. Diagnosis of dermatomyositis and polymyositis: a study of 102 cases. *Arq Neuropsiquiatr* 2000; 58(3B): 789–799.
16. Tanimoto K, Nakano K, Kano S, et al. Classification criteria for polymyositis and dermatomyositis. *J Rheumatol* 1995; 22: 668–674.
17. Sontheimer RD. Dermatomyositis: an overview of recent progress with emphasasis on dermatologic aspects. *Dermatol Clin* 2002; 20: 387–408.
18. Thune P. The coexistence of amyopathic dermatomyositis and fibromyalgia. *Acta Derm Venerol* 2000; 80: 453–454.
19. Caro I. Dermatomyositis as a systemic disease. *Med Clin North Am* 1989; 73(5): 1181–1192.
20. Price CJ, Frankel JP, Hammans SR. Palatal palsy in dermatomyositis. *Eur J Neurol* 2001; 8(2): 197–198.
21. Bowyer SL, Blane CE, Sullivan DB, et al. Childhood dermatomyositis: factors predicting functional outcome and development of dystrophic cacification. *J Pediatr* 1983; 103: 882–888.

9 Joint Involvement

As a multisystem disorder, dermatomyositis also affects joints. Arthralgia is an early symptom of DM in about one third of the cases; however, its severity seems to diminish as weakness becomes more prominent [1]. Arthralgia and arthritis are not prominent features of DM patients from the USA [2], but in Japan they are important signs, and are even included as new criteria for diagnosis [3]. According to various clinical studies in a large group of patients with IIMs, arthralgia has been present in between 17% and 47% of cases in Canada [4, 5], 26% in Brazil [6], 28% in UK [7], 29% in the USA [8], 35% in Singapore [9], 45% in Sweden [10], 47% in Bulgaria [11], and 65% in Australia [12]. Joint involvement of the hands, wrists, and ankles is most common in patients with overlap syndrome, and is a feature of so-called "antisynthetase" or "Jo-1 syndrome" [13]. Arthralgias, arthritis, or both are accompanied by morning stiffness. In the first study by Bohan et al. (1977) of 153 patients with PM/DM, 26% of all groups and 53% of the overlap syndrome had arthralgias [14]. In another series of 105 cases, Tymms and Webb [12] observed that 65% of all IIM patients and 100% of those with overlap syndrome had arthritis. Hochberg et al. [8] have found that 29% of all 76 IIM patients and 67% of those from overlap group had arthralgias or arthritis. In a study by Citera et al. [15], of 29 patients with PM/DM, 27.5% had arthritis.

From studies performed to date, joint involvement was more common in males. The mean age was 30 years and the mean disease duration was 5.3 years. PM patients, especially those with antisynthetase antibodies, frequently develop a nonerosive arthralgia or arthritis. The inflammation involves predominantly small joints, including the proximal interphalangeals, metocarpophalangeals, wrists, elbows, ankles, and knees. The anti-Jo-1 antibody is associated with both a deforming, predominantly nonerosive subluxing arthropathy [13], and erosive polyarthritis with soft-tissue calcification [15, 16]. Joint affection precedes the muscle disease [17] or occurs simultaneously [18]. Usually the patients are seronegative, and diagnostic radiographs are normal. The analysis of joint fluid shows normal or minimally elevated leukocyte counts [19]. Synovial biopsy shows some fibrin coating and mild proliferation of the synovial lining cells.

Arthritis has been noted to occur in 20–65% of juvenile DM patients [20]. This is a nonerosive arthritis involving knees, wrists, elbows, and fingers, and is seen early in the course of the disease. For some patients this can be a major symptomatic problem. Surprisingly,

L.A. Dourmishev and A.L. Dourmishev, *Dermatomyositis: Advances in Recognition, Understanding and Management,*

9

it has also been observed in patients with juvenile amyopathic DM [21]. The frequency of arthritis in juvenile amyopathic DM is similar to that in classic juvenile DM. In a study, three of five juvenile amyopathic DM patients (60%) and 49 of 80 children with classic juvenile DM (61%) were reported to have arthritis which appeared an average of 4.9 years after the disease onset [20].

Joint contractures occur mostly in classic and juvenile dermatomyositis. Cutaneous calcinosis is frequently located on the elbows, knees, and other joints, and can cause considerable disability with severe pain and skin ulcers resulting in joint contractures, which require surgical treatment [22].

Joint pain and swelling are recognised features of myositis, but the use of aggressive immunosuppressive agents to treat IM may result in arthritic complications, as exemplified by three cases of mycobacterial infection published over the past year [23]. Two cases with PM and one with DM complicated by mycobacterial infection in or around the left knee in men with IM have been reported [23]. Atypical mycobacterial infection is commonly seen in immunosuppressed DM patients. Cases of *Mycobacterium avium-intracellulare* complex infection in DM presenting as tenosynovitis [24] and deep cutaneous infection [25] have been reported. Other atypical mycobacterial infections reported in patients with DM include a case of cutaneous *M. chelonae* infection [26].

In a study of 30 cases of *M. tuberculosis* infection in patients with autoimmune rheumatic disease, five had IIMs [27]. A 50-year-old woman with definite DM under immunosuppressive therapy who died from generalized miliary *M. tuberculosis* infection has been observed [28]. A case series in 1987 reported two patients with dermatomyositis who developed muscular tuberculosis [29]. Recently, another rare case of extraspinal musculoskeletal tuberculosis associated with DM has been reported [30].

References

1. Mills JA. Dermatomyositis. In: *Dermatology in General Medicine*. Fitzpatrick TB, Eisen AZ, Wolff K, et al. (eds), McGraw-Hill, New York, 1993; 2148–2155.
2. Provost TT, Flyn JA. Dermatomyositis. In: *Cutaneous Medicine, Cutaneous Manifestations of Systemic Diseases*, Provost TT, Flynn JA (eds), BC Decker, Hamilton/London, 2001; 82–103.
3. Tanimoto K, Nakano K, Kano S. Classification criteria for polymyositis and dermatomyositis. *J Rheumatol* 1995; 22: 668–674.
4. Holden DJ, Brownell AKW, Fritzler MJ. Clinical and serological features of patients with polymyositis and dermatomyositis. *Can Med Assoc J* 1985; 132: 649–653.
5. Uthman I, Vazquez-Abad D, Senexal JL. Distinctive features of idiopathic inflammatory myopathies in French Canadians. *Semin Arthritis Rheum* 1996; 26: 447–458.
6. Scola RH, Werneck LC, Prevedello DMS, et al. Diagnosis of dermatomyositis and polymyositis: a study of 102 cases. *Arq Neuropsiquiatr* 2000; 58: 789–799.
7. Ramirez G, Asherson RA, Khamashta MA, et al. Adult onset polymyositis/dermatomyositis: description of 25 patients with emphasis of treatment. *Semin Arthritis Rheum* 1990; 20: 114–120.
8. Hochberg MC, Feldman D, Stevens MB. Adult onset polymyositis/dermatomyositis: an analysis of clinical and laboratory features and survival in 76 patients with a review of the literature. *Semin Arthritis Rheum* 1986; 15: 168–178.

9. Koh ET, Seow A, Ong B, et al. Adult onset polymyositis/dermatomyositis: clinical and laboratory features and treatment response in 75 patients. *Ann Rheum Dis* 1993; 52: 857–861.
10. Lundberg I, Nennesmo I, Hedfors E. A Clinical serological, and histopathological study of myositis patients with and without anti-RNP antibodies. *Semin Arthritis Rheum* 1992; 22: 127–138.
11. Dourmishev LA. Dermatomyositis: current aspects. PhD Thesis, Sofia 2002; 140.
12. Tymms KE, Webb J. Dermatomyositis and other connective tissue disease: a review of 105 cases. *J Rheumatol* 1985; 12: 1140–1148.
13. Oddis CV, Medsger TA, Cooperstein LA. A subluxing arthropathy associated with the anti-Jo-1 antibody in polymyositis/dermatomyositis. *Arthritis Rheum* 1990; 33: 1640.
14. Bohan A, Peter JB, Bowman RL, et al. A computer-assisted analysis of 153 patients with polymyositis and dermatomyositis. *Medicine* 1977; 56: 255–286.
15. Citera G, Goni MA, Maldonado Cocco JA, et al. Joint involvement in polymyositis/dermatomyositis. *Clin Rheumatol* 1994; 13: 70–74.
16. Cohen MG, Ho KK, Webb J. Finger joint calcinosis followed by osteolysis in a patient with multisystem connective tissue disease and anti-Jo-1 antibody. *J Rheumatol* 1987; 14: 605–608.
17. Wasko CM, Carlson GW, Tomaino MM, Oddis CV. Dermatomyositis with erosive arthropathy: associaction with anti-PL-7 antibody. *J Rheumatol* 1999; 26: 2693–2694.
18. Schumacher HR, Schimmer B, Gordon GV, et al. Articular manifestation of polymyositis and dermatomyositis. *Am J Med* 1979; 67: 287–292.
19. Caro I. Dermatomyositis as a systemic disease. *Med Clin North Am* 1989; 73(5): 1181–1192.
20. Tse S, Lubelsky S, Gordon M, et al. The arthritis of inflammatory childhood myositis syndromes. *J Rheumatol* 2001; 28: 192–197.
21. Sontheimer RD. Dermatomyositis: an overview of recent progress with emphasasis on dermatologic aspects. *Dermatol Clin* 2002; 20: 387–408.
22. Guven M, Gholve PA, Blyakher A, et al. Juvenile dermatomyositis with bilateral progressive knee flexion contracture. *Clin Orthop* 2007; 464: 238–241.
23. Haq I, Isenberg DA. Myositis and swollen knees: disease or treatment complication? *Ann Rheum Dis* 2002; 61: 544–546.
24. Barcat D, Mercie P, Constans J, et al. Disseminated Mycobacterium avium complex infection associated with bifocal synovitis in a patient with dermatomyositis. *Clin Infect Dis* 1998; 26: 1004–1005.
25. Bedlow AJ, Vittay G, Stephenson J, et al. Deep cutaneous infection with Mycobacterium avium-intracellulare complex in an immunosuppressed patient with dermatomyositis. *Br J Dermatol* 1998; 139: 920–922.
26. Banuls J, Ramon R, Pascual E, et al. Mycobacterium chelonae infection resistant to clarithromycin in a patient with dermatomyositis. *Br J Dermatol* 2000; 143: 1345.
27. Hernandez-Cruz B, Sifuentes-Orsonio J, Ponce-de-Leon Rosales S, et al. Mycobacterium tuberculosis infection in patients with systemic rheumatic diseases. A case series. *Clin Exp Rheumatol* 1999; 17: 289–296.
28. Durmischev A, Lazarova A, Krasteva M, et al. Dermatomyositis und tuberculosis (Fall Beobachtung mit exitus letalis). *Z Hautkrh* 1988; 63: 62–63.
29. Camus JP, Koeger AC, Nahoul K, et al. Isolated muscular tuberculosis treated with corticosteroids. Developing outbreak of dermatomyositis under rifampicin treatment. 2 cases. *Ann Med Interne* (Paris) 1987; 138: 524–526.
30. Liu CH, Liu WC, Chen LW, et al. Tuberculous myofasciitis in dermatomyositis. *Clin Rheumatol* 2008. Early online, doi: 10.1007/s10067-007-0799-3.

Cardiac Manifestations of Dermatomyositis

10

First cardiac involvement in PM was described in 1899 by Oppenheim [1]. In the remote past it was noted that in DM patients "the heart does not suffer," or that "the heart muscle is spared" [2]. However, based on the limited autopsy studies, cardiac involvement is probably common though in general clinically asymptomatic. Although uncommon, significant cardiac involvement may be the major source of morbidity and event of disease mortality [3, 4]. The myocardium is affected in DM patients with a frequency that varies in different series, depending on the care with which cardiac features have been sought [5]. In spite of the different pathogeneic mechanisms involved in most studies of cardiac manifestations DM and PM were combined, because of the similarity of symptoms and the low incidence of both diseases [6]. Up to 50% of DM patients with noninvasive studies have asymptomatic cardiac manifestations [3, 7]. Noninvasive studies in DM/PM have shown that up to 85% of patients have abnormalities on Holter-ECG, 57% in cardial technetium-99m-pyrophosphate scintigraphy, and 15% in radionucleotide ventriculography [8, 9]. Cardiac manifestations of DM have included arrythmias, hyperkinetic state, conduction abnormalities, congestive heart failure, pericarditis, pericardial effusions, pericardial tamponade and myocarditis with secondary fibrosis of the myocardium [10–14]. In addition to the myocardial inflammatory diseases, a proliferation of smooth muscle cells of the small vessels may occur, resulting in a decrease in capillary blood flow [5]. This so-called "small-vessel disease" is inconsistently found in DM, and causes clinical symptoms like arrhythmia and angina pectoris [15]. Conduction abnormalities are the most common features and include ST-T changes, abnormal Q waves, bundle branch block, and congestive heart failure [16]. Cardiac palpitations have been more prevalent in PM than in DM patients [17]. Arrhythmias and myocarditis leading to congestive heart failure rarely occur in patients with an acute disease [18, 19] However, in patients with chronic DM, the heart failure is commonly related to hypertension as an adverse effect of the long-term corticosteroid treatment [20]. Clinically significant arrythmias are infrequent, but may be life-threatening when they appear [21]. Autopsies from 20 patients with DM/PM revealed myocarditis in six patients, whereas four of them had small-vessel disease [22]. The coincidence of Raynaud's phemoenon, small-vessel disease, and Prinzmetal's angina has also been described in DM patients [6, 23]. Autopsy material has demonstrated the presence of interstitial and perivascular mononuclear cell infiltrates in heart muscle, similar to those

10

seen in the skeletal muscle [24]. Fibrosis may be extensive [14]. Pericardial involvement in DM is very rare, usually with asymptomatic manifestation. Since the pericardial tamponada can be fatal for DM/PM patients, ECG study of every case is recommended [13]. Pulmonary edema can result from the above-mentioned cardiac complications, and can present as interstitial infiltrates on chest radiograph, and/or hypoxia.

Clinically symptomatic cardiac involvement in DM and PM patients is not common, but when present it is associated with a poor prognosis [25].

Association between cardiac involvement and anti-signal recognition particle (SRP) antibodies has been reported [17, 26]. More recent evidence suggests that anti-SRP antibodies may not contribute to cardiac involvement to the degree that was once suspected [27].

References

1. Oppenheim H. Zur Dermatomyositis. *Ber Kil Wochenschr* 1899; 38: 805–807.
2. Reich NE, Reinchard JB. Dermatomyositis associated with hypertrichosis. *Arch Dermatol Syphilol* 1948; 57: 725–732.
3. Gottdiener JS, Sherber HS, Hawley RJ, et al. Cardiac manifestations in polymyositis. *Am J Cardiol* 1978; 41: 1141–1149.
4. Drachev I, Shishmanov D. Dermatopolymyositis with heart involvement. *Savr Med* 1953; 4: 103–106 [Bulgarian].
5. Askari AD. The heart in polymyositis and dermatomyositis. *Mt Sinai J Med* 1988; 55(6): 479–482.
6. Riemekasten G, Opitz C, Audring H, et al. Beware of the heart: the multiple picture of the cardiac involvement in myositis. *Rheumatology* 1999; 38: 1153–1157.
7. Miller OF, Newman ED. Dermatomyositis and polymyositis. In: *Cutaneous Medicine and Surgery*, Arndt KA, Leboit PC, Robinson JK, et al. (eds), W.B. Saunders, Philadelphia, 1996; 283–290.
8. Taylor AJ, Worthman DC, Burge JR, et al. The heart in polymyositis: a prospective evolution of 26 patients. *Clin Cardiol* 1993; 16: 802–806.
9. Buchpiguel CA, Roizemblatt S, Pastor EH, et al. Cardiac and skeletal muscle scintigraphy in dermato- and polymyositis: clinical implications. *Eur J Nucl Med* 1996; 23: 199–203.
10. Askari AD. Inflammatory disorders of muscle. Cardiac abnormalities. *Clin Rheum Dis* 1984; 10(1): 131–149.
11. Yale SH, Adlakha A, Stanton MS. Dermatomyositis with pericardial tamponade and polymyositis with pericardial effusion. *Am Heart J* 1993; 126(4): 997–999.
12. Lie JT. Cardiac manifestations in polymyositis/dermatomyositis: how to get to the heart of the matter. *J Rheumatol* 1995; 22: 809–811.
13. Chraibi S, Ibnadeljalil H, Habbal R, et al. Pericardial tamponade as the first manifestation of dermatopolymyositis. *Ann Med Intern* 1998; 131: 205–208.
14. Anders HJ, Wanders A, Rihl M, et al. Myocardial fibrosis in polymyositis. *J Rheumatol* 1999; 26: 1840–1842.
15. Peng SK, French WJ. Morphological changes in small vessels on endomyocardial biopsies. *Ann Clin Lab Sci* 1986; 16: 180–188.
16. Bohan A, Peter JB, Bowman RL, et al. A computer-assisted analysis of 153 patients with polymyositis and dermatomyositis. *Medicine* 1977; 56: 255–286.

17. Love LA, Leff RL, Fraser DD, et al. A new approach to the classification of idiopathic inflammatory myopathy: myositis-specific autoantibodies define useful homogeneous patient groups. *Medicine* 1991; 70: 360–374.
18. Haupt HM, Hutchins GM. The heart and cardiac conduction system in polymyositis-dermatomyositis: a clinicopathologic study of 16 autopsied patients. *Am J Cardiol* 1982; 50: 998–1006.
19. Quartier P, Bonnet D, Fournet JC, et al. Severe cardiac involvement in children with systemic sclerosis and myositis. *J Rheumatol* 2002; 29: 1767–1773.
20. Dalakas MC, Hohlfeld R. Polymyositis and dermatomyositis. *Lancet* 2003; 362: 971–982.
21. Mills JA. Dermatomyositis. In: *Dermatology in General Medicine*, Fitzpatrick TB, Eisen AZ, Wolff K, et al. (eds), McGraw-Hill, New York, 1993; 2148–2155.
22. Denbow CE, Lie T, Trancredi RG, et al. Cardiac involvement in polymyositis: a clinicopathologic study of 20 autopsied patients. *Arthritis Rheum* 1979; 22: 1088–1092.
23. Botker HE, Sonne HS, Sorensen KE. Frequency of systemic microvascular dysfunction in syndrome X and in variant angina. *Am J Cardiol* 1996; 78: 182–186.
24. Provost TT, Flyn JA. Dermatomyositis. In: *Cutaneous Medicine, Cutaneous Manifestations of Systemic Diseases*, BC Decker, Hamilton/London, 2001; 82–103.
25. Gonzalez-Lopez L, Gamez-Nava JI, Sanchez L, et al. Cardiac manifestations in dermato-polymyositis. *Clin Exp Rheumatol* 1996; 14: 373–379.
26. Targoff IN, Johnson AE, Miller FW. Antibody to signal recognition particle in polymyositis. *Arthritis Rheum* 1990; 33: 1361–1370.
27. Hengstman GJ, van Engelen BG, Vree Egberts WT, et al. Myositis-specific autoantibodies: overview and recent developments. *Curr Opin Rheumatol* 2001; 13: 476–482.

Complications of Dermatomyositis

Pulmonary Complications of Dermatomyositis

11

In addition to the primary disturbance of the skeletal muscles, extramuscular manifestations may be prominent in patients with idiopathic inflammatory myopathy [1]. Pulmonary complications of PM/DM are divided into primary and secondary. PM and DM may be associated with a diffuse interstitial lung disease (ILD). Initially described by Mills and Mathews in 1956, ILD has been reported as a PM/DM complication in between 5% and 30% of the cases [2]. The presence of ILD in patients with myositis affects the prognosis, and often has an influence on the choice of immunosuppressive treatment [3]. Recent studies show that lung involvement in PM/DM varies between 9% and 46%, depending on the diagnostic method [3–5], but pulmonary function is abnormal in about 40% of DM patients [6, 7]. Chest computed tomography (CT) scan can identify earlier lung involvement than a routine chest radiography [3, 6]. Interstitial lung disease is a primary process seen in DM and PM, and is more frequent in patients with esophageal involvement [8].

Six different entities have been described in patients with ILDs: bronchiolitis obliterans organizing pneumonia (BOOP); diffuse alveolar damage (DAD); nonspecific interstitial pneumonia (NSIP); usual interstitial pneumonia (UIP); pulmonary capillaritis and alveolar hemorrhage (PCAH); and acute interstitial pneumonia (AIP). Early descriptions of the ILD associated with PM/DM suggested that it shared many features with idiopathic pulmonary fibrosis (IPF) [9, 10], although some patients had histological findings described as DAD, BOOP, UIP, or a nonclassifiable interstitial pneumonia (NCIP) [11, 12]. The frequency of the HLA-DRB1*1302-DQA1*0102-DQB1*0604 haplotype in Japanese DM patients was significantly higher than in healthy controls (42.1% vs 17.7%), and in PM patients (42.1% vs 9.4%). Furthermore, the frequency of the HLA-DRB1*0405-DQA1*03-DQB1*0401 haplotype was higher in PM patients with ILD than in controls (50.0% vs 17.7%), and in PM without ILD (50.0% vs 5.5%) [13].

Pulmonary disease in DM patients has been recognized for many years, but was not considered as a common manifestation of the disease [14]. In a retrospective study of PM/DM, only ten of 213 patients (4.7%) had radiologic evidence of parenchymal lung disease [15]. In the study by Bohan et al. of 153 computer-analyzed PM/DM patients, pulmonary disease was not reported [16]. In another study of 42 patients with PM/DM, the radiologic evidence of ILD [UIP, AIP] was found in 10% of the cases [10]. Reviewing the 65 published cases of ILD, including their own data, they concluded that ILD were associated

11

with IIMs in 55% of the cases with PM and 45% with DM [10], which was confirmed later by others [7].

Reliable epidemiological data [7, 10] for association of ILD and DM can be summarized as follow:

1. ILD is associated in 45% of the cases with DM.
2. The average age of the patients is 50 years, and the female to male ratio is 1.6:1.
3. The ILD associated with DM is indistinguishable from idiopathic pulmonary fibrosis or lung disease associated with other connective tissue diseases.
4. The development of ILD occurs early in the course of DM, and frequently precedes skin and muscle manifestations.
5. Joint symptoms are more frequent in patients with an association of DM and ILD.
6. There is a high correlation between ILD associated with DM and the presence of autoantibodies to tRNA synthetases [7, 17–19] or a mucin-like glycoprotein (KL-6) [20].
7. Lung involvement appears to be responsive to corticosteroid therapy [10]; however, recently Takada et al. reported patients with PM/DM with steroid-resistant ILD [21].
8. Characteristic features of DM patients with accompanying rapidly progressive interstitial lung disease (RP-ILD) include lesser complaints of muscle weakness, a lack of elevation of serum CK, and negative tests for autoantibodies [22–25].
9. Pathohistology of the lung disease in these patients mostly reveals DAD [12, 25, 26].
10. Pathohistologic findings of biopsed muscles has revealed mild myositis [25].
11. An increased CD4 + to CD8 + T lymphocyte ratio in the peripheral blood seems to participate in the lung damage induced in DM patients with RP-ILD [25].

Early studies describing the histopathology of ILD in PM/DM have recognized several patterns including DAD, BOOP, cellular interstitial pneumonia (not otherwise specified), and UIP [11, 12].

The clinical manifestations of ILD occurring in PM/DM are variable. The majority of patients with ILD have experienced respiratory symptoms such as cough or dyspnea, but ILD has also been present in patients without any clinical signs of pulmonary disease. Recently, in a study by Douglas et al., the initial presentations were either musculoskeletal (myalgias, weakness, and arthralgias) or pulmonary (cough, dyspnea, and fever) alone; and both syndromes occurred simultaneously in only a quarter of patients [27]. According to Tazelaar et al. [12], three types of lung disease are found in PM/DM patients: interstitial pneumonia or ILD (41%), diffuse alveolitis (36.2%), and a broncheolitis obliterans organizing pneumonia (22.8%). This complication presents clinically with symptoms of nonproductive cough and exertional dyspnea that are accompanied by bibasilar fine crackling rales. Pulmonary function tests show a restrictive pattern with reduced diffusion test capacity. The interstitial lung disease associated with PM/DM usually takes the form of NSIP with characteristic histopathology, radiographic findings, responsiveness to therapy, and survival [27]. In a study by Tansey et al., nonspecific interstitial pneumonia was the most common pattern, with an overall biopsy prevalence of 39% from 54 lung biopsies and patient prevalence of 41% from 37 patients with PM/DM [28]. In a study by Cottin et al., NSIP was the most common histological pattern of interstitial pneumonia in patients with amyopathic DM (100%) and in patients with respiratory symptoms as the initial clinical manifestation of the connective tissue disease (75%). Five-year survival in these patients was 50% [29]. Occasionally, the disease may present as acute interstitial pneumonia with diffuse alveolar damage with rapid progression to respiratory failure or bronchiolitis obliterans organizing pneumonia. Diffuse alveolar damage has also been reported in three patients with amyopathic DM and acute respiratory failure [30].

In general, ILD in DM patients is an insidious process occurring over months. The presentation of pulmonary involvement can be acute, chronic, or as an incidental finding on chest imaging [31] and it correlates with the underlying histopathologic disease. Frazier and Miller [15] divided their patients with ILD into three groups. The clinical manifestations in the first group initiated acute febrile onset, nonproductive cough and progressive dyspnea (hypoxemia); radiographs of the chest showed a granular shadowing superimposed on a reticulo-nodular pattern. Such patients are often treatment-resistant and at risk for death. The second group had a more insidious onset of dyspnea and cough with or without myositis, and a diffuse interstitial fibrosis (DIF) more prominent at the lung bases. The third group presented with either PM or DM and without pulmonary symptoms, but pathological chest radiograph revealed evidence of ILD [15]. In addition, intimal thickening of small pulmonary arteries and arterials can be seen, resulting in pulmonary hypertension. Other investigators divided ILD into two clinical patterns: an acute–subacute type and a chronic type. The chronic type presented with a much slower pace of progressive dyspnea [32]. The severity of the lung affection, like the skin disease, is unrelated to the severity of the muscle syndrome. It has been suggested that ILD associated with the MSAs (particulary antisynthetases) can occur occasionally in the absence of skin and muscle disease. In some individuals however, ILD presents before the clinical appearence of myositis. ILD has been observed in patients having only cutaneous manifestations of DM for prolonged periods of time [32]. In a retrospective study with 20-year follow-up, it was shown that patients with pulmonary involvement (i.e., with either ILD, subclinical alveolitis, or ventilatory insufficiency-related respiratory striated muscle weakness) had higher mortality rates than those without lung involvement [6]. The serum aspartat aminotransferase and ferritin levels were higher in the group of patients with pulmonary involvement, and both characteristic nailfold changes and anti-Jo-1 antibody were present [7].

The most common CT findings in lung disease associated with PM/DM have been irregular linear opacities with areas of consolidation and ground-glass attenuation [33–35]. Diffusion capacity and the findings on high-resolution computed tomography (HRCT) were especially sensitive in detecting this disease. In patients with ILD, abnormalities on HRCT were more common than on chest X-ray examination and lung function test [3]. A recent retrospective review of the CT scan findings of 14 patients with NSIP associated with PM/DM over an average duration of follow-up of 27.6 months (range 3–61 months) concluded that, during the treatment, serial CT scans of PM/DM patients with NSIP showed limited radiographic progression of the fibrosis and an improvement in ground-glass and/or reticular opacities [36].

An association between anti-Jo-1 antibodies and arthritis with ILD has earlier been reported [10, 17, 18] and it is suggested that this constitutes a distinct subgroup of myositis, which is named "antisynthetase syndrome" [37, 38]. The presence of the Jo-1 antibody in association with ILD was initially reported in 11 cases from a Japanese study of 324 patients with connective tissue disease [17]. Ten of the patients had PM and one had DM. All eleven patients had radiographic evidence of ILD. In a US study of 44 patients with PM/DM it was found that ten cases(23%) had Jo-1 antibodies in sera, and five of them

(50%) had ILD [18]. These [17, 18, 39] and other studies [40, 41] have concluded that there is a high correlation between PM/DM with the Jo-1 antibody and the presence of ILD. Anti-Jo-1 antibody is found in 25% of patients with myositis, especially in those with cryptogenic fibrosing alveolitis, Raynaud's phenomenon, sicca syndrome, and mild arthritis [39]. PM and pulmonary fibrosis associated with anti-Pl-7 antibody has been also reported [41]. It is suggested that patients with classic DM who have the antisynthetase syndrome have increased risk of developing ILD [32]. These patients tend to have an acute onset of severe myositis in the spring, the human leukocyte antigen haplotypes HLA-DR3, HLA-DRw52, and HLA-DQA1*0501, an exacerbation of myositis with tapering of medications, moderate response to therapy, a 5-year survival rate of 70%, and a fatal outcome due to pulmonary complications [37, 38].

A new class of autoantibodies to aminoacyl-tRNA synthetases, termed anti-KS, that recognized asparaginyl-tRNA synthetase, was recently described [42]. Unlike other antisynthetases, anti-KS antibodies were detected only in patients with ILD without myositis [42] (see Chapter 31).

Antibodies directed against endothelial cells have also been reported to have a statistically significant increase in patients with ILD [43]. Antibodies against 62 kD antigen (anti-ADAM 10 – A disintegrin and metalloprotease) in bronchial epithelial cells have been determined in the serum of a Japanese woman with pulmonary fibrosis associated with DM [44].

One of the findings of special interest is the elevation of KL-6 level in the serum. KL-6 is a pulmonary glycoprotein, preferentially expressed on type II pneumocysted, which acted as a marker of clinically active lung disease [20]. KL-6 concentrations in sera of patients with interstitial pneumonia associated with PM/DM were significantly higher than those of PM/DM without IP, and healthy nonsmokers [45]. It has been proposed to be a sensitive indicator of interstitial pneumonia in patients with classic DM in adults and children [45–47]. In a small study, serum surfactant protein D (SP-D) was found to be increased in patients with PM/DM-associated ILD and to be inversely correlated with the vital capacity and the diffusing capacity of the lung for carbon monoxide in those patients [48].

Interstitial pneumonitis and pulmonary fibrosis can complicate classic and amyopathic DM [20, 26, 29, 49–51]. In the initial description of six cases with DM without muscle involvement by Krain [52], one patient had "pulmonary fibrosis," which persisted despite corticosteroid treatment. High percentage of ILD in amyopathic DM has been reported from Japan. In many cases, ILD occurred in amyopathic DM patients in the absence of antisynthetase autoantibodies, which are considered to be markers for ILD risk in classic DM patients [32]. The acute pattern of ILD presentation with rapidly progressive dyspnea, progressive hypoxemia, treatment-resistance, and fatal outcome has been observed in a high percentage of amyopathic DM patients developing pulmonary disease in Japanese [32, 51]. NSIP was found to be the most common histological pattern of interstitial pneumonitis encountered in DM/PM, particularly in patients with amyopathic DM and in DM/PM patients with respiratory symptoms as the initial clinical manifestation of the connective tissue disease [29]

The five major causes of pulmonary disease in patients with DM are:

1. **Restrictive ventilatory defects.** These defects develop from severe weakness of the respiratory muscles (diaphragm and the intercostal muscles) and lead to hypoventilation. They occur in less than 10% of patients, and may require intubation and mechanical ventilation in such patients.

2. **Pharyngo-esophageal dysfunction.** All DM patients have weakened cough mechanism, slower protective movements with vomiting, and pharyngeal dysfunction. Dysphagia, nasal regurgitation, and aspiration pneumonia may occur because of the affection of the striated muscles of the pharynx and the upper esophagus and gastrointestinal reflux.
3. **Underlying autoimmune processes** are related to the ILD, or interstitial pneumonia (IP). An increased CD4 + to CD8 + T lymphocyte ratio in the peripheral blood has been reported in DM patients with RP-ILD [25]. Recently, the activation markers and cytokine profiles of pulmonary T cells in bronchoalveolar lavage fluids (BALF) from patients with corticosteroid-resistant (six cases) and corticosteroid-sensitive (16 cases) interstitial pneumonia and DM/PM have been reported [53]. CD25 + CD4 + T cells in BALF were significantly increased in corticosteroid-resistant IP compared with those in corticosteroid-sensitive IP. Moreover, CD25 + CD8 + T cells in BALF were significantly increased only in corticosteroid-resistant IP, but not in corticosteroid-sensitive IP or in healthy controls IP. IFN-γ mRNA was detected in BALF T cells in corticosteroid-resistant and corticosteroid-sensitive IP but not in controls. IFN-γ activates macrophages to produce proinflammatory cytokines such as IL-1 and TNF-γ, and superoxide that causes tissue damage. IFN-γ also induces the expression of adhesion molecules intercellular adhesion molecule-1 (ICAM-1) and vascular cell adhesion molecule-1 (VCAM-1) on vascular endothelial cells, which allows migration of inflammatory cells into alveolar spaces [53]. These results indicate that activated Th1-type pulmonary T cells play an important role in the development of corticosteroid-resistant IP in DM/PM, and that the increase in CD25 + CD8 + T cells in BALF is a useful indicator for corticosteroid-resistant IP in DM/PM [53]. All patients with DM showed increased RP105 negative B cell populations (activated B cells) in the peripheral blood compared with patients with PM and normal subjects [54]. Bronchoalveolar lavage fluid from a patient with DM and active IP contained a large number of RP105-negative B cells [54]. Several studies have provided findings implying that T cells, especially activated CD8 + cells, may play essential roles, and thus could be therapeutic targets in this disease [21].
4. **Antisynthetase autoantibodies**. ILD is most commonly seen in PM patients possessing antisynthetase antibodies [Jo-1, Pl-7, Pl-12, OJ, and KS], and also occurs in patients with classic DM.
5. **Pulmonary complications of the disease from immunosuppressive therapy**. ILD has usually taken the form of acute to subacute antibiotic-resistant community-acquired pneumonia [27]. The use of potent immunosuppressive drugs in patients with inflammatory diseases has been linked to opportunistic infections, including *Nocardia* [55] and *Pneumocystis carinii* [56, 57]. Some DM patients with ILD show steroid resistance [21]. Infectious pneumonitis can occur as a complication of high-dose steroid and/or immunosuppressive therapy, particularly after methotrexate treatment (i.e., drug-induced hypersensitivity pneumonitis) or might be a result of opportunistic infections. Methotrexate causes lung disease in 3–5% of treated patients [58]. The presentation can mimic the myositis-induced IP and thus be indistinguishable from it. The presence of eosinophilia is suggestive for methotrexate lung injury, as well as the presence of granulomas on lung biopsy [59]. Discontinuing methotrexate and adding steroids is the mainstay of the treatment. Usually this complication carries a favorable prognosis [57]. Cyclophosphamide-induced pulmonary disease is similar in presentation,

11

course, and treatment to methotrexate-induced pulmonary disease, but it occurs less frequently [2].

Bronchiolitis obliterans (BO) has also been described.

Secondary complications of PM/DM have included aspiration pneumonia/ pneumonitis, muscle weakness, infection, drug-induced disease, pulmonary congestion secondary to heart failure, pulmonary hypertension, pneumomediastinum, pneumothorax, and massive subcutaneous emphysema [60, 61].

Recurrent aspiration pneumonia due to esophageal involvement and ventilatory failure secondary to muscle weakness is uncommonly associated with diffuse lung disease [27].

Infectious pneumonitis can occur as a complication in DM patients. It is characterized by dyspnea, cough, fever, and interstitial infiltrates. The case of Jang et al. [61] supports the model of pulmonary rupture secondary to interstitial lung disease, and subpleural pulmonary infarctions due to vasculitis.

Pneumomediastinum occurs in DM but not in PM patients, usually DM patients who are on corticosteroids and with normal creatine kinase levels. Pneumomediastinum complicates 7.4% of cases among patients with ILD, but has been described in patients with no underlying lung pathology. The pathophysiology is unclear, but it is thought to be secondary to the vasculopathy associated with DM, which causes a disruption of the bronchial mucosal barrier [62], or to ILD-induced cysts, which can rupture, especially when the interstitium is weakened by steroids.

Other respiratory manifestations of DM have included ventilatory insufficiency, opportunistic infections, pleural effusions, drug-induced reaction, malignancy, pulmonary hypertension, and pulmonary alveolar proteinosis [10, 12, 26, 63].

Only a few cases of pulmonary hypertension have been reported in patients with DM, most of which were associated with ILD [24–26]. A 36-year-old man with severe pulmonary hypertension and features of DM and monoclonal gammopathy has been reported [26]. The patient responded to treatment with cyclophosphamide and prostacyclin, and remained asymptomatic for more than 5 years after the discontinuation of the therapy [26].

Long-term prognosis of the disease in PM/DM patients with lung involvement is serious, and the death rate is higher (27%) than in the patients without pulmonal damage (9%) [7, 64, 65]. Five-year survival rate is about 50% [29]. Pulmonary disease similar to malignancy is a potentially life-threatening complication of the DM pattern of the disease presentation.

Cutaneous signs predicting severe pulmonary involvement and poor prognosis are lacking. Atypical skin lesions such as "mechanic's hands" and cuticular hyperplasia have been seen more often in DM patients with ILD [66]. The nailfold changes were higher in this group of patients with pulmonary involvement [7]. Adult DM patients with associated RP-ILD who had multiple digital infarcts and histopathological evidence of inflammatory microangiopathy in the early course of their illness have been reported, and it has been suggested that digital infarcts are features of severe pulmonary involvement and poor prognosis [67]. However, the better survival associated with NSIP [68–73] undoubtedly accounts for favorable prognosis for patients with PM/DM-ILD in comparison with patients with classic idiopathic pulmonary fibrosis (IPF) [27]. Clinically, NSIP can present as chronic progressive symptoms of cough and dyspnea on exertion in a patient known to have PM/DM, as a radiographic infiltrate in an established case, or as an abnormal

PFT or high-resolution computed tomography (HRCT), in a patient with normal chest radiograph [30].

Several recent reviews have shed new light on pulmonary disease. Recently, Douglas et al. [27] reported findings in 70 PM/DM patients with diffuse ILD gathered from 973 patients evaluated at the Mayo Clinic. In the initial presentations of only 15 patients (21.4%) did either musculoskeletal (arthralgias, myalgias, and weakness) and pulmonary (cough, dyspnea, and fever) symptoms occur simultaneously. Pulmonary disease usually took the form of acute to subacute antibiotic-resistant community-acquired pneumonia. Chest radiographs and computed tomography commonly demonstrated bilateral irregular linear opacities involving the lung bases; occasionally with consolidation. Jo-1 antibody was present in 19 of 50 tested patients (38%). Associated malignancy was found in 4 of 70 patients (5.7%). Surgical lung biopsies disclosed NSIP in 18 of 22 patients (81.8%), organizing DAD in two, BOOP in one, and UIP also in one patient. The treatment usually included prednisone in 40–60 mg/day dosages for initial control, followed by lower dose prednisone plus an immunosuppressive agent such as azathioprine or methotrexate for disease suppression. Survival was significantly better than that observed for historical control subjects with idiopathic UIP, and was more consistent with survival previously reported for idiopathic NSIP. There was no difference in survival between Jo-1-positive and Jo-1-negative groups. In a series of 156 patients in France, 36 demonstrated pulmonary involvement [74]. A high morbidity and mortality, including five deaths, was notable. In this series, a substantial proportion of patients (19.2%) improved or even showed a resolution of their lung disease [74].

The majority of patients with ILD experienced respiratory symptoms such as cough or dyspnea, but ILD was also present in patients without any clinical signs of pulmonary disease; thus, neither cough nor dyspnea are a valid indicator of pulmonary involvement in DM/PM, and cannot be used for selection of patients who should undergo radiological and lung function assessments [3].

References

1. Dalakas M. Polymyositis, dermatomyositis and inclusion body myositis. *N Engl J Med* 1991; 325(21): 1487–1498.
2. Aoun NY, Velez E, Aggarwal A, et al. Fatal acute interstitial pneumonitis complicating polymyositis in a 41-year-old man. *Respir Care* 2004; 49: 1515–1521.
3. Fathi M, Dastmalchi M, Rasmussen E, et al. Interstitial lung disease, a common manifestation of newly diagnosed polymyositis and dermatomyositis. *Ann Rheum Dis* 2004; 63: 297–301.
4. Schwarz MI. Pulmonary and cardiac manifestations of polymyositis-dermatomyositis. *J Thorac Imag* 1992; 7: 46–54.
5. Ikezoe J, Johkoh T, Kohno N, et al. High-resolution CT findings of lung disease in patients with polymyositis and dermatomyositis. *J Thorac Imag* 1996; 11: 250–259.
6. Marie I, Hatron PY, Hachulla E, et al. Pulmonary involvement in polymyositis and in dermatomyositis. *J Rheumatol* 1998; 25: 1336–1343.
7. Marie I, Hatron PY, Hachulla E, et al. Survival of patients with polymyositis/dermatomyositis and pulmonary involvement. *J Rheumatol* 1999; 26: 1852–1854.
8. Callen JP. Dermatomyositis. *Lancet* 2000; 355: 53–57.
9. Duncan PE, Griffin JP, Garcia A, et al. Fibrosing alveolitis in polymyositis: a review of histologically confirmed cases. *Am J Med* 1974; 57: 621–626.

11

10. Dickey BF, Myers AR. Pulmonary disease in polymyositis and dermatomyositis. *Sem Arthritis Rheum* 1984; 14: 60–76.
11. Schwarz MI, Matthay RA, Sahn SA, et al. Interstitial lung disease in polymyositis and dermatomyositis: analysis of six cases and review of the literature. *Medicine* 1976; 55: 89–104.
12. Tazelaar HD, Viggiano RW, Pichersgill J, et al. Interstitial lung disease in polymyositis and dermatomyositis: clinical features and prognosis as correlated with histologic findings. *Am Rev Resp Dis* 1990; 29: 727–733.
13. Horiki T, Ichikawa Y, Hoshina Y, et al. HLA class II haplotypes associated with pulmonary interstitial lesions of polymyositis/dermatomyositis in Japanese patients. *Tissue Antigens* 2002; 59: 25–30
14. Caro I. Dermatomyositis as a systemic disease. *Med Clin North Am* 1989; 73(5): 1181–1192.
15. Frazier AR, Miller RD. Interstitial pneumonitis in association with polymyositis and dermatomyositis. *Chest* 1974; 66: 403–407.
16. Bohan A, Peter JB, Bowman RL, et al. A computer-assisted analysis of 153 patients with polymyositis and dermatomyositis. *Medicine* 1977; 56: 255–286.
17. Yoshida S, Akizuki M, Mimori T, et al. The precipitating antibody to an acidic nuclear antigen protein, the Jo-1, in connective tissue diseases: a marker for a subset of polymyositis with interstitial pulmonary fibrosis. *Arthritis Rheum* 1983; 26: 604–611.
18. Hochberg MC, Feldman D, Stevens MB. Antibody to Jo-1 in polymyositis/dermatomyositis: association with interstitial pulmonary disease. *J Rheumatol* 1984; 11: 663–665.
19. Philips TJ, Leigh IM, Wright J. Dermatomyositis and pulmonary fibrosis associated with anti-Jo-1 antibody. *J Am Acad Dermatol* 1987; 17: 381–382.
20. Hirakata M, Nagai S. Interstitial lung disease in polymyositis and dermatomyositis. *Curr Opin Rheumatol* 2000; 12: 501–508.
21. Takada T, Suzuki E, Nakano M, et al. Clinical features of polymyosiytis/ dermatomyositis with steroid-resistent interstitial lung disease. *Intern Med* 1998; 37: 669–673.
22. Fudman EJ, Schnitzler TJ. Dermatomyositis without creatine kinase elevation: a poor prognostic sign. *Am J Med* 1986; 80: 329–332.
23. Takizawa H, Shiga J, Moroi Y, et al. Interstitial lung disease in dermatomyositis. *J Rheumatol* 1987; 14: 102–107.
24. Hashimoto Y, Nawata Y, Kurasawa K, et al. Investigation of EB virus and cytomegalovirus in rapidly progressive interstitial pneumonitis in polymyositis/dermatomyositis by in situ hybridization and polymerase chain reaction. *Clin Immunol Immunopathol* 1995; 77: 298–306.
25. Ito M, Kaise S, Suzuki S, et al. Clinico-laboratory characterisyics of patients with dermatomyositis accompanied by rapid progressive interstitial lung disease. *Clin Rheumatol* 1999; 18: 462–467.
26. Toyoshima M, Sato A, Chida M, et al. Clinicopathological features of interstitial pneumonia associated with amyopathic dermatomyositis. *Jpn J Thor Dis* 1997; 35: 281–287 [abstract].
27. Douglas WW, Tazelaar HD, Hartman TE, et al. Polymyositis/dermatomyositis associated interstitial lung disease. *Am J Respir Crit Care Med* 2001; 164: 1182–1185.
28. Tansey D, Wells AU, Colby T, et al. Variations in histological patterns of interstitial pneumonia between connective tissue disorders and their relationship to prognosis. *Histopathology* 2004; 44: 585–596.
29. Cottin V, Thivolet-Bejoui F, Reynaud-Gaubertz M, et al. Interstitial lung disease in amyopathic dermatomyositis, dermatomyositis and polymyositis. *Eur Respir J* 2003; 22: 245–250.
30. Lee CS, Chen TL, Tzen CY, et al. Idiopathic inflammatory myopathy with diffuse alveolar damage. *Clin Rheumatol* 2002; 21: 391–396.
31. Schwarz MI. The lung in polymyositis. *Clin Chest Med* 1998; 19: 701–712.

32. Sontheimer RD. Dermatomyositis: an overview of recent progress with emphasasis on dermatologic aspects. *Dermatol Clin* 2002; 20: 387–408.
33. Mino M, Noma S, Taguchi Y, et al. Pulmonary involvement in polymyositis and dermatomyositis: sequential evaluation with CT. *Am J Radiology* 1997; 169: 83–87.
34. Akira M, Hara H, Sakatani M. Interstitial lung disease in association with polymyositis-dermatomyositis: long-term follow-up CT evaluation in seven patients. *Radiology* 1999; 210: 333–338.
35. Hartman TE, Swensen SJ, Hansell DM, et al. Nonspecific interstitial pneumonia: Variable appearance at high-resolution chest CT. *Radiology* 2000; 217: 701–705.
36. Arakawa H, Yamada H, Kurihara Y, et al. Nonspecific interstitial pneumonia associated with polymyositis and dermatomyositis: Serial high-resolution CT findings and functional correlation. *Chest* 2003; 123: 1096–1103.
37. Love LA, Leff RL, Fraser DD, et al. A new approach to the classification of idiopathic inflammatory myopathy: myositis-specific autoantibodies define useful homogeneous patient groups. *Medicine* 1991; 70: 360–374.
38. Miller F. Myositis-specific autoantibodies. Touchstones for understanding the inflammatory myopathies. *J Am Med Assoc* 1993; 270: 1846–1849.
39. Bernstein RM, Morgan SH, Chapman J, et al. Anti-Jo-1 antibody: a marker for myositis with interstitial lung disease. *Br J Med* 1984; 289: 151–152.
40. Walker EJ, Tymms KE, Webb J, et al. Improved detection of anti-Jo-1 antibody, a marker for myositis, using purified histityl-tRNA synthetase. *J Immunol Methods* 1987; 96: 149–156.
41. Lamedica G, Parodi A, Peris G, et al. Polymyositis and pulmonary fibrosis associated with anti-PL-7 antibody. *J Am Acad Dermatol* 1988; 19: 567–568.
42. Hirakata M, Suwa A, Nagai S, et al. Anti KS. Identification of autoantibodies to asparginyl-transfer RNA synthetase associated with interstitial lung disease. *J Immunol* 1999; 162: 2315–2320.
43. Cervera R, Ramirez G, Fernandez-Sola J, et al. Antibodies to endothelial cells in dermatomyositis: Association with interstitial lung disease. *BMJ* 1991; 302: 880–881.
44. Fujita J, Takeuchi T, Dobashi N, et al. Detection of anti-ADAM 10 antibody in serum of a patient with pulmonary fibrosis associated with dermatomyositis. *Ann Rheum Dis* 1999; 58: 770–772.
45. Bandoh S, Fujita J, Ohtsuki Y, et al. Sequential changes of KL-6 in sera of patients with interstitial pneumonia associated with polymyositis/dermatomyositis. *Ann Rheum Dis* 2000; 59: 257–262.
46. Kubo M, Ihn H, Yamane K, et al. Serum Kl-6 in adult patients with polymyositis and dermatomyositis. *Rheumatology (Oxford)* 2000; 39: 632–636.
47. Kobayashi I, Ono S, Kawamura N, et al. Kl-6 is a potential marker for interstitial lung disease associated with juvenile dermatomyositis. *J Pediatr* 2001; 138: 274–276.
48. Ihn H, Asano Y, Kubo M, et al. Clinical significance of serum surfactant protein D (SP-D) in patients with polymyositis/dermatomyositis: correlation with interstitial lung disease. *Rheumatology (Oxford)* 2002; 41: 1268–1272.
49. Mijailovi B, Karadagli D, Dostani I, et al. Amyopathic dermatomyositis with interstitial lung disease. *Vojnosanit Pregl* 1997; 54(3): 269–271 [Serbian].
50. el-Azhary R, Pakzad SY. Amyopathic dermatomyositis: retrospective review of 37 cases. *J Am Acad Dermatol* 2002; 46: 560–565.
51. Sontheimer RD, Miyagawa S. Potentially fatal interstitial lung disease can occur in clinically amyopathic dermatomyositis. *J Am Acad Dermatol* 2003; 48: 797–798.

52. Krain LS. Dermatomyositis in six patients without initial muscle involvement. *Arch Dermatol* 1975; 111: 241–245.
53. Kurasawa K, Nawata Y, Takabayashi K, et al. Activation of pulmonary T cells in corticosteroid-resistant and -sensitive interstitial pneumonitis in dermatomyositis/polymyositis. *Clin Exp Immunol* 2002; 129: 541–548.
54. Kikuchi Y, Koarada S, Tada Y, et al. Difference in B cell activation between dermatomyositis and polymyositis: analysis of the expression of RP105 on peripheral blood B cells. *Ann Rheum Dis* 2001; 60: 1137–1140.
55. La Civita L, Battiloro R, Celano M. Nocardia pleural empyema complicating anti-Jo1 positive polymyositis during immunoglobulin and steroid therapy. *J Rheumatol* 2001; 28: 215–216.
56. Bachelez H, Schremmer B, Cadranel J, et al. Fulminant *Pneumocystis carinii* pneumonia in 4 patients with dermatomyositis. *Arch Intern Med* 1997; 157: 1501–1503.
57. Ward MM, Donald F. Pneumocystis carinii pneumonia in patients with connective tissue diseases. *Arth Rheum* 1999; 42(4): 780–789.
58. Zitnik RJ, Cooper JA Jr. Pulmonary disease due to antirheumatic agents. *Clin Chest Med* 1990; 11: 139–150.
59. Miller M. Pulmonary disease in dermatomyositis and polymyositis. *UpToDate 2003*. Available at http://uptodate.com. Accessed September 21, 2004.
60. Jansen TL, Barrera P, Van Engelen BG, et al. Dermatomyositis with subclinical myositis and spontaneous pneumo-mediastinum with pneumothorax: case report and review of the literature. *Clin Exp Rheumatol* 1998; 16: 733–735.
61. Jang KA, Kim SH, Choi JH, et al. Subcutaneous emphysema with spontaneous pneumomediastinum and pneumothorax in adult dermatomyositis. *J Dermatol* 1999; 26: 125–127.
62. Kono H, Inokuma S, Nakayama H, et al. Pneumomediastinum in dermatomyositis: association with cutaneous vasculopathy. *Ann Rheum Dis* 2000; 59: 372–376.
63. Kovacs SO, Kovacs SC. Dermatomyositis. *J Am Acad Dermatol* 1998; 39: 899–920.
64. Lakhanpal S, Lie JT, Conn DL, et al. Pulmonary disease in polymyositis/dermatomyositis: a clinicopathological analysis of 65 autopsy cases. *Ann Rheum Dis* 1987; 46: 23–29.
65. Maugars YM, Berthelot JM, Abbas AA, et al. Long-term prognosis of 69 patients with dermatomyositis. *Clin Exp Rheumatol* 1996; 14: 263–274.
66. Grau JM, Miro O, Pedrol E, et al. Interstitial lung disease related to dermatomyositis. Comparative study with patient without lung involvement. *J Rheumatol* 1996; 23: 1921–1926.
67. Tjiu JW, Lin SJ, Wang LF, et al. Digital infarcts showing microangiopathy in adult dermatomyositis suggest severe pulmonary involvement and poor prognosis. *Br J Dermatol* 2004; 150: 1214–1226.
68. Katzenstein AA, Fiorelli RF. Nonspecific interstitial pneumonia/fibrosis: histological features and clinical significance. *Am J Surg Pathol* 1994; 18: 136–147.
69. Bjoraker JA, Ryu JH, Edwin MK, et al. Prognostic significance of histopathological subsets in idiopathic pulmonary fibrosis. *Am J Respir Crit Care Med* 1998; 157: 199–203.
70. Nagai S, Kitaichi M, Itoh H, et al. Idiopathic nonspecific interstitial pneumonia/fibrosis: comparison with idiopathic pulmonary fibrosis and BOOP. *Eur Respir J* 1998; 12: 1010–1019.
71. Daniil ZD, Gilchrist FC, Nicholson AG, et al. A histologic pattern of non specific interstitial pneumonia is associated with a better prognosis than interstitial pneumonia in patients with cryptogenic fibrosing alveolitis. *Am J Respir Crit Care Med* 1999; 160: 899–905.
72. Nicholson AG, Colby TV, Du Bois RM, et al. The prognostic significance of the histologic pattern of interstitial pneumonia in patients presenting with the clinical entity of cryptogenic fibrosing alveolitis. *Am J Respir Crit Care Med* 2000; 162: 2213–2217.
73. American Thoracic Society International Consensus Statement. Idiopathic pulmonary fibrosis: diagnosis and treatment. *Am J Respir Crit Care Med* 2000; 161: 646–664.
74. Marie I, Hachulla E, Cherin P, et al. Interstitial lung disease in polymyositis and dermatomyositis. *Arthritis Rheum* 2002; 47: 614–622.

Gastrointestinal Complications of Dermatomyositis 12

Gastrointestinal manifestations of DM in adults have included dysphagia, esophageal reflux, esophageal dysmotility, delayed gastric emptying, decreased intestinal motility, and rectal incontinence [1, 2]. The most common gastrointestinal symptom in juvenile DM is dysphagia, as a result of pharyngeal and upper esophageal involvement [3]; however, occasionally ulceration and perforation of the gastrointestinal tract [4, 5], and pneumatosis intestinalis [6, 7] have been reported. Although dysphagia results from inflammation and atrophy of esophageal muscle, ulceration is the consequence of vasculitis and thromboses of both esophageal and small bowel blood vesels [1, 5, 8, 9].

Dysphagia occurs in approximately 25–50% of DM patients. According to various clinical studies in a large group of patients with IIMs, dysphagia has been present in 29% of cases in Australia [10], 30% in Brazil [11], 31–43% in Canada [12, 13], 45% in the USA [14], 47% in Bulgaria [15], and 52% in Sweden [16]. Low frequency of dysphagia has been reported in Singapore – 11% of IIM patients [17] (Table 12.1).

The dysphagia can be of two types: proximal or distal [18]. Proximal dysphagia is caused by the involvement of striated muscle of the pharynx or proximal esophagus. This involvement correlates with the severity of the muscle disease, and is responsive to steroids. Distal dysphagia is related to the involvement of non-striated muscle, and seems to be more common in patients with overlap with SSc or another connective tissue disease. Two different types of abnormalities are encountered in cricopharyngeal (CP) sphincter muscle [19]: (1) the duration of CP-sphincter pause is shortened, or (2) it is prolonged during water swallowing. These two findings are interpreted respectively as hyperreflexic and hyporeflexic sphincter behavior. In the first case, hyperreflexic sphincter behavior may indicate the inflammation and/or edema in the muscle during the acute stage of PM/DM. However, in chronic disease course it may be related with muscle fibrosis [20]. In the second case, sphincter hyporeflexes could be related with the muscle weakness and the low muscle tonous of CP sphincter. Dysphagia generally signifies a rapidly progressive course, and is associated with the presence of pulmonary disease. It may also be associated with a poor prognosis.

In some patients, involvement of the muscles of the upper esophagus, the cricopharyngeal muscle, and other muscles in the hypopharynx may produce difficulty in swallowing and dysphonia (nasal speech and hoarseness] [21]. The difficulty in swallowing has been

L.A. Dourmishev and A.L. Dourmishev, *Dermatomyositis: Advances in Recognition, Understanding and Management,*

12

Table 12.1 Degree of dysphagia in DM [19]

Grade 1	No complaint and no clinical findings related to oropharyngeal dysphagia
Grade 2	Dysphagia is suspected from the patient's complaints; however, the clinical examination does not support the presence of dysphagia
Grade 3	Dysphagia is clinically evident, but the patient could manage swallowing by measures other than non-oral feeding
Grade 4	Dysphagia is so severe that non-oral feeding (i.e., nasogastric tube) is needed

reported in 12–54% of patients with PM/DM [20, 22, 23]. It is more commonly observed in the acute inflammatory phase of these conditions [20, 24]. In patients with PM/DM, the triggering time of the pharyngeal phase of swallowing determined by EMG is found normal [19]. On the other hand, the pharyngeal transit time of the bolus from the oral cavity to the upper esophageal sphincter is significantly prolonged [19, 25]. The sensation of food sticking in the back of the throat, esophageal reflux, and heartburn may become prominent. Aspiration, especially in patients with compromised pulmonary functions, is potentially lethal. In patients with any of these symptoms, a swallowing study should be performed to evaluate for aspiration. If such risk is demonstrated, a gastric feeding tube should be passed to allow proper nutrition without risk of aspiration. Monitoring handling of secretions during eating is especially important in children [21].

Distal esophageal dysmotility has been reported in up to two thirds of adult DM patients, and delayed gastric emptying and dysmotility are also commonly seen [26]. Radiographic abnormalities such as a dilated atonic esophagus, delayed gastric emptying, inflammatory bowel disease and the thickening of the small bowel wall, or "stacked coin" appearance have been reported in adult patients [27–29] and in juvenile DM [7]. In a recent study of 48 patients with DM/PM, severe gastrointestinal tract manifestations were identified in three patients (6%) with DM [30]. The prominent clinical symptoms included recurrent abdominal pain and bloody diarrhea, which despite the aggressive therapy ended with fatal gastrointestinal perforations in two patients. Edematous hyperemic bowel wall with multiple erosions and ulcerous lesions were the prominent findings on endoscopy. Histology revealed diffuse mucosal inflammation and multiple vascular ectasias without microscopic signs of vasculitis [30].

Gastrointestinal manifestations of juvenile DM include intractable abdominal pain which aggravates after steroid and NSAID therapies, with accompanying vomiting, constipation, hematemesis, ulceration, and perforation [9, 31–33]. Gastrointestinal findings may occur later in the course of the illness, even if the associated juvenile DM is improving [33]. Thromboses of the bowel blood vessels are part of the pathology of gastrointestinal ulcerations in juvenile DM [8, 9, 32]. Large-bowel infarction secondary to vasculopathy has occurred in juvenile patients with myositis. Furthermore, children with DM, much more than adults, may develop a vascular insult along the gastrointestinal tract, which on occasions may produce perforation. However, adult-onset DM complicated with life-threatening gastrointestinal ischemia and perforation has rarely been reported [5, 34]. Some patients with DM have exhibited life-threatening gastrointestinal complications, including duodenal perforation [34], intestinal pseudo-obstruction [35], multiple ulcerations with gastrointestinal hemorrhage [36], and rhabdomyolysis and paralytic ileus [37], all of which have been reported to be refractory to corticosteroid but responsive to IVIG therapy.

Pancreatitis associated with juvenile DM is very rare [38–40]. The pancreatitis may have been due to juvenile DM activity or its therapy prior to the development of pancreatitis [39]. Heckmatt et al. [40] reported two out of 14 children with JDM who had developed pancreatitis preceding the treatment of cyclosporin A, although the relation to the disease activity or other reason remains unclear.

Malabsorption can occur in patients with juvenile DM. The radiographic finding is thickening of the intestinal folds as determined by barium study [41].

References

1. DeMerieus P, Verity MA, Clements PJ, et al. Esophageal abnormalities and dysphagia in polymyositis and dermatomyositis: clinical, radiographic and pathologic features. *Arthritis Rheum* 1983; 26: 961–968.
2. Vitali C, Scuito M, Rossi B. Rectal incontinence due to unusual localization of the myositis process in the external sphincter of a patient with dermatomyositis. *Arthritis Rheum* 1991; 34: 1337.
3. Pachman LM. Juvenile dermatomyositis: pathophysiology and disease expression. *Pediatr Clin North Am* 1995; 42: 1071–1097.
4. Schullinger JN, Jacobs JC, Berdon WE. Diagnosis and management of gastrointestinal perforations in childhood dermatomyositis with particular reference to perforations of the duodenum. *J Pediatr Surg* 1985; 20: 521–524.
5. Chen GY, Liu MF, Lee J, et al. Combination of massive mucinosis, dermatomyositis, pyoderma gangrenosum-like ulcer, bullae and fatal intestinal vasculopathy in a young female. *Eur J Dermatol* 2005; 15: 396–400.
6. Fischer TJ, Cipel L, Stiehm ER. Pneumatosis intestinalis associated with fatal childhood dermatomyositis. *Pediatrics* 1978; 61: 127–130.
7. Laskin BL, Choyke P, Keenan GF, et al. Novel gastrointestinal tract manifestations in juvenile dermatomyositis. *J Pediatr* 1999; 135: 371–374.
8. Banker B, Viktor M. Dermatomyositis (systemic angiopathy) of childhood. *Medicine* 1966; 45: 261–289.
9. Michailov G, Vlasov V. Upon visceral changes in dermatomyositis: case report. *Savr Med* 1974; 12: 47–50 [Bulgarian].
10. Tymms KE, Webb J. Dermatopolymyositis and other connective tissue diseases: a review of 105 cases. *J Rheumatol* 1985; 12: 1140–1148.
11. Scola RH, Werneck LC, Prevedello DS, et al. Diagnosis of dermatomyositis and polymyositis: a study of 102 cases. *Arq Neuropsiquiatr* 2000; 58: 789–799.
12. Holden DJ, Brownell AKW, Fritzler MJ. Clinical and serological features of patients with polymyositis and dermatomyositis. *Can Med Assoc J* 1985; 132: 649–653.
13. Uthman I, Vazquez-Abad D, Senexal JL. Distinctive features of idiopathic inflammatory myopathies in French-Canadians. *Semin Arthritis Rheum* 1996; 26: 447–458.
14. Hochberg MC, Feldman D, Stevens MB. Adult-onset polymyositis/dermatomyositis: an analysis of clinical and laboratory features and survival in 76 patients with review of the literature. *Semin Arthritis Rheum* 1986; 15: 168–178.
15. Dourmishev LA. Dermatomyositis: Current aspects. Ph.D. thesis, Sofia, 2002; 140.
16. Lundberg I, Nennesmo I, Hedfors E. A clinical serological, and histopathological study of myositis patients with and without anti-RNP antibodies. *Semin Arthritis Rheum* 1992; 22: 127–138.
17. Koh ET, Seow A, Ong B, et al. Adult-onset polymyositis/dermatomyositis: clinical and laboratory features and treatment response in 75 patients. *Ann Rheum Dis* 1993; 52: 857–861.
18. Callen JP. Dermatomyositis. *Lancet* 2000; 355: 53–57.

19. Ertekin C, Seçil Y, Yüceyar N, et al. Oropharyngeal dysphagia in polymyositis/dermatomyositis. *Clin Neurol Neurosurg* 2004; 107(1): 32–37.
20. Sonies BC. Evaluation and treatment of speech and swallowing disorders associated with myopathies. *Curr Opin Rheumatol* 1997; 9: 486–495.
21. Provost TT, Flyn JA. Dermatomyositis. In: *Cutaneous Medicine, Cutaneous Manifestations of Systemic Diseases*, Provost TT, Flynn JA (eds), BC Decker, Hamilton/London, 2001; 82–103.
22. Bohan A, Peter JB, Bowman RL, Pearson CM. A computer-assisted analysis of 153 patients with polymyositis and dermatomyositis. *Medicine* 1977; 56: 255–286.
23. Cunningham Jr JD, Lowry LD. Head and neck manifestations of dermatomyositis-polymyositis. *Otolaryngol Head Neck Surg* 1985; 93: 673–677.
24. Plotz PH, Dalakas M, Leff RL, et al. Current concepts in the idiopathic inflammatory myopathies: polymyositis, dermatomyositis and related disorders. *Ann Intern Med* 1989; 111: 143–157.
25. Vencovsky J, Rehák F, Pafko P, et al. Acute cricopharyngeal obstruction in dermatomyositis. *J Rheum* 1988; 15: 1016–1018.
26. Horowitz M, Mc Neil JD, Maddern GJ, et al. Abnormalities of gastric and esophageal emptying in polymyositis and dermatomyositis. *Gastroenterology* 1986; 90: 434–439.
27. Kleckner FS. Dermatomyositis and its manifestations in the gastrointestinal tract. *Am J Gastroenterol* 1970; 53: 141–146.
28. Kulkarni A, Ravi TJ, Brodmerkel GJ Jr, et al. Inflammatory myositis in association with inflammatory bowel disease. *Dig Dis Sci* 1997; 42(6): 1142–1145.
29. Boardman P, Nolan DJ. Case report: small intestine pseudo-obstruction: an unusual manifestation of polymyositis. *Clin Radiol* 1998; 53: 706–707.
30. Tweezer-Zaks N, Ben-Horin S, Schiby G, et al. Severe gastrointestinal inflammation in adult dermatomyositis: characterization of a novel clinical association. *Am J Med Sci* 2006; 332(6): 308–313.
31. Sullivan DB, Cassidy JT, Petty RT. Dermatomyositis in pediatric patient. *Arthritis Rheum* 1977; 20: 327–331.
32. Wang IJ, Hsu WM, Shun CT, et al. Juvenile dermatomyositis complicated with vasculitis and duodenal perforation. *J Formos Med Assoc* 2001; 100: 844–846.
33. Mamyrova G, Kleiner DE, James-Newton L, et al. Late-onset gastrointestinal pain in juvenile dermatomyositis as a manifestation of ischemic ulceration from chronic endarteropathy. *Arthritis Rheum* 2007; 57(5): 881–884.
34. Eshraghi N, Farahmand M, Maerz LL, et al. Adult-onset dermatomyositis, with severe gastrointestinal manifestations: case report and review of the literature. *Sugery* 1998; 123: 356–358.
35. Rigby SP, Schott JM, Bliss P, et al. Dilated stomach and weak muscles. *Lancet* 2000; 356: 1898.
36. Marie I, Levesque H, Cailleux N, et al. Intravenous immunoglobulin for treatment of gastrointestinal haemorrhage in dermatomyositis. *Ann Rheum Dis* 2001; 60: 723–724.
37. Fukunaga E, Kunishigea M, Mitsuia T, et al. Severe dermatomyositis with rhabdomyolysis and paralytic ileus: a case successfully treated with plasmapheresis and intravenous immunoglobulin. *EFNS Eur J Neurol* 2002; 9: 687–702.
38. Barr HS, Wolff OH. Pancreatic necrosis in cortisone-treated children. *Lancet* 1957; 272(6973): 812–815.
39. See Y, Martin K, Rooney M, et al. Severe juvenile dermatomyositis complicated by pancreatitis. *Br J Rheumatol* 1997; 36(8): 912–916.
40. Heckmatt J, Hasson N, Saunders C, et al. Cyclosporin in juvenile dermatomyositis. *Lancet* 1989; 1(8646): 1063–1066.
41. Ryan M, Carr J. Malabsorption, immunodeficiency, and miscellaneous disorders of the small bowel. In: *Alimentary Tract Radiology*, Freeny PC, Stevenson GW (eds), 5th ed., Mosby, St. Louis, 1994; 659–688.

Ophthalmic Complications of Dermatomyositis 13

The heliotrope eyelid eruption is considered as a hallmark of DM. The associated periorbital redness and edema, producing ptosis, chemosis, and exophthalmos may initially be mistaken for infective orbital cellulitis. Ocular muscles in DM remain normal, even in advanced, untreated cases. If the ocular muscles are affected, the diagnosis of inflammatory myopathy should be in doubt [1], and the diagnosis of orbital myositis should be discussed [2]. Involvement of the extraocular muscles is extremely rare, and can cause pain and ophthalmoplegia [3]. Ptosis of the eyelids, diplopia, and strabismus due to extraocular muscle involvement can be observed in some DM patients [4].

Ocular manifestations have included conjunctival edema, nystagmus, extraocular muscle imbalance, iritis, cotton wool spots, optic atrophy, and conjunctival pseudopolyposis [5, 6]. Eyelid and lens abnormalities are frequently observed in patients with JDM, while retinopathy is rare [7]. The bulbar conjunctiva shows areas with dilated vessels and areas that look white and avascular [8]. In addition, vasculitis involving the conjunctival vessels can produce infarction. Additional features seen in DM are iritis [9], episcleritis [10], and uveitis with glaucoma [11]. Thromboses of the vessels at the margin of the eyelid have been detected in juvenile DM patients. Also, as a reflection of the vasculopathy these patients may develop transient "cotton wool" spots in the retina [12]. The cotton wool spots are nonspecific and indicate arteriolar obstruction or capillary damage, mediated by nerve fiber layer infarction, which produces axonal swelling and rupture [13]. Retinopathy associated with DM is initially described by Bruce [14] in 1938. Later, a few cases and studies have been reported in both adults and children [7, 15–19]. Retinopathy, leading to persistent and profound visual loss, has also been reported [17, 20–22]. More commonly, retinopathy associated with DM completely resolves without lasting complications [13] or with the development of retinal neovascularization [19]. Rarely, areas of pigment clumping are left, some surrounded with lighter halos (Elschnig's spots) indicating choriocapillary infarction [21]. Later still, there may be diffuse pallor of the optic disc resulting from retinal neuronal atrophy, producing irreversible visual impairment, which is very rare [21]. It has been postulated that children are more likely to have associated retinopathy because of the increased systemic vasculitis seen in juvenile DM [23]. Profound visual loss in DM is caused by macular hemorrhage or macular edema, which produces central scotomas. Visual recovery is usually complete [24, 25]. Over subsequent months the hemorrhages

L.A. Dourmishev and A.L. Dourmishev, *Dermatomyositis: Advances in Recognition, Understanding and Management*,

13

and cotton wool spots will be expected to resolve completely. The retinal infarctive events are felt to be similar to the arteriolar endothelial damage and platelet thrombi seen in muscle biopsy specimens [26].

Optic neuropathy has been described in patients with DM, but only in association with retinopathy [10]. A relative afferent pupillary defect, dyschromatopsia, visual field defects and pallid optic disc edema in the absence of retinopathy are evidence that the visual loss was from an optic neuropathy and not a retinopathy [27]. Recently, a 58-year-old woman with visual loss from optic neuropathy without retinopathy in DM has been reported [27]. She had no history of vascular disease, simultaneously swollen optic nerves and a relatively large cup-to-disc ratio in each eye. All clinical features would be extremely unusual for another cause of optic neuropathy such as non-arteritic ischemic optic neuropathy [28]. Retinal artery inflammation also can produce optic atrophy.

References

1. Dalakas M. Polymyositis, dermatomyositis and inclusion body myositis. *N Engl J Med* 1991; 325(21): 1487–1498.
2. Stevens AW, Grossman ME, Barr ML. Orbital myositis, vitiligo and giant cell myocarditis. *J Am Acad Dermatol* 1996; 35: 310–312.
3. Scopetta C, Morante M, Casali C, et al. Dermatomyositis spares extra-ocular muscles. *Neurology* 1985; 35: 141.
4. Beloev Z, Teodosieva E, Kantarev I. Damage of V and VII cranial nerves in dermatomyositis. *Neurol Psychiatr Neurosurgery* (Sofia) 1977; 1: 60–62 [Bulgarian].
5. Ibanez HE, Bardenstein DS, Korman NJ, et al. Exuberant conjunctival pseudopolyposis in a patient with dermatomyositis. *Ann Ophtalmol* 1993; 25: 326–327.
6. Migliaresi S, Ambrosone L, Tirri G. Eye involvement in dermatomyositis/polymyositis. *J Rheumatol* 1996; 23: 2006–2007.
7. Akikusa JD, Tennankore DK, Levin AV, et al. Eye findings in patients with juvenile dermatomyositis. *J Rheumatol* 2005; 32(10): 1986–1991.
8. Van Nouhuys CE, Sengers RC. Bilateral avascular zones of the conjunctiva in a patient with juvenile dermatomyositis. *Am J Ophtalmol* 1987; 104: 440–442.
9. Oppenheim H. *Lehrbuch der Nervenkrankheiten für Arzte und Studierende*, 7th ed. Karger, Berlin, 1923; 840.
10. Cohen B, Sedwick L, Burde R. Retinopathy of dermatomyositis. *J Clin Neuro-ophthalmol* 1985; 5: 177–179.
11. Tuovinen E, Raudasoja R. Poikilodermatomyositis with retinal haemorrhages and secondary glaucoma. *Acta Ophthalmol* 1965; 43: 669–672.
12. Mileva E. Macular changes in dermatomyositis. *Med Letopisi* 1947; 39: 1134 [Bulgarian].
13. Backhouse O, Griffiths B, Henderson T, et al. Ophthalmic manifestations of dermatomyositis. *Ann Rheum Dis* 1998; 57: 447–449.
14. Bruce G. Retinitis in dermatomyositis. *Trans Am Ophthalmol Soc* 1938; 36: 282–292.
15. Lisman J. Dermatomyositis with retinopathy. *Arch Ophthalmol* 1947; 37: 155–159.
16. De Vries S. Retinopathy in dermatomyositis. *Arch Ophthalmol* 1951; 46: 432–435.
17. Munro S. Fundus appearance in a case of acute dermatomyositis. *Br J Ophthalmol* 1959; 43: 548–558.
18. Liebman S, Cook C. Dermatomyositis with retinopathy. *Arch Ophthalmol* 1965; 74: 704–705.

19. Venkatesh P, Bhaskar VM, Keshavamurthy R, et al. Proliferative vascular retinopathy in polymyositis and dermatomyositis with scleroderma (overlap syndrome). *Ocul Immunol Inflamm* 2007; 15(1): 45–49.
20. Nutt A. Ophthalmic manifestation in paediatric practice. *Trans Ophthalmol Soc UK* 1959; 79: 315–334.
21. Klein B. Comments on cotton-wool lesions of the retina. *Am J Ophthalmol* 1965; 59: 17–23.
22. Yeo LM, Swaby DS, Situnayake RD, et al. Irreversible visual loss in dermatomyositis. *Br J Rheumatol* 1995; 34(12): 1179–1181.
23. Harrison S, Frenkel M, Grossman B, et al. Retinopathy in childhood dermatomyositis. *Am J Ophthalmol* 1973; 76: 786–790.
24. Fong LP, Yeung J. Spontaneous regression of retinal neovascularisation in juvenile dermatomyositis. *Aust N Z J Ophthalmol* 1990; 18: 107–108.
25. Chu-Lee A, Stroller G, Jaffe IA. Retinopathy in adult dermatomyositis. *J Rheumatol* 1995; 22: 2372–2373.
26. Crowe W, Bove K, Levinson J, et al. Clinical and pathological implications of histopathology in childhood polydermatomyositis. *Arthritis Rheum* 1982; 25: 126–139.
27. Foroozon R. Visual loss from optic neuropathy in dermatomyositis. *Rheumatology* 2004; 43: 391–393.
28. Buono LM, Foroozan R, Sergott RC, et al. Nonarteritic anterior ischemic optic neuropathy. *Curr Opin Ophthalmol* 2002; 13: 357–361.

Renal Complications of Dermatomyositis

14

Both DM or PM relatively rarely cause renal involvement [1]. To date, few reports have described renal manifestations in patients with either PM or DM [2–4]. Dyck et al. described five patients with biopsy-proven primary idiopathic PM, normal kidney function and 24 h urine protein excretions ranging from 2.1 to 4.1 g. Four of the five patients underwent a renal biopsy, and all four were found to have mesangial proliferative glomerulonephritis. Three of the four biopsies underwent immunofluorescent staining showing diffuse mesangial deposits of IgG and IgM, and rare IgA and C3 immunoreactants with the same distribution. Only one of the five patients had decreased C3 levels. Pasquali et al. [3] prospectively studied the renal manifestations of 12 patients with DM and eight with PM. Eleven of the 20 patients had a protein excretion rate of more than 500 mg/24 h. The two patients with DM were found to have minimal change disease and mesangial proliferative glomerulonephritis, while another three patients with PM were found to have minimal change disease, amyloidosis, and membranoproliferative glomerulonephritis [3]. A recent retrospective study of 65 Taiwanese patients with PM/DM hospitalized between 1992 and 2002 has found a varying degree of renal involvement in 14 (21.5%) of them [4]. All the 14 patients had from mild to prominent hematuria and proteinuria, and in four patients with PM and in five patients with DM acute tubular necroses with renal failure were found. Renal biopsy in two DM patients with overt proteinuria revealed IgA nephropathy in one and membranous nephropathy in the other [4]. Corticosteroids, with or without other immunosuppressive agents, may ameliorate the glomerulonephritis [2, 3, 5]. In the study by Dyck et al. [2], four of the five patients were followed for 2–7 years after treatment, and none had a recurrence of their renal disease or of their PM, while two of the four patients were on maintenance steroids for approximately 4½ years. One patient, who was in remission within 3 months after the initiation of corticosteroid and methotrexate therapy, underwent a repeat renal biopsy 18 months latter, the results of which were normal. As demonstrated in the study by Dyck et al. [2], both the myositis and proteinuria improved in concert with corticosteroid therapy.

Isolated case reports have noted the presence of various glomerulopathies with PM [5, 6]. Recently, a 28-year-old male with PM and nephrotic-range proteinuria has been reported [7]. Muscle biopsy confirmed the diagnosis of PM, and a renal biopsy demonstrated IgM mesangial glomerulonephritis. Following a short-course of prednisone, both the myositis and proteinuria resolved.

L.A. Dourmishev and A.L. Dourmishev, *Dermatomyositis: Advances in Recognition, Understanding and Management*,

14

Acute renal failure due to PM or DM has also been observed [8, 9]. Acute tubular necrosis with renal failure related to myoglobulinemia and myoglobulinuria resulting from extensive muscle fiber necrosis is a well-recognized feature of acute rhabdomyolysis [4]. Well-documented cases of PM with myoglobuinuria are rare [1, 8, 10]. No patient with typical DM had ever been reported to have myoglobulinuria before 1964 [11]. After that, nine patients of DM with myoglobulinuria or anuric renal failure in eight case reports have been announced in English literature [9, 12–18]. Reliable data for myoglobinuric renal failure associated with DM are summarized below:

(i) In eight patients, CK levels were markedly elevated (except the case reported by Park et al. [9]) more than 500 U/l; renal failure was not related to the CK level, but depended on the urinary myoglobin concentrations [19].
(ii) Five of eight patients had visible myoglobulinuria with oliguric or anuric renal failure [18].
(iii) Only one third of the patients with urinary myoglobin concentrations exceeding the quoted threshold of 1 mg/ml had renal failure [19], or developed it [20].
(iv) A 24-year-old heroin user with traumatic myoglobinuria developed typical skin and muscle features of DM a few weeks afterwards, suggesting that DM may result from, rather than cause myoglobinuria [15].
(v) In two patients there was a fatal outcome.
(vi) One patient failed to respond to immunosuppressant treatment with corticosteroids, methotrexate, and plasmapheresis [17].
(vii) The other case relapsed during the reduction of steroid therapy [14].

It is suggested, however, that myoglobin in concentration of greater than 0.25 mg/ml may cause urine darkening, and may provoke renal failure due to acute tubular necrosis [4, 18]. The myoglobin clearance, as determined from the urine volume and the serum to urinary myoglobin concentration, is suggested as a better predictor for the development of acute renal failure [20]. Elevated serum myoglobin levels usually resolve within 1–2 days in a monophasic illness caused by trauma, infection, or drugs, and their persistent presence implies a metabolic myopathy with ongoing muscle fiber destruction [21].

References

1. Bohan A, Peter JB. Polymyositis and dermatomyositis. *N Engl J Med* 1975; 292: 344–347.
2. Dyck RF, Katz A, Gordon DA, et al. Glomerulonephritis associated with polymyositis. *J Rheumatol* 1979; 6(3): 336–344.
3. Pasquali JL, Meyer P, Christmann D, et al. Renal changes in dermatomyositis and polymyositis. *Ann Med Intern* 1987; 138: 109–113.
4. Yen TH, Lai PC, Chen CC, et al. Renal involvement in patients with polymyositis and dermatomyositis. *Int J Clin Pract* 2005; 59(2): 188–193.
5. Frost NA, Morand EF, Hall CL, et al. Idiopathic polymyositis complicated by arthritis and mesangial proliferative glomerulonephritis: case report and review of the literature. *Br J Rheum* 1993; 32: 929–931.
6. Picco P, Gattorno M, Barbano GC, et al. Mesangial glomerulonephritis and transient SLE manifestations in an adolescent with dermatomyositis. *Lupus* 1997; 6: 72–73.

7. Valenzuela OF, Reiser IW, Porush JG. Idiopathic polymyositis and glomerulonephritis. *J Nephrol* 2001; 14: 120–124.
8. Sloan MF, Franks AJ, Exely KA, et al. Acute renal failure due to polymyositis. *Br Med J* 1978; 1: 1457.
9. Park SK, Cho KH, Kang SK. Acute renal failure associated with dermatomyositis and colon cancer. *Nephron* 1990; 55: 225–226.
10. Ditzian-Kadanov R, Reinhard JD, Thomas C, et al. Polymyositis with myoglobinuria in pregnancy: a report and review of the literature. *J Rheumatol* 1988; 15: 513–514.
11. Rowland LP, Fahn S, Hirschberg E, et al. Myoglobulinuria. *Arch Neurol* 1964; 18: 141–150.
12. Kagen LJ. Myoglobinemia and myoglobinuria in patient with myositis. *Arthritis Rheum* 1971; 14: 457–464.
13. Marks AD. Myoglobinuria. *Am J Med Sci* 1971; 261: 350–358.
14. Kessler E, Weinberger I, Rosenfeld JB. Myoglobinuric acute renal failure in a case of dermatomyositis. *Isr J Med Sci* 1972; 8: 978–983.
15. Marks SH, McShane DJ, Mitchell DM. Dermatomyositis following rhabdomyolysis. *J Rheum* 1976; 3: 224–226.
16. Singhal PC, Narayanan-Nampoory MR, Visweswaran RK, et al. Myoglobinuric renal failure associated with dermatomyositis. *J Assoc Phys India* 1985; 33: 672–673.
17. Caccamo DV, Keene CY, Durham J, et al. Fulminant rhabdomyolysis in a patient with dermatomyositis. *Neurology* 1993; 43: 844–845.
18. Rose MR, Kissel JT, Bickley LS et al. Sustained myoglobinuria: the presenting manifestation of dermatomyositis. *Neurology* 1996; 47: 119–123.
19. Feinfeld DA, Cheng JT, Beysolow TD, et al. A prospective study of urine and serum myoglobin levels in patient with acute rhabdomyolysis. *Clin Nephrol* 1992; 38: 193–195.
20. Wu AHB, Laios I, Green S, et al. Immunoasssays for serum and urine myoglobin: myoglobin clearance assessed as a risk factor for acute renal failure. *Clin Chem* 1994; 40: 796–802.
21. Rose JD. Membranous glomerulonephritis, dermatomyositis and bronchial carcinoma. *Br Med J* 1979; 2(6191): 641.

Complications of Central Nervous System in Dermatomyositis

15

The association of DM or PM and nervous system involvement is a very rarely observed and controversial entity. In their report, O'Leary and Waisman noted an asymmetry of the face due to facial nerve palsy in patients with DM [1]. Later, Karajashev et al. [2] reported a 72-year-old man with acute form of DM associated with gastric cancer, in whom the autopsy found morphologic changes in the central nervous system. Histology from brain and spinal cord specimen revealed a dystrophic injury of ganglial cells in brain, loss of dendrites, reduction of the number of Purkinje's cells in the cerebellum, lysis of tigroid substance and lymphocitic infiltrates in the spinal cord [3]. Recently a 50-year-old man with an overlap syndrome of DM and SLE was reported, whose magnetic resonance image of the brain showed a rapidly increasing large tumor in the left frontal lobe [4]. The pathological finding from the brain biopsy was fibrinoid necrosis, inflammatory cell aggregation around blood vessels and many myelin-laden macrophages with central necrosis. Neurologic symptoms in the patient such as paresis were mild and the lesion responded well to steroid treatment [4].

Beloev et al. [5] reported a 42-year-old man with typical cutaneous features of DM, degenerative changes in muscle biopsy, and normal serum enzymes who in the course of the disease developed unilateral damage of right V and VII cranial nerves, presenting with one-sided pains, hypasthesia, and painfulness to the touch in the area of n. trigeminus and facial nerve palsy. Laraki R et al. [6], in their study of four cases, proposed the following criteria of primary nerve involvement in DM/PM patients: early abolition of tendinous reflexes in a patient without notable muscular atrophy and with little or no myalgia, sensitive abnormalities in areas other than those of muscular involvement, early weakness of distal muscles, decrease in nerve conduction speed, target fibers and lesions of nerve trunks. They reported two DM cases with peripheral neuropathy, and two other patients with polyradiculoneuritis and vasculitis [6]. One of the patients had HTLV-I infection confirmed by polymerase chain reaction (PCR), suggesting the direct pathogenic role of certain viruses in those patients [6].

Price et al. [7] reported a 68-year-old woman with typical cutaneous rash and DM confirmed by EMG and muscle biopsy, who developed nasal speech, nasal regurgitation of fluids, dysphagia, and palatal palsy. Authors concluded that DM may cause palatal palsy in addition to more widely recognized features, and that such a presentation may occur in the context of occult malignancy [7].

15

Central nervous system involvement in juvenile DM has been reported in a few cases with seizures or organic brain disorder, reflecting the underlying vasculopathy prominent in this disorder [8]. The complications in juvenile DM may occur for a number of reasons. These include vasculopathy as a part of dermatomyositis, true cerebral vasculitis of small or medium-sized vessels, hypoxic ischemic encephalopathy secondary to cerebral hypoperfusion, and hypertensive encephalopathy, possibly as a consequence of drug treatment [8]. Cyclosporin-associated encephalopathy is a possible cause of seizures, since the drug is highly lipid-soluble and crosses the blood–brain barrier with toxic levels, especially in combinations of high-dose steroids [9].

Later pseudoseizures may occurred, associated with emotional lability and depressive symptoms, probably constituting an organic brain syndrome effect, secondary to high-dose steroids [8].

References

1. O'Leary PA, Waisman M. Dermatomyositis: a study of 40 cases. *Arch Dermatol Syphilol* 1940; 41: 1001.
2. Karajashev G, Angelov A, Slavov M. Acute dermatomyositis in association with gastric cancer and morphologic changes in central nervous system. *Dermatol Venereol* (Sofia), 1973; 1: 64–68 [Bulgarian].
3. Bojinov C, Manolov C, Lolova I, et al. Polymyositis. In: *Myopathies* [Clinical, Biochemical, Histologic and Electron-Microscopic Study], Bojinov C, Galabov G. Sofia (eds), *Med I Physk* 1973; 183–230 [Bulgarian].
4. Kano S, Nakamori T, Imafuku I, et al. Overlap syndrome of systemic lupus erythematosus and dermatomyositis presented a large demyelinating subcortical lesion mimicking brain tumor and high level of CSF antineuronal and serum anti-ribosomal P antibodies. *Rinsho Shinkeigaku* 2002; 42(3): 197–201 [Japanese].
5. Beloev Z, Teodosieva E, Kantarev I. Damage of V and VII cranial nerves in dermatomyositis. *Neurol Psychiatr Neurosurgery*, Sofia 1977; 1: 60–62.
6. Laraki R, Blétry O, Agbalika F, et al. Do neuromyosites exist? *Ann Med Interne (Paris)* 1994; 145(2): 88–97 [French].
7. Price CJ, Frankel JP, Hammans SR. Palatal palsy in dermatomyositis. (Letter). *Eur J Neurol* 2001; 8: 197–198.
8. Ramanan AV, Sawhney S, Murray KJ Central nervous system complications in two cases of juvenile onset dermatomyositis. *Rheumatology* 2001; 40; 1293–1298.
9. Koh MK, Habib N. Neurological complications following cyclosporin therapy – a case report. *Clin Transplant* 1993; 7: 216–217.

Pregnancy Complicated by Dermatomyositis

16

Pregnancy complicated by DM is rare. There are a limited number of case reports on the debut of DM during pregnancy. It is not clear whether the association of pregnancy with DM is actually low, because the rarity of pregnancy-associated DM may reflect a low incidence of DM in young adult women. There are no available epidemiological data on pregnancy and DM/PM. The association of PM/DM and pregnancy is very rare, and this has been attributed to the low percentage (14%) of cases in which the disease begins during the reproductive period of a woman's life [1]; it is also probable that family planning policy after the clinical manifestation of the disease lowers the association of PM/DM and pregnancy [2]. In one hospital-based myositis study of 22 women, myositis developed during the childbearing years in eight of them (36%) and three (13.6%) presented with PM within 3 months of delivery [3]. A relationship between pregnancy and DM has rarely been documented, and most cases have been reported from the viewpoint of the management of high-risk pregnancy [4–6].

There are at least two types of pregnancy-related DM. In the first type, the disease activity is provoked during pregnancy and tends to improve after delivery, while in the other type the onset is in the postpartum period [6]. The onset of DM has been reported during all three trimesters of pregnancy. The initial symptoms are usually nonspecific and include slight fatigue, which is common during pregnancy, and periungal erythema on the backs of the fingers, which could easily be overlooked by other than dermatologists. The uterus is unaffected by the myositic progression of the disease, athough England et al. [7] described a patient with a hypotonic uterus. In most cases the myositis of the mother improved after delivery, and occasionally remission was observed immediately postpartum [5, 6]. In other cases the myositis in the mother worsened after delivery [6, 8]. In order to find common features of DM/PM with pregnancy-associated onset Kanoh et al. [6] have summarized 15 case reports. In 12 of the 15 patients, the disease developed during pregnancy. In the majority of those cases the disease was active and resistant to steroid therapy during pregnancy but improved after delivery [6]. Apparent high risk for both premature delivery and fetal mortality in these cases is also shown. If the onset was in the first trimester, fetal mortality was very high (83%), and even with onset in the second or third trimester, the risk for premature delivery remained high, although all infants were alive. In contrast, postpartum onset of DM is extremely rare, and only three cases have been reported [6].

L.A. Dourmishev and A.L. Dourmishev, *Dermatomyositis: Advances in Recognition, Understanding and Management,* © Springer-Verlag Berlin Heidelberg 2009

16

As DM with onset during pregnancy tends to improve after delivery, the role of pregnancy in cases with postpartum onset seems to be different. It is impossible to answer whether pregnancy could be a triggering factor for the development of DM. Premature labor is common in cases with onset during pregnancy [6]. In a study of 18 women with PM/DM, 77 pregnancies before the onset of the disease were analyzed [9]. Seven of them (9%) ended in abortion and two (2.5%) with perinatal death [9]. Three premature infants however survived. There were ten pregnancies in seven of the PM/DM patients who had active disease at the time of the pregnancy: three (30%) ended in abortion, three of the remainder ended in prenatal death (25%), and a half of the infants were born prematurely. Total fetal loss was 11.5% before and 55% after development of PM/DM. Four of the seven patients had the onset of PM/DM during pregnancy and three others had exacerbation of disease during pregnancy [10]. In another series of three patients with five successful pregnancies associated with DM, the authors concluded that women with DM in remission can have successful pregnancy and delivery [11]. One report shows that exacerbation or relapse occurs during the course of pregnancy and immediately postpartum in 25–60% of cases [12]. Papapetropoulus et al. [2] reported a 35-year-old woman with PM and with three pregnancies. The PM in the patient was confirmed at the age of 17 years with blood biochemistry investigations, EMG, and muscle biopsy. After 3 years of steroid treatment she recovered completely, and 5 years later she delivered a normal male baby without any relapse of her illness. During the second pregnancy she developed relapse of the disease, and pregnancy was terminated by cesarian section at the end of 16 weeks. The steroid treatment was initiated, and continued on a reducing dose schedule for about 2 years. Thirty months after the last pregnancy and without any clinical or laboratory evidence of relapse, she had her second normal baby by cesarian section.

Amyopathic DM presenting during pregnancy has also been reported [13]. A 34-year-old woman with pathognomonic cutaneous manifestations of DM, but without associated skeletal muscle involvement, was observed from the third month of pregnancy to the delivery. The patient was treated with potent topical steroids. She delivered a healthy newborn, and the rash reached complete resolution 2 weeks later.

Some authors suggest that the outlook for the fetus is unfavorable when DM is first diagnosed during pregnancy [8]. Other consider that fetal prognosis parallels the activity of maternal diseases [14]. In patients with pre-existing static disease, little apparent risk to the mother or fetus is observed. This is in contrast to the new onset of the disease during pregnancy or exacerbation in the first trimester, for which the prognosis is unfavorable [6, 11, 14].

Various factors have been considered as triggers for development of DM/PM during pregnancy: (i) the exposure of mater to fetal antigens [15], (ii) changes in maternal hormonal status [12]; and (iii) the reactivation of certain viruses by pregnancy [16]. However, the peak incidence of DM is not within reproductive years, making estrogens less likely to be a causative factor [17].

Recently it has been proposed that microchimerism may contribute to the pathogenesis of autoimmune diseases or DM and PM respectively. Bauer et al. [18] first speculated that the fetus and its complement of foreign antigens might be involved in the development of DM during pregnancy. Microchimerism is defined by the presence within a specimen of a low level of cells derived from a different person. The main, natural source of microchimerism is pregnancy. Bidirectional cell trafficking between a mother and fetus during pregnancy has become an accepted fact. It has been demonstrated that during the course of pregnancy fetal cells (predominantly lymphocytes) pass routinely into the maternal circulation [19]. Production of antibodies to fetal (paternal) HLA antigens also has been confirmed. Such immunological changes in the mother may be potentially relevant to the development of the autoimmune disease [20]. In adult PM/DM, fetal microchimerism was found in an occasional patient out of 18 women investigated [21]. During this period there are also hormonal changes such as altered progesterone and cortisone concentrations, which could affect susceptibility to the development of autoimmune disease [17]. The clinical course of the cases with postpartum onset in relation to pregnancy suggests that once the disease has developed, subsequent activity of DM is independent of the pregnancy [6].

In conclusion, pregnancy could be a trigger for the development of DM. If exacerbation of DM occurs, corticosteroid therapy should minimize fetal loss. Pregnancy should be avoided during active disease but is not absolutely contraindicated during remission.

References

1. Rinheiro GRC, Goldenberg J, Atra E, et al. Juvenile dermatomyositis and pregnancy. Report and literature review. *J Rheumatol* 1992; 19: 1798–1801.
2. Papapetropoulus T, Kanellakopoulus N, Tsibri E, et al. Polymyositis and pregnancy: report of a case with three pregnancies. *J Neurol Neurosurg Psychiatry* 1998; 64: 406.
3. Steiner I, Averbuch-Heller L, Abramsky O, et al. Postpartum idiopathic polymyositis. *Lancet* 1992; 339: 256.
4. Ishii N, Ono H, Kawaguchi T, et al. Dermatomyositis and pregnancy. Case report and review of the literature. *Dermatologica* 1991; 183: 146–149.
5. Harris A, Webley M, Usherwood M, et al. Dermatomyositis presenting in pregnancy. *Br J Dermatol* 1995; 133: 783–785.
6. Kanoh H, Izumi T, Seishima M, et al. A case of dermatomyositis that developed after delivery: the involvement of pregnancy in the induction of dermatomyositis. *Br J Dermatol* 1999; 141: 897–900.
7. England MJ, Perlmann T, Veriava Y. Dermatomyositis in pregnancy. *J Reprod Med* 1986; 31: 633–636.
8. Rosenzweig BA, Rotmentsch S, Binette SP, et al. Primary idiopathic polymyositis and dermatomyositis complicating pregnancy: diagnosis and management. *Obstet Gynecol Surv* 1989; 44: 162–170.
9. Gutierrez G, Daguino R, Mintz G. Polymyositis, dermatomyositis and pregnancy. *Arthritis Rheum* 1984; 27: 291–294.
10. Caro I. Dermatomyositis as a systemic disease. *Med Clin North Am* 1989; 73: 1181–1192.
11. King CR, Chow S. Dermatomyositis and pregnancy. *Obstet Gynecol* 1985; 66: 589–592.
12. Tsai A, Lindheimer MD, Lamberg SI. Dermatomyositis complicating pregnancy. *Obstet Gynecol* 1973; 41: 570–573.
13. Morihara K, Katoh N, Hirano S, et al. Amyopathic dermatomyositis presenting during pregnancy. *J Am Acad Dermatol* 2004; 51(5): 838–840.
14. Silva CA, Sultan SM, Isenberg DA. Pregnancy outcome in adult-onset idiopathic inflammatory myopathy. *Rheumatology* 2003; 42: 1168–1172.

15. Katz AL. Another case of polymyositis in pregnancy. *Arch Intern Med* 1980; 140:1123.
16. Satoh M, Ajamani AK, Hirakata M, et al. Onset of polymyositis with autoantibodies to threonyl-tRNA synthetase during pregnancy. *J Rheumatol* 1994; 21: 1564–1566.
17. Dorph C, Lundberg IE. Idiopathic inflammatory myopathies — myositis. *Best Pract Res Clin Rheum* 2002; 16: 817–832.
18. Bauer KA, Siegler M, Lindheimer MA. Polymyositis complicating pregnancy. *Arch Intern Med* 1979; 139: 449.
19. Artlett CM, Rames R, Jiminez SA, et al. Chimeric cells of maternal origin in juvenile idiopathic inflammatory myopathies. Childhood Myositis Heterogeneity Collaborative Group. *Lancet* 2000; 356: 2155–2156.
20. Nelson JL. Pregnancy immunology and autoimmune disease. *J Reprod Med* 1998; 43: 335–340.
21. Selva-O'Caalaghan A, Boeckh-Behrens TM, Balada-Prades E, et al. Fetal microchimerism and inflammatory myopathies. *Lancet* 2001; 357: 887.

Calcinosis in Dermatomyositis 17

Calcinosis is a distressing late complication of juvenile DM [1, 2], but may appear early in the disease course [3] or be a consequence of externed therapy with corticosteroids [1, 4]. It may be expected in most long-term survivors of juvenile DM [1], but it occurs also in adults [5]. Calcinosis occurs in 30% [6] to 70% [7] of juvenile DM, and is two to three times more common than in adult DM [8]. In a large retrospective study was found cutaneous calcification in 20% of adults and 74% of children [9]. Approximately 25% of juvenile-onset classic DM patients have dystrophic calcification at the time of diagnosis, and 40–50% develop calcinosis sometime during the course of their disease [10]. Calcinosis is a late manifestation, with average duration of the disease in adults being 3.8 years prior to the clinical diagnosis. In both children and adults, the severity of calcinosis often correlates with the level of long-term disability [1]. It is usually a sign of "burned-out" myositis; it contributes to muscle atrophy and joint contractures [11]. Cutaneous calcinosis in DM usually appears between 4 months and 12 years after the onset of the disease, with an average time interval of 2–5 years between the disease onset and calcium deposition [8]. Calcium deposit in the skin is a common cause of cutaneous ulceration [11] and sterile necrotic abcesses [12].

Calcification associated with DM has been categorized into five different subtypes: (i) superficial calcifications present as small and hard plaques or nodules that can be felt just below the skin surface, (ii) subcutaneous calcifications — large tumorous deposits of calcium, which often appear "popcorn-like" on X-ray examination, (iii) intermuscular calcifications — deposits in the intermuscular fascia with limitation of movement in the involved muscle group, (iv) dystrophic calcification — a severe form, which resembles an exoskeleton, (v) a mixed form of calcinosis [1], and (vi) calcinosis universalis, which is loosely defined as numerous large deposits of calcium in the skin, subcutaneous tissue, muscles, and tendons [13]. Calcification of the muscles is generally asymptomatic, and may be seen only on radiological assesment [14]. Bone resorption markers, serum ionized Ca and urinary Ca levels point to the increased bone turnover and reduced excretion in patients with extensive calcinosis [15]. Complete regression of calcium deposits is not usually expected except in the first subtype [2].

Subcutaneous calcifications occur only in DM, in some cases extruding on the skin and causing ulcerations, infections, and pain, especially at sites of compression (elbows, buttocks, back) [16]. MRI abnormalities indicating skin, subcutaneous, or fascial edema

L.A. Dourmishev and A.L. Dourmishev, *Dermatomyositis: Advances in Recognition, Understanding and Management,* © Springer-Verlag Berlin Heidelberg 2009

17

were observed in approximately 80% of 26 children with classic juvenile DM [17]. The development of soft-tissue calcification in areas previously found to be edematous by MRI was found in five of the children within a 4- to 9-month follow-up period [17]. Subcutaneous calcinosis over the extensor surfaces of extremities frequently leads to chronic and difficult-healing ulcers. [5].

Calcification may be classified as metabolic or dystrophic in type [18]. The precise mechanism of calcium deposit in DM is unclear. In dystrophic calcification, which by definition occurs in injured tissue, when the muscles are involved, the calcificates are generally found in those muscles that are most severely affected by myositis [1, 9]. However, Olhoffers et al. [13] reported a 69-year-old woman with amyopatic DM, who developed calcinosis universalis 18 months prior to the appearance of classic DM.

Although the mechanism of calcification in the lesions is unclear, it has been suggested that denatured proteins preferentially bind phosphate ions, which in turn react with calcium ions to form a precipitate of calcium phosphate [8]. The nucleus of calcinosis consists of hydroxyapatite. High levels of gamma-carboxyglutamic acid have been found in involved tissue, and urine excretion of γ-carboxyglutamate was increased in patients with calcinosis and juvenile DM in comparison to children with juvenile DM without calcifications or to cases with other connective tissue diseases [19]. This calcium-binding amino acid is increased in patients with SSc and DM, and its level correlates with the extent of calcium deposit [20]. Large subcutaneous deposits can contain a liquid suspension of calcium crystals called "milk of calcium." The presence of macrophages, interleukin 6 (IL6), IL1, and TNF-α in the milk of calcium, and detectable levels of IL1 in the serum, suggest a major role of the activated macrophages in the process of calcinosis [21]. It has been suggested that TNF-α-308A promoter polymorphism might represent a risk factor for developing calcinosis [22]. It has been observed that lipodystrophy in juvenile DM was associated with calcinosis [23].

Some authors presume that calcinosis is a good prognostic factor. In the study by Muller et al., out of 75 adult DM patients without calcinosis, 26 died, usually in about 2 years, whereas of 12 adults with calcinosis, no one died [9]. But others have supposed that this treatment-resistant complication can be a major contributor to morbidity and occasionally mortality in such patients.

References

1. Bowyer SL, Blane CE, Sullivan DB, et al. Chilhood dermatomyositis factors predicting functional outcome and development of dystrophic calcification. *J Pediatr* 1983; 103: 882–888.
2. Ichiki Y, Akiyama T, Shimozawa N, et al. An extremely severe case of cutaneous calcinosis with juvenile dermatomyositis, and successful treatment with diltiazem. *Br J Dermatol* 2001; 144: 894–897.
3. Pachman LM, Cooke N. Juvenile dermatomyositis: a clinical and immunologic study. *J Pediatr* 1980; 96: 226–234.
4. Miller G, Heckmatt JZ, Dubowitz V. Drug treatment of juvenile dermatomyositis. *Arch Dis Child* 1983; 58: 445–450.
5. Dasgeb B, Phillips TJ. Adult-onset dermatomyositis complicated by calcinosis cutis. *Wounds* 2004; 16(12): 364–370.

6. Pachman LM, Friedman JM, Maryjowski-Sweeney ML, et al. Immunogenetic studies of juvenile dermatomyositis. III. Study of antibody to organ-specific and nuclear antigens. *Arthritis Rheum* 1985; 28(2): 151–157.
7. Bowyer SL, Clark RAF, Ragsdale CG, et al. Juvenile dermatomyositis: histological findings and pathogenic hypothesis for the associated skin changes. *J Rheumatol* 1986; 13: 753–758.
8. Wananukul S, Pongprasit P, Wattanakrai P. Calcinosis cutis presenting years before other clinical manifestations of juvenile dermatomyositis: report of two cases. *Aust J Dermatol* 1997; 38: 202–205.
9. Muller SA, Winkelmann RK, Brunsting LA. Calcinosis in dermatomyositis. *Arch Dermatol* 1959; 79: 669–673.
10. Sontheimer RD. Dermatomyositis: an overview of recent progress with emphasasis on dermatologic aspects. *Dermatol Clin* 2002; 20: 387–408.
11. Sewell JR, Liyanage B, Ansell BM. Calcinosis in juvenile dermatomyositis. *Skeletal Radiol* 1978; 3: 137–143.
12. Wedgewood RJ, Cook CD, Cohen J. Dermatomyositis: report of 26 cases in children with a discussion of endocrine therapy in 13. *Pediatrics* 1953; 12: 447–466.
13. Olhoffers IH, Carroll C, Watsky K. Dermatomyositis sine myositis with calcinosis universalis. *Br J Dermatol* 1999; 141: 365–366.
14. Callen JP. Dermatomyositis. *Lancet* 2000; 355: 53–57.
15. Murphy E, Freaney R, Bresnihan B, et al. Increased bone resorption and failure to respond to antiresorptive therapy in progressive dystrophic calcification. *Calcif Tissue Int* 2003; 73(5): 433–440.
16. Dalakas MC. Calcifications in dermatomyositis. *N Engl J Med* 1995; 333: 978.
17. Kimball AB, Summers RM, Turner M, et al. Magnetic resonance imaging detection of occult skin and subcutaneous abnormalities in juvenile dermatomyositis: implications for diagnosis and therapy. *Arthritis Rheum* 2000; 43: 1866–1873.
18. Halbert AR. Juvenile dermatomyositis. *Aust J Dermatol* 1996; 37: 106–108.
19. Lian J, Pachman L, Gunberg C, et al. Gamma carboxyglutamate excretion and calcinosis in juvenile dermatomyositis. *Arthritis Rheum* 1982; 25: 1094–1100.
20. Lian J, Pachman L, Gunberg C, et al. Gamma carboxyglutamate excretion: a marker on patients with ectopic calcification disorders. *Arthritis Rheum* 1979; 22: 634–635.
21. Mukamel M, Horev G, Mimouni M. New insight into calcinosis of juvenile dermatomyositis: a study of composition and treatment. *J Pediatr* 2001; 138(5): 736–766.
22. Pachman LM, Liotta-Davis MR, Hong DK, et al. TNF-α-308A allele in juvenile dermatomyositis: association with increased production of tumor necrosis factor alpha, disease duration, and pathologic calcifications. *Arthritis Rheum* 2000; 43: 2368–2377.
23. Rider L, Ruiz-Hidalgo M, Labora J, et al. Lipodystrophy in juvenile dermatomyositis is associated with calcinosis, but not with hepatocyte differentiation factor DLK levels [abstract]. *Arthritis Rheum* 2001; 44: S264.

18 Internal Malignancy Associated with Dermatomyositis

Although all the inflammatory myopathies can have a coincidental association with malignant disease, especially in older age-groups, the frequency of cancer is definitely increased in DM [1]. DM is an idiopathic inflammatory myopathy with diagnostic cutaneous manifestations, which often heralds paraneoplastic features of underlying internal malignancy [2].

The first reported association of DM with malignancy was by Stertz in 1916 [3], who described a patient with proximal muscle weakness, eyelid changes, and muscle biopsy evidence of myositis, and who had a coexisting gastric cancer. In the same year, Kankeleit [4] described a patient with DM and breast cancer, and the seeds of the controversy were thus sown [5]. From 1916 to 1975, 258 similar cases were published in the literature and analyzed by Barnes and Mawr [6]. Before 1951, only case reports of DM associated with malignancy appeared in the literature. In a larger series, Schuerman estimated that the incidence of malignancy in DM patients was five-fold that of the general population [7]. Curtis et al. [8] reported an 18% incidence of malignancy in theier series of 45 DM patients, and Christianson et al. [9] from the Mayo Clinic retrospectively studied 270 patients of whom only 7% had such an association. Arundell et al. [10] from the Cleveland Clinic found an associated malignant tumor in 12 of their 23 DM patients (52%) over the age of 40. Batschwarov and Minkov [11] from the Plovdiv Clinic investigated 18 DM patients, 12 of them over 40 years of age, and found malignancy in 6 (50%). In two cases, the surgical removal of the tumor was followed by tremporary remission of the DM. They concluded that there is considerable variation in the incidence of malignancy in different series; the selection of patients, the diagnostic facilities available and the length of follow-up are significant factors, and the patient's age is of fundamental importance. All of these studies were done prior to the criteria for diagnosis set forth by Bohan and Peter, and therefore many of the studied groups of patients were heterogeneous. Bohan et al. [12] reported an analysis of 153 patients with DM, and found 8/60 (13%) with malignancy. They had been criticized because of the inclusion in this analysis of patients with overlap syndrome, who did not have an increased risk for malignancy [5], and for the lack of a control group from the general population [13]. Callen et al. [14] studied 58 patients with definite or probable DM/PM and found a significantly increased risk for malignancy in seven of 27 DM patients (26%) in comparison to one of 31 PM patients (3%)

18

and a control group of other connective tissue diseases. Manchul et al. [15] investigated three groups of patients — two of 71 myositis patients (31 DM and 40 PM) and a control group of 42 patients with rheumatic and myopathic diseases. They found association of malignancy in 32% of DM patients, compared to 18% in PM patients and 7% in control group. Hidano et al. [16] collected 569 DM patients and found an associated malignancy in 112 of them (20%).

Other reports, however, have not arrived at the same conclusions. Lakhanpal et al. [17] from the Mayo Clinic studied 115 myositis patients (50 DM and 65 PM), and demonstrated no difference in malignancy incidence between these groups and controls. This work has been criticized because of the high incidence (17%) of malignancy in their control group [5].

The findings of the work by Richardson and Callen (1989), summarized since Bohan and Peter's criteria were put forward, concluded that there appears an increased incidence of malignancy in myositis patients; and that the incidence of malignancy in DM is greater than that in PM [5].

Numerous studies regarding association of cancer and DM have been carried out, with partially conflicting results [13]. A lot of independent, multicentric, and national retrospective investigations of different duration (from 5 to 20 years) concerning the association of DM and malignancy have been implemented, and a frequency range between 4.4% and 43% in the Caucasian population has been established [13] (Table 18.1).

In spite of all this, many authors suggest that this association of DM and malignancy is accidental. They have proposed the provision of new bigger multicentric epidemiological investigations to be compared with control groups to prove the assertion of an increased risk of carcinomas in patients with DM.

Table 18.1 Frequency of malignancy in dermatomyositis [29]

Author	Year	Design	Frequency of neoplasy
Cox et al.	1990	Re, Mu	23/53 (43%)
Basset-Seguin et al.	1990	Re, In	13/32 (41%)
Bonnethblanc et al.	1990	Re, Mu	34/118 (28%)
Duncan et al.	1991	In	10/39 (26%)
Hidano et al.	1992	Re, Mu	47/182 (26%)
Lifermann et al.	1993	Re	25/76 (33%)
Al Ballaa et al.	1993	Re	5/22 (23%)
Rose et al.	1994	Re	10/29 (35%)
Whitmore et al.	1994	In	5/15 (30%)
Whitmore et al.	1996	In	6/19 (31%)[a]
Dourmishev	1999	Re, In	12/50 (24%)

Re – retrospective; In – from single institute; Mu – multicenter
[a]DM + amyopathic DM.

18.1 Population-Based Epidemiologic Studies

The idea of DM and occult malignancy association provoked considerable controversy in the past [14, 18, 19]. Several population-based epidemiologic studies of this issue have clearly confirmed the existence of such a relationship in European whites having classic DM [1, 19–22] and in Australians with biopsy-proven IM [23]. Using a retrospective population-based survey of data from the Swedish Cancer Registry from 1958 through 1987, Sigurgeirsson et al. [1] calculated that the average incidence of cancer in a cohort of 788 patients with DM was 15%. No cancers were found in children with DM under 16 years of age. There was a 17-fold increase in ovarian cancer; and the mortality was increased in men and doubled in women [1]. These studies indicate marginal to no increased risk of malignancy in PM patients. A population-based study from Sweden implied a relative risk of associated malignancy of 2.4–3.4 in DM patients and 1.7–1.8 in those with PM [1]. In a study of 788 patients, the death rate was higher in those with DM owing to the presence of malignancy [1]. The association of malignancy with PM may result from diagnosis bias, with a heightened surveillance for cancer when this condition is diagnosed, whereas the increased risk with DM appears to be real (Table 18.2).

A population-based, retrospective study of 246 patients in Finland deduced that there was a 6.5-fold risk of malignancy in DM patients (mainly with ovarian, stomach, lung, nonmelanoma skin, and male genitalia neoplasy), but no increased risk in PM patients and for those treated with cytotoxic agents [20].

A comprehensive 20-year follow-up of 392 DM patients in Denmark also implied an increased risk of malignancy in these patients, and showed that the increased risk for

Table 18.2 Comparative data of malignancy and DM/PM

Author	No of patients	DM/PM	sir DM	sir DM 1 year	sir DM >5 years
Sigurgeiersson et al. (1992) (Sweden)	788	392/396	F = 3.9 M = 2.2	–	–
Zantos et al. (1994) (Denmark)	1,078	513/565	4.4	–	–
Chow et al. (1995)	539	336/203	3.8		1.5
Airio et al. (1995) (Finland)	246	71/175	6.5	3.0	4.4
Buchbinder et al. (2001) (Australia)	537	85/321	6.2	4.3	–
Stockton et al. (2001) (Scotland)	705	286/419	3.3	–	–
Hill et al. (2001) (Sweden, Denmark, Finland)	1,532	618/914	3.0	13.5	1.4

sir – standardized incidence ratio

malignancy disappeared by the third year after diagnosis [24]. In one Australian study, the IIM–malignancy association was ascertained in a group of 537 patients with biopsy-proven inflammatory myopathy [23]. In this retrospective, population-based study, the unadjusted incidence of malignancy associated with DM was 42% versus 18% for PM. After adjusting for age and gender, there was a sixfold increase in the cancer risk among DM patients compared with the general population (standardized incidence ratio 6.2, 95% CI 3.9–10.0); a twofold increase was observed in PM patients (standardized incidence ratio 2.0, 95% CI 1.4–2.7), although the relative risk for malignant disease in DM compared with PM was 2.4 (CI, 1.3–4.2). In these large studies and in the combined analysis of three large Scandinavian studies [22], the increased incidence declined over the years following the diagnosis, but was still measurable as long as 5 years after the disease onset in DM patients. However, the results applicable for the Scandinavian population could not be applied to the general population or to people of African or Asian descent [22].

18.2 Is DM a Paraneoplastic Phenomenon?

Cancer and DM could be related through different mechanisms, e.g., by sharing risk factors [25]. Such a hypothesis would be supported by a cancer preceding the diagnosis of DM or occurring at the same time. In that case, DM may be considered to be a paraneoplastic phenomenon [25]. In the meta-analysis an increased risk of antecedent cancer indicating a paraneoplastic phenomenon for DM with odds ratio of 4.4 (9.5% CI 3.0, 6.6), but not for PM, has been reported [26]. Similar data were noted in the Finnish population study [20]. In the pooled analysis of the three Scandinavian population studies, an increased cancer incidence was recorded in patients 2 years before DM diagnosis [22]. The increased risk for developing cancer in DM patients has been convincingly demonstrated in several studies, mainly from northern Europe and Australia. The persistently increased risk of developing malignancy 5 years after DM diagnosis suggests a true association which could indicate that there could be a shared susceptibility, or that DM or its treatment could induce neoplasma [26].

18.3 Age

The frequency of the association of DM and malignancy increases with the age of patients [27]. Associated malignancy with DM is most frequent after 40 years of age [11, 28, 29]. In one series of 38 patients with adult DM, 30 of them (79%) were about the age of 40 years, and 12 (31.6%) were found to have an associated malignancy [28]. DM associated with cancer has rarely been reported in childhood [30, 31].

18.4 Temporal Relationship between Dermatomyositis and Malignancy

The relationship in time between the onset of DM and the discovery of malignancy is quite variable [14, 29]. Dermatomyositis may precede the malignancy by years, might be discovered concurrently with the cancer, or could become evident years after the tumor is diagnosed and antineoplastic therapy is initiated [11, 15, 29]. It has been suggested that diagnoses of DM and malignancy separated widely in time are probably coincidental findings, whereas those temporally related perhaps share a causal rather than a casual relationship [5].

The same variability holds true for the clinical courses of DM and associated malignancy. There are many reports of improvement in myositis and cutaneous lesions following successful treatment of malignancy [8, 10, 11, 32]. Others authors, however, do not share this observation [12, 14]. There is no solid evidence from a large group of patients that argues strongly in favor of either view. It thus appears reasonable to suggest that in some patients, treatment of malignancy may have a beneficial effect on muscular and/or cutaneous components of their disease, while in others no such benefit is seen [5].

18.5 Tumor Types of Occult Malignancy in DM

The association of DM and the discovery of tumor types in different studies is quite variable. Many different types of malignancy, usually carcinoma rather than sarcoma, have been observed in patients with DM. Barnes and Mawr [6] reported that the breast was the most frequent tumor site in a study of 258 DM cases (17.8%). Sigurgeirsson et al. [1] reported that the colon (including the rectum) and the lungs were the most frequent cancer sites in a study of 750 patients with PM or DM in Sweden. Hatada et al. [33] mentioned that gastric cancer was the most frequent cancer site in DM in Japan (25.4%). The tumor types seem to be roughly commensurate with those of the general population [14, 17]. Gynecologic tumors (particulary ovarian carcinoma) are seen more frequently in white women with DM than would be expected in the general population [29, 34–39], and poses essentially a practical problem. Because the frequency of DM is higher in females, the incidence of ovarial and breast tumors in DM patients is also elevated. Other malignant diseases have also been described, such as lymphoma [16, 17, 40], Hodgkin disease [40], myeloma, or tymoma [16] that generally involve immunologic disturbances. Most recently, urachal adenocarcinoma, anaplastic thyroid carcinoma and recurrent adrenal gland carcinoma have been observed in association with DM [41–43].

Scandinavian and Scottish epidemiological data gives the conclusion that DM and PM are associated with specific cancer types: ovarian, lung, stomach, colon, pancreas, and bladder carcinomas, and non-Hodgkin lymphoma (NHL) for DM, and NHL, lung, and bladder cancer for PM [19, 22]. It is difficult to determine which lymphomas are most commonly associated with DM, since most epidemiologic studies just use the term "non-Hodgkin's lymphoma," which includes about 30 different diseases.

In Southeastern Asia, the incidence of nasopharyngeal carcinoma is elevated in the male population with or without DM [28, 44, 45]. In a recent study of 143 patients from Taiwan, nasopharyngeal cancer was the most common form of malignancy, with predisposing factors of an older age at onset (odds ratio 9.10) and male gender (odds ratio 4.06) [18]. Hepatocellular carcinoma (HCC) is endemic in Taiwan. The association of DM with HCC was first reported by Wong [46]. Only ten such cases have been reported in the past 30 years in the literature [47].

18.6 Malignancy in Different Clinical Variants of DM

Association of internal malignancy with DM has been reported mainly in the classic form of the disease, but also in patients with amyopathic DM, juvenile DM, drug-induced DM, polymyositis, and inclusion body myositis [48]. The patients with overlap syndrome, however, do not have an increased risk for malignancy [49].

Increasing age, the extent of cutaneous manifestations, and skin disease severity (i.e., blistering, ulceration), and the elevation of serum CPK levels seem to enhance the risk of malignancy in patients with classic DM. It has been suggested that the presence of other systemic complications of DM, such as ILD, is correlated with a decreased risk for internal malignancy [18].

There are many reports of patients with amyopathic DM (DM sine myositis) who developed an associated cancer. The coexistence of internal malignancy in patients with amyopathic DM was reported for the first time in 1993. Stonecipher et al. [50, 51], in a series of 13 cases with amyopathic DM, found two patients with adenocarcinoma of the breast. Whitmore et al. [52] reported a series of 12 patients with amyopathic DM, and 25% of them had underlying malignancy which was fatal in all cases: in three women ovarian cancers, and in one man squamous cell carcinoma. Finger et al. [53] also observed a case of amyopathic DM associated with adenocarcinoma of colon. Other authors reported the association of amyopathic DM with lymphoma [54] and with transitional cell carcinoma of the bladder [55]. Although the diagnostic criteria guidelines for distinguishing amyopathic DM from classic DM are not standardized, no separation should be made to await evidence of a myositis and to evaluate patients for underlying occult malignancy [56]. In a recent systemic review of the literature, from about 300 published cases of amyopathic DM it was determined that approximately 10% of them were associated with internal malignancy [57]. In a retrospective analysis of 746 DM patients seen at the Mayo Clinic between 1976 and 1994, it was revealed that 32 (4%) had amyopathic DM [58]. Four of 16 patients (25%) with amyopathic DM who were followed up between 2 and 10 years were found to have an internal malignancy [58]. In another retrospective study in Hong Kong between 1988 and 1996, six patients who fulfilled the criteria of amyopathic DM were found [45], and five of them, all male had associated malignancy (83.3%). Three patients suffered from nasopharyngeal carcinoma (60% of the total paraneoplastic cases); the other two developed non-small-cell carcinoma of the lung and metastatic carcinoma of unknown origin [45].

Other reports from Southeastern Asia found different results and did not share the same conclusions. In a 3-year retrospective review of DM patients seen at the National Skin Centre of Singapore, it was concluded that amyopathic DM is a common presentation in the ethnic population, and that patients with this disease were carriers of a lower risk of associated malignancy than classic DM [59]. In another retrospective study of 143 Taiwan DM patients, 20 of them with amyopathic DM, no malignancy-associated cases were found [18].

A few case reports have been published of juvenile DM associated with malignant tumors, such as lymphoid tumors [60], acute lymphoblastic leukemia [61], neuroblastoma [62], nasopharyngeal carcinoma [63], and hepatocarcinoma [64]. These case reports suggest that even in children with DM a careful medical evalution for cancer is needed.

The simultaneous arising of malignancy and DM as a paraneoplastic phenomenon; the beginning of DM during the treatment with medicines or ionizing therapy for cancer, and the arising of reversible leukaemia and lymphoma during the treatment of DM with immunosuppressive drugs, are the evidence deserving especially attention.

It is being increasingly recognized that certain drugs used for the treatment of malignancy can induce the cutaneous or systemic manifestations of DM or PM — i.e., drug-induced DM [65]. Such drugs as hydroxyurea, used for the treatment of chronic myelogenous leukemia continuously for up to 10 years [66–68], tamoxifen [69], tegafur [70], cyclophosphamid, and etoposid and after total body irradiation [68] or radiotherapy [71] applied for medication of malignant tumors have been reported to produced a DM-like cutaneous eruption indistinguishable from classic DM in adults or amyopathic DM.

The clinical manifestations of drug-induced paraneoplastic DM could be divided into two groups: (a) in patients with cancers treated with chemotherapeutic agents who later on could develop signs of DM [66–68, 72], and vice versa (b) in DM patients treated with antineoplastic drugs, who later develop malignancy [73–75].

Eleven cases of inclusion body myositis (IBM) associated with malignancy have been published [32]. Polymyositis and IBM are clinically presented with myositis syndrome only. A 62-year-old patient with transitional cell carcinoma of the bladder with the histological and other signs of IBM has been observed. Myositis syndrome in this patient was associated with clinical features of DM and normal serum creatine kinase, suggestive of cancer-associated DM [76].

18.7 Regional Association

The review of case reports of patients from the Asia-Pacific region presents probably a unique regional association of DM and a specific type of malignancy, reflecting a possible genetic predisposition [46] or the influence of environmental factors. Over the years, publications from the region have highlighted the significant association of DM and nasopharyngeal carcinoma [28, 44–46, 77].

Many authors have stressed the importance of measures for early malignancy discovery; however, the best cancer-screening regimen necessary for patients with a recently diagnosed myositis, as well as the interval needed between screenings, remains uncertain.

18

Conclusion

(i) DM is associated with an increased incidence of malignancy.
(ii) The association is more frequent in adults after the age of 40, but can be seen in childhood.
(iii) The neoplasma can precede, occur simultaneously with, or follow the diagnosis of DM.
(iv) The cancer type frequency corresponds to that in the general population.
(v) Internal malignancy may be associated with all clinical variants of DM.
(vi) The treatment of associated cancer may or may not have any effect on the myositis or cutaneous manifestations activity.
(vii) In DM patients, a search for malignancy should be carried out during the first 3–5 years after the disease onset.

References

1. Sigurgeirsson B, Lindelöf B, Edhag O, Allander E. Risk of cancer in patients with dermatomyositis or polymyositis: a population-based study. *N Engl J Med* 1992; 326: 363–367.
2. Drake L, Dinehart SM, Farmer ER, et al. Guidelines of care for dermatomyositis. *J Am Acad Dermatol* 1996; 34: 824–829.
3. Stertz G. Polymyositis. *Berl Klin Wochenschr* 1916; 53: 489.
4. Kankeleit H. Uber primaire nichteitrige polymyositis. *Dtsch Arch Klin Med* 1916; 120: 335–339.
5. Richardson J, Callen J. Dermatomyositis and malignancy. *Med Clin North Am* 1989; 73: 1211–1220.
6. Barnes BE, Mawr B. Dermatomyositis and malignancy. A review of the literature. *Ann Intern Med* 1976; 84: 68–76.
7. Schuerman H. Zür Klinik und Pathogenese der Dermatomyositis [Polymyositis]. *Arch Dermatol Syph* 1939; 178: 414–468.
8. Curtis AC, Blaylock HC, Harell ER. Malignant lesions associated with dermatomyositis. *JAMA* 1952; 150(9): 844–846.
9. Christianson HB, Brunsting LA, Perry HO. Dermatomyositis: unusual features, complications and treatment. *Arch Dermatol* 1954; 74: 581–589.
10. Arundell FD, Wilkinson RD, Haserick JR. Dermatomyositis and malignant neoplasm in adults: an survey of twenty years' experience. *Arch Dermatol* 1960; 82: 772–775.
11. Batschwarov B, Minkov D. Dermatomyositis and carcinoma. (A study based on an 18 years follow-up in Bulgaria). *Br J Dermatol* 1968; 80: 84–85.
12. Bohan A, Peter JB, Bowman RL, et al. A computer-assisted analysis of 153 patients with polymyositis and dermatomyositis. *Medicine* 1977; 56: 255–286.
13. Bernard P, Bonnetblanc JM. Dermatomyositis and malignancy. *J Invest Dermatol* 1993; 100(1): 128S–132S.
14. Callen JP, Hyla JF, Bole GG Jr, et al. The relationship of dermatomyositis and polymyositis to internal malignancy. *Arch Dermatol* 1980; 116(3): 295–298.
15. Manchul L, Jin A, Pritchard KI, et al. The frequency of malignancy in patients with dermatomyositis/polymyositis. *Arch Intern Med* 1985; 145: 1835–1839.
16. Hidano A, Kaneko K, Arai Y, et al. Survey of the prognosis for dermatomyositis, with special reference to its association with malignancy and pulmonary fibrosis. *J Dermatol* 1986; 13(4): 233–241.

17. Lakhanpal S, Bunch TW, Ilstrup DM, et al. Polymyositis-dermatomyositis and malignant lesions: Does an association exist? *Mayo Clin Proc* 1986; 61: 645–653.
18. Chen YJ, Wu CY, Shen JL. Predicting factors of malignancy in dermatomyositis and polymyositis: a case-control study. *Br J Dermatol* 2001; 144: 825–831.
19. Stockton D, Doherty VR, Brewster DH. Risk of cancer in patients with dermatomyositis or polymyositis, and follow-up implications: a Scottish population-based cohort study. *Br J Cancer* 2001; 85: 41–45.
20. Airio A, Pukkala E, Isomäki H. Elevated cancer incidence in patients with dermatomyositis: a population-based study. *J Rheumatol* 1995; 22: 1300–1303.
21. Yazici Y, Kagen LJ. The association of malignancy with myositis. *Curr Opin Rheumatol* 2000; 12(6): 498–500.
22. Hill CL, Zhang Y, Sigurgeirsson B, et al. Frequency of specific cancer types in dermatomyositis and polymyositis: a population-based study. *Lancet* 2001; 357: 96–100.
23. Buchbinder R, Forbes A, Hall S, et al. Incidence of malignant disease in biopsy-proven inflammatory myopathy. *Ann Intern Med* 2001; 134: 1087–1095.
24. Chow WH, Gridley G, Mellemkjaer L, et al. Cancer risk following polymyositis and dermatomyositis: a nationwide cohort study in Denmark. *Cancer Causes Control* 1995; 6: 9–13.
25. Dorph C, Lundberg IE. Idiopathic inflammatory myopathies – myositis. *Best Pract Res Clin Rheumatol* 2002; 16(5): 817–832.
26. Zantos D, Zhang Y, Felson D. The overall and temporal association of cancer with polymyositis and dermatomyositis. *J Rheumatol* 1994; 21(10): 1855–1859.
27. Rose C, Hatron PY, Brouillard M, et al. Signes prédicatifs de cancers au cours de la dermatomyosite. Etude de 29 observations. *Rev Med Int* 1994; 15(1): 19–24.
28. Leow YH, Goh CL. Malignancy and adult dermatomyositis. *Int J Dermatol* 1997; 36: 904–907.
29. Dourmishev LA. Dermatomyositis associated with malignancy. 12 case reports. *Adv Exp Med Biol* 1999; 455: 193–199.
30. Sherry DD, Haas JE, Milstein JM. Childhood polymyositis as a paraneoplastic phenomenon. *Pediatr Neurol* 1993; 9: 155–156.
31. Léaute-Labrèze C, Perel Y, Taïeb A. Childhood dermatomyositis associated with hepatocarcinoma. *N Engl J Med* 1995; 333(16): 1083.
32. Jansen ML, Weiting JM, Andary MT, et al. Inclusion body myositis and transitional cell carcinoma of the bladder: significant resolution of symptoms after tumour excision. *Arch Phys Med Rehabl* 1997; 78: 237–239.
33. Hatada T, Aoki I, Ikeda H, et al. Dermatomyositis and malignancy: case report and review of the Japanese literature. *Tumori* 1996; 82: 273–275.
34. Verducci MA, Malkasian GD, Friedman SJ, et al. Gynecologic carcinoma associated with dermatomyositis–polymyositis. *Obstret Gyncol* 1984; 64: 695.
35. Callen JP. Dermatomyositis and female malignancy. *J Surg Oncol* 1986; 32: 121–124.
36. Mordel N, Margalioth EJ, Harats N, et al. Concurrence of ovarian cancer and dermatomyositis. A report of two cases and literature review. *J Reprod Med* 1988; 33(7): 649–655.
37. Cherin P, Piette JC, Herson S, et al. Dermatomyositis and ovarian cancer: a report of 7 cases and literature review. *J Rheumatol* 1993; 20: 1897–1899.
38. Kubo M, Sato S, Kitahara H, et al. Vesicle formation in dermatomyositis associated with gynecologic malignancies. *J Am Acad Dermatol* 1996; 34: 391–394.
39. Davis MD, Ahmed I. Ovarian malignancy in patients with dermatomyositis and polymyositis: a retrospective analysis of fourteen cases. *J Am Acad Dermatol* 1997; 37: 730–733.
40. Tymms KE, Webb J. Dermatomyositis and other connective tissue diseases: a review of 105 cases. *J Rheumatol* 1985; 12: 1140–1148.

18

41. Sekine H, Ohya K, Kojima S, et al. Dermatomyositis associated with urachal adenocarcinoma. *J Urology* 2002; 168: 1488–1489.
42. Smith CJ, Staniland JR. A difficult case of inflammatory myositis. *Age Ageing* 2003; 32: 351–352.
43. Lingor P, von Boetticher D, Bahr M, et al. Paraneoplastic polymyositis in recurring adrenal gland carcinoma. *Lancet Neurology* 2003; 2: 435–436.
44. Chan HL. Dermatomyositis and cancer in Singapoore. *Int J Dermatol* 1985; 24: 447–450.
45. Fung WK, Chan HL, Lam WM. Amyopathic dermatomyositis in Hong Kong – association with nasopharyngeal carcinoma. *Int J Dermatol* 1998; 37: 659–663.
46. Wong KO. Dermatomyositis: a clinical investigation of 23 cases in Hong Kong. *Br J Dermatol* 1969; 81: 544–547.
47. Cheng TI, Tsou MH, Yang PS, et al. Dermatomyositis and erythrocytosis associated with hepatocellular carcinoma. *J Gastroenterol Hepatol* 2002; 17: 1239–1242.
48. Dourmishev LA, Dourmishev AL, Schwartz RA. Dermatomyositis: cutaneous manifestations of its variants. *Int J Dermatol* 2002; 41(10): 625–630.
49. Callen JP. Dermatomyositis. *Neurol Clin* 1987; 5: 379–403.
50. Stonecipher MR, Jorizzo JR, White WL, et al. Cutaneous changes of dermatomyositis in patients with normal muscle enzymes: Dermatomyositis sine myositis? *J Am Acad Dermatol* 1993; 28: 951–956.
51. Stonecipher MR, Jorizzo JR, Monu J, et al. Dermatomyositis with normal muscle enzyme concentration. A single-blind study of the diagnostic value of magnetic resonance imaging and ultrasound. *Arch Dermatol* 1994; 130: 1294–1299.
52. Whitmore S, Anhalt G, Provost T, et al. Serum CA-125 screening for ovarian cancer in patients with dermatomyositis. *Gynecol Oncol* 1997; 65: 241–244.
53. Finger DR, Dunn CL, Gilliland WR, et al. Amyopathic dermatomyositis associated with malignancy. *Int J Dermatol* 1996; 35: 663–664.
54. Osman Y, Narita M, Kishi K, et al. Case report: amyopathic dermatomyositis associated with transformed malignant lymphoma. *Am J Med Sci* 1996; 311: 240–242.
55. Russ BW, English JC, King DH, et al. Amyopathic dermatomyositis associated with transitional cell carcinoma of the bladder. *Cutis* 1999; 63: 73–76.
56. Kagen LJ. Amyopathic dermatomyositis. *Arch Dermatol* 1995; 131: 1458–1459.
57. Sontheimer RD. Dermatomyositis: an overview of recent progress with emphasasis on dermatologic aspects. *Dermatol Clin* 2002; 20: 387–408.
58. el-Azhary R, Pakzad SY. Amyopathic dermatomyositis: retrospective review of 37 cases. *J Am Acad Dermatol* 2002; 46: 560–565.
59. Ang P, Sugeng MW, Chua SH. Classic and amyopathic dermatomyositis seen at the National Skin Centre of Singapore: a 3-year retrospective review of their clinical characteristics and association with malignancy. *Ann Acad Med Singapore* 2000; 29: 219–223.
60. Taieb A, Guichard C, Salamon R, et al. Prognosis in juvenile dermatopolymyositis: a cooperative retrospective study of 70 cases. *Pediatr Dermatol* 1985; 2: 275–281.
61. Falcini F, Taccetti G, Trapani S, et al. Acute lymphoblastic leukemia associated with dermatomyositis in a child. *Pediatr Dermatol* 1993; 10: 199–200.
62. Kalmanti M, Athanasiou A. Neuroblastoma occurring in a child with dermatomyositis. *Am J Pediatr Hematol Oncol* 1985; 7: 387–388.
63. De Bersques J. Deux cas de dermatomyosite chez des adolescentes. *Nouv Dermatol* 1987; 6: 499.
64. Leaute-Labreze C, Perel Y, Taieb A. Childhood dermatomyositis associated with hepatocarcinoma. *N Engl J Med* 1995; 333: 1083–1084.
65. Dourmishev A, Dourmishev L. Dermatomyositis and drugs. *Adv Exp Med Biol* 1999; 455: 187–191.

66. Rocamora V, Puig L, Alomar A. Dermatomyositis-like eruption following hydroxyurea therapy. *J Eur Acad Dermatol Venereol* 2000; 14: 227–228.
67. Marie I, Joly P, Levesque H, et al. Pseudo-dermatomositis as a complication of hydroxyurea therapy. *Clin Exp Rheumatol* 2000; 18: 536–537.
68. Ruiz-Genao DP, Sanz-Sánchez T, Bartolomé-González B, et al. Dermatomyositis-like reaction induced by chemotherapeutical agents. *Int J Dermatol* 2002; 41: 885–887.
69. Harris AL, Smith IE, Snaith M. Tamoxifen-induced tumor regression associated with dermatomyositis. *Br Med J* 1982; 284: 1674.
70. Akiyama C. Osada A, Sou K, et al. A case of dermatomyositis triggered by tegafur. *Acta Derm Venereol (Stockh)* 1997; 77: 490.
71. Monk BE, Pembroke AC. Dermatomyositis following radiotherapy. *Br J Dermatol* 1983; 109 (Suppl 24): 103.
72. Richard M, Truchetet F, Friedel J, et al. Skin lesions simulating chronic dermatomyositis during long-term hydroxyurea therapy. *J Am Acad Dermatol* 1989; 21: 797–799.
73. Krishnan K, Adams P, Silveira S, et al. Therapy-related acute myeloid leukaemia following immunosuppression with azathioprine for polymyositis. *Clin Lab Haematol* 1994; 16: 285–289.
74. Arnold JA, Ranson SA, Abdalla SH. Azathioprine-associated acute myeloid leukaemia with trilineage dysplasia and complex karyotype: a case report and review of the literature. *Clin Lab Haematol* 1999; 21(4): 289–292.
75. Roddy E, Courtney PA, Morris A. Non-Hodgkin's lymphoma in a patient with refractory dermatomyositis which had been treated with infliximab. *Rheumatology (Oxford)* 2002; 41(10): 1194–1195.
76. Talanin NY, Bushore D, Rasberry R, et al. Dermatomyositis with the features of inclusion body myositis associated with carcinoma of the bladder. *Br J Dermatol* 1999; 141: 926–930.
77. Goh CL, Rajan VS. Dermatomyositis in a skin centre. *Ann Acad Med Singapore* 1983; 12: 6–12.

Clinical Variants of Dermatomyositis

Adult inflammatory myopathies (or myositis) includes the three most common diseases: polymyositis (PM), dermatomyositis (DM), and inclusion body myositis (IBM), and a number of much rare entities. For clinicians, the criteria proposed by Bohan and Peter remain the most familiar and accepted definitions of the first two of these immunomediated myopathies. They combine clinical, laboratory, and pathological features, and have been used in almost all clinical trials. Additional idiopathic inflammatory myopathies, including giant cell myositis, focal/localized myositis, granulomatous myositis, macrophagic myofasciitis, pipestem capillary disease, and myositis related to other connective tissue diseases will be explored in the next section of monography.

DM has a number of clinical variants, with characteristic clinical manifestations and laboratory constellations that may require complex methods and techniques for diagnosis. Cutaneous findings in such inflammatory myopathies are useful to facilitate accurate diagnosis and suggest the necessary therapy. In the recent years, skin features typical of DM have been described in many patients with PM variants (inclusion body myositis, drug-induced polymyositis). The various forms of this disease require distinction, as they have different prognoses and may require different therapeutic approaches.

19 Classic Dermatomyositis in Adults

"Classic" DM in adults has various clinical and pathological features, which do not always appear simultaneously or with the same severity. Dermatomyositis is identified by a characteristic rash, which appeared simultaneously or, more commonly, preceded muscle weakness. In addition to manifesting clinical and laboratory evidence of myositis, adult patients with classic DM develop the hallmark cutaneous findings. Cutaneous manifestations of DM could be classified as photosensitive, hyperkeratotic, and vascular (see Table 6.2). Photosensitive lesions consist of heliotrope rash, a periorbital, dusky, violaceous erythema of one or both eyelids. Heliotrope rash could be a component of a more confluent erythema involving the entire face in many cases associated with edema, and erythematous exanthemas on discrete areas of the body: the neck, and anterior chest (in a V-sign) or the nape of the neck and the posterior aspect of the shoulders (shawl-sign), knees, elbows, and malleoli [1–3]. An erythematous rash may also be found on the face in a limited malar distribution, or more extensively with perioral sparing [4]. This erythema can extend to the ears and scalp [5]. The lesions are pruritic, and can be exacerbated after exposure to the sunlight. Gottron rash is a characteristic feature, with violaceous to dusky, red, flat-topped papules and plaques prominent on dorsal interphalangeal joints, elbows, and knees and, rarely, the malleoli. These papules evolve over time to have depressed, atrophic, porcelain white centers and prominent telangiectasias known as Gottron's sign over bony prominences.

A rare subgroup of patients have follicular hyperkeratosis, which may occur as a pityriasis rubra pilaris-like eruption (Wong-type DM). The lateral and palmar areas of the fingers may become rough with cracked, "dirty" horizontal lines, resembling "mechanic's hands", and dilated capillary loops with punctate infarcts at the base of the fingernails with irregular, thickened, and distorted cuticles could be prominent. Scalp involvement is frequently evident as a diffuse, erythematous, scaly, atrophic dermatosis with mild-to-moderate alopecia. Cutaneous vasculitis is seen as palpable purpura and digital or oral ulcerations. Panniculitis may be a characteristic component of classic DM in adults.

Several case reports have described DM with vesicular and bullous lesions, but without immunofluorescence studies, and it is difficult to predict whether these patients had associated autoimmune bullous dermatosis. Rare cutaneous findings described in patients with classic DM in adults include also the flagellate erythema [6], erythroderma [7], and cutaneous mucinosis.

19

19.1 Association of DM with Other Dermatoses

Extremely rare associations with DM include localized lipoatrophy not clinically preceded by panniculitis [8]. Dermatitis herpetiformis [9, 10], bullous pemphigoid [11–13], and bullous pemphigoid with PM and contact dermatitis have also been described in DM patients [14].

Patients having hallmark skin manifestations of DM in typical locations have findings of other skin diseases such as urticarial lesions [15], lichen planus, [16], nasal septal perforation [17], acquired ichthyosis, [18, 19], malacoplakia, [20], porphyria cutanea tarda [21, 22], pityriasis rubra pilaris [23], malignant atrophic papulosis — Degos disease [24], pyoderma gangrenosum-like ulcers [25, 26], Sweet syndrome [27], chondrodermatitis nodularis helices in childhood DM [28], porokeratosis [29], pemphigus foliaceus [30], sarcoidosis [31, 32], deep cutaneous infection with *Mycobacterium avium-intracellulare* complex [33], and *M. tuberculosis* [34], disseminated cutaneous infection with *M. chelonae* mimicking panniculitis [35], calcific myonecrosis [36], etc. (Table 19.1).

Table 19.1 Association of DM with other dermatoses

Disease	Reference
Dermatitis herpetiformis	White and Tesar (1982), Kalovidouris et al. (1989)
Bullous pemphigoid	Glover and Leigh (1992), Iwai et al. (1996), Tsukada et al. (2003)
Porphyria cutanea tarda	Belaich et al. (1989), Bauza et al. (2003)
Pemphigus foliaceus	Narbutt et al. (2003)
Linear IgA bullous dermatosis	Barrows-Wade et al. (1992)
Localized lipoatrophy	Commens et al. (1990)
Acquired lypodystrophy	Huemer et al. (2001), Rider et al. (2001)
Palmar mucinosis	Del Pozo et al. (2001), Sontheimer (2002)
Reticular erythematous mucinosis	Kock et al. (1994)
Plaque-like mucinosis	Requena et al. (1990), Kaufmann et al. (1998)
Cellulite-like mucinosis	Igarashi et al. (1985), Chen et al. (2005)
Scleromyxedema (lichen myxedematosus)	Von Nagy et al. (1962), Johnson et al. (1973), Launay et al. (2001)
Sarcoidosis	Ogawa et al. (1976), Itoh et al. (1980), Hart et al. (1988), Lipton et al. (1988), Takano et al. (1996), Brateanu et al. (2000), Ito et al. (2003)
Urticaria	Payne and Thomas (1984)
Lichen planus	Al-Najjar et al. (1985)
Pityriasis rubra pilaris	Requena et al. (1997), Lupton et al. (2000)
Malignant atrophic papulosis (Degos disease)	Tsao et al. (1997)

(continued)

Table 19.1 (continued)

Disease	Reference
Chondrodermatitis nodularis helices	Sasaki et al. (1999)
Porokeratosis	Monteagudo-Sánchez et al. (2006), Valverde et al. (2007)
T-cell lymphoma	Rybojad et al. (2001)
Malacoplakia	Singh et al. (1987)
Pyoderma gangrenosum	Shah et al. (1996), Chen et al. (2005)
Nasal septal perforation	Martinez-Cordero et al. (1986)
Acquired hypertrichosis	Turner (1937), Reich and Reinchard (1948), Pope et al. (1994), Faure Fontanela (1995), Piantanila et al. (1999)
Acquired ichthyosis	Urrutia et al. (1987), Inuzuka et al. (2001)
Sweet syndrome	Yoo et al. (1999)
Antiphospholipid syndrome	Sherer et al. (2000)
Hemophagocytic syndrome	Yasuma et al. (1998), Madaule et al. (2000)
Skin infection with	
Mycobacterium avium-intracellulare	Bedlow et al. (1998)
M. chelonae	Leung et al. (2005)
Calcific myonecrosis	Batz et al. (2005)
Angiokeratomas	Shannon and Ford (1999)
Keratoses	See et al. (1997), Caporali et al. (2004)
Acanthosis nigricans	Randle and Winkelmann (1979), Tuna Castro M and García Kutzbach (1996)

19.2 Muscle Disease in DM

The muscle weakness varies from mild to severe, even to quadriparesis [37]. Although the cases of dermatomyositis sine dermatomyositis with skin limited affection are accepted as a separate clinical variant, some authors still believe that amyopathic and myopathic DM are part of the range of DM affecting skin and muscle to a varying degree.

Progressive weakness is the major clinical manifestation of DM. It is always symmetric and bilateral, and affects different muscle groups such as the abductors or adductors of the arms, flexors, or extensors of the thigh, or neck flexors. Dermatomyositis presents with a varying degree of muscle weakness that develops slowly, over weeks to months, but rare cases with acute course are also reported in literature.

Half of the patients complain of myalgia or have some muscle tenderness. Pain is rarely a prominent symptom of the disease. Arthralgia and arthritis occur in 20–25% of DM patients [1].

19

In addition to skin and muscle, the disease can also involve other internal organs, especially the lungs, heart, intestines, and eyes. Dysphagia, nasal regurgitation, and aspiration pneumonia may occur because of the esophageal dysfunction. Lung involvement in DM and pulmonary function is abnormal in about 40% of the patients [38]. Patients with classic DM have ECG alterations in 40% of the cases, such as nonspecific ST-T changes, arrhythmia, abnormal Q waves, bundle branch block, and congestive heart failure [1]. Pericardial involvement in DM is very rare, usually with asymptomatic manifestation. Sarcoplasmic membrane muscle enzymes (CK, ASAT, LDH, ALAT, aldolase) are often elevated [1, 39]. Changes of the levels of serum enzymes depend on the form, severity of disease and the treatment.

General symptoms of DM include fever, malaise, weight loss, arthralgia, and Raynaud's phenomenon (Table 19.2).

Table 19.2 Diagnostic cutaneous and muscle manifestations of DM

Cutaneous manifestations		
1. Photosensitive features	**2. Keratotic (trauma-induced) features**	**3. Vascular features**
(a) "Heliotrope" (palpebral, periorbital, facial) rash with or without edema	(a) Gottron's papules	(a) Proximal nailfold erythema, telangiectasias, and periungual infarcts
(b) "Shawl" or "V"-sign and other erythemas on the extensor aspects	(b) Scalp scaly disease	(b) Cutaneous vasculitis (palpable purpura, urticaria-vasculitis lesions, livedo reticularis)
(c) Poikiloderma atrophicans	(c) Cuticular hypertrophy (Keining's-sign)	(c) Epidermal necrosis (eschares)
	(d) Follicular hyperkeratosis (Wong sign);	(d) Ulcers (digital or oral)
	(e) Mechanic's hands	(e) Telangiectasias (mucosal, skin)
	(f) "Holster" sign (Sontheimer sign)	
	(g) "Callosity feet" (Dourmishev's sign)	
4. Increased photosensitivity against UV-B light	**5. Pathological findings compatible with DM**	
Features of the muscle damage (Bohan and Peter's criteria, 1975)		
1. Subjective complaints		
(a) Proximal muscle weakness		
(b) Myalgia or muscle pain		
(c) Arthralgias or nondestructive arthritis		

(continued)

Table 19.1 (continued)

2. Evidence of myositis by
(a) EMG
(b) Imaging techniques (MRI, 31P-MR-spectroscopy)
(c) Ultrasound
3. Elevated muscle enzymes (CK, aldolase, transaminases, LDH)
4. Myositis-specific antibodies (Jo-1, Mi-2)
5. Pathologic findings compatible with inflammatory myositis
Laboratory features for active muscle inflammatory disease
1. ESR — accelerated ≥ 20 mm/h (by Westergren)
2. Neopterin and factor VIII-related antigen (von Willebrand factor)
3. C reactive protein
4. Other

19.3 Autoantibody Defined Syndromes in DM

19.3.1 Anti-Mi-2 Antibody Syndrome

The first case with anti-Mi-2 antibody syndrome was a 60-year-old patient with classic DM in whom the antibody was initially detected [40]. The anti-Mi-2 autoantibodies are found strongly associated with a tryptophan at position 9 of the HLA-DRbeta chain [41].

Patients with anti-Mi-2 antibodies have classic forms of DM: pronounced "V-sign" and "shawl-sign" rashes and cuticular overgrowth (Table 19.3). HLA-DR7, HLA-DRw53, and HLA-DQA1*0201 genotypes predominate in those patients, as well as the relatively good response to therapy, and the favorable prognosis [42–45]. However, a Mi-2-positive DM patient with fatal hemophagocytic syndrome was recently reported [46]. An 83-year-old man with DM and anti-Mi-2 antibodies in sera developed marked febrile pancytopenia with fatal outcome from hemophagocytic syndrome [47]. Bone marrow aspiration showed decreased number of megakaryocytes, erythroblasts, and macrophages with cytophagocytosis.

Juvenile DM patients with anti-Mi-2 autoantibodies and clinical features similar to those seen in adults have also been reported. However, in contrast to adult patients, they often do not routinely manifest the V-sign, shawl-sign, or cuticular overgrowth [48]. These children usually demonstrate a monocyclic course and a good response to treatment [48–50].

19.3.2 Antisynthetase Syndrome [Anti-Jo-1 Antibody Syndrome]

[See Chapter 25].

Table 19.3 Relationship between cutaneous manifestations of DM/PM and MSA

Disease	Cutaneous manifestations	Features	MSA or MAA	References
DM	**Photosensitive**	Heliotrope rash V-sign Shawl sign	Anti-Mi-2 antibody	Lowe et al. (1991), Miller (1993), Nilasena et al. (1995)
DM (PM, SSc)	**Hyperkeratotic**	Mechanic's hands (71%)	Anti-Jo-1 antibody	Mitra et al. (1994), Moder et al. (1993), Perret et al. (1996), Herrero et al. (2000)
		Callosity feet	Anti-Jo-1 antibody	Dourmishev and Dourmishev (2004)
		Keining's-sign	Anti-Jo-1 antibody	Marie et al. (1999)
		Gottron's papules (42%)	Anti-Jo-1 and other antisynthetases	Jablonska and Blaszcyk (1999)
Sclero–myositis		Mechanic's hands	Anti-PM-Scl antibody	Genth et al. (1990), Oddis et al. (1992), Rider et al. (1994), Genth and Mireau (1995), Török et al. (2004)
DM	**Vascular**	Nailfold signs	Anti-Jo-1 and other antisynthetases	Marie et al. (1999)
		Gingival telangiectasia	Anti-Jo-1 antibody	Dourmishev and Dourmishev (2004)
		Nonhealing cutaneous ulcers	Anti-Jo-1 antibody	Rider et al. (1994)
PM/SSc/OS	**Edematous**	Sclerodactily	Anti-P7 antibody	Sato et al. (2005)
DM/PM		Finger swelling	Anti-7SL RNA autoantibody	Satoh et al. (2005)

19.3.3 Anti-Signal Recognition Particle Syndrome [Anti-SRP Syndrome]

[See Chapter 25].

Whereas the overwhelming majority of patients with anti-SRP until now were reported to have PM [42, 49], and anti-Mi-2 was almost completely specific for DM [40–42], Brouwer et al. [50] mentioned several anti-SRP positive patients with DM and anti-Mi-2 positive PM cases, and even some patients with these autoantibodies and IBM.

19.3.4 Association of DM with Internal Diseases

Other less common internal diseases observed and possibly linked to DM include antiphospholipid syndrome [51], hemophagocitic syndrome [46, 47], T-cell lymphoma [52, 53], tuberculosis infection [34, 54], and toxoplasmosis [54].

Although a case of Coombs-positive hemolytic anemia or immune thrombocytopenia associated with DM has been previously reported [55, 56], Evans' syndrome with DM is very rare [57, 58]. Recently, a 59-year-old woman, with DM associated with Evans' syndrome (Coombs-positive hemolytic anemia and immune thrombocytopenia with positive antiplatelet antibody) has been reported [58]. Thrombocytopenia responded to intravenous immunoglobulin (IVIG) for a short time. However, the patient was successfully treated with cyclophosphamide in addition to oral prednisolone [58].

References

1. Bohan A, Peter JB, Bowman RL. A computer-assisted analysis of 153 patients with polymyositis and dermatomyositis. *Medicine* 1977; 56: 255–286.
2. Kovacs SO, Kovacs SC. Dermatomyositis. *J Am Acad Dermatol* 1998; 39: 899–920.
3. Dourmishev LA, Dourmishev AL, Schwartz RA. Dermatomyositis: cutaneous manifestations of its variants. *Int J Dermatol* 2002; 41(10): 625–630.
4. Santmyire-Rosenberger B, Dugan EM. Skin involvement in dermatomyositis. *Curr Opin Rheumatol* 2003; 15(6): 714–722.
5. Sontheimer RD. Dermatomyositis: an overview of recent progress with emphasis on dermatologic aspects. *Dermatol Clin* 2002; 20: 387–408.
6. Kimyai-Asadi A, Tausk FA, Nousari HC. A patient with dermatomyositis and linear streaks on the back. *Archiv Dermatol* 2000; 136(5): 667–670.
7. Maruani A, Armingaud P, Nseir A, et al. Erythroderma and cutaneous necrosis in patient with dermatomyositis. *Ann Dermatol Venereol* 2003; 150: 353–356.
8. Commens C, O'Neill P, Walker G. Dermatomyositis associated with multifocal lipoatrophy. *J Am Acad Dermatol* 1990; 22: 966–969.
9. White SW, Tesar JT. Dermatomyositis and dermatitis herpetiformis. *Arch Dermatol* 1982; 118: 599–601.
10. Kalovidouris AE, Miller FW, Lawley TJ. Polymyositis/dermatomyositis associated with dermatitis herpetiformis. *Arthritis Rheum* 1989; 32: 1179–1181.
11. Glover M, Leigh I. Dermatomyositis pemphigoides: a case with coexistent dermatomyositis and bullous pemphigoid. *J Am Acad Dermatol* 1992; 27: 849–852.
12. Iwai T, Muro Y, Ohashi M. Two cases of dermatomyositis with vesicular and bullous lesions. *Hifubyo Rinsho (Tokyo)* 1996; 18: 903–906 [Japanese].
13. Tsukada Y, Kawase MK, Murashima A, et al. Bullous pemphigoid associated with dermatomyositis successfully controlled with minocycline. *Clin Exp Dermatol* 2003; 28: 554–564.
14. Peck SM, Lefkovits AM. Bullous pemphigoid with polymyositis and co-existing contact dermatitis. *Arch Dermatol* 1966; 94: 672–674.
15. Payne CM, Thomas RH. Dermatomyositis with urticated lesions. *J R Soc Med* 1984; 77(2): 137–138.
16. Al-Najjar A, Reily GD, Harrington CI. Dermatomyositis and lichen planus: an association or manifestation? *Clin Exp Dermatol* 1985; 10: 174–178.
17. Martinez-Cordero E, Katona G. Nasal septal perforation in dermatomyositis. *J Rheumatol* 1986; 13: 231–232.
18. Urrutia S, Vazquea F, Requena L, et al. Acquired ichthyosis associated with dermatomyositis. *J Am Acad Dermatol* 1987; 16: 627–629.
19. Inuzuka M, Tomita K, Tokura Y, et al. Acquired ichthyosis associated with dermatomyositis in a patient with hepatocellular carcinoma. *Br J Dermatol* 2001; 144: 415–448.
20. Singh M, Kaur S, Vajpayee BK, et al. Cutaneous malacoplakia with dermatomyositis. *Int J Dermatol* 1987; 26: 190.

19

21. Belaich S, Crickx B, Picard C, et al. Porphyria cutanea tarda associated with pure cutaneous dermatomyositis. *Ann Dermatol Venereol* 1989; 116: 826–827.
22. Bauzá A, España A, Lloret P. Porphyria cutanea tarda, dermatomyositis and non-Hodgkin lymphoma in virus C infection. *Eur J Dermatol* 2003; 13(3): 302–304.
23. Requena L, Grilli R, Soriano L, et al. Dermatomyositis with a pityriasis rubra pilaris-like eruption: a little-known distinctive cutaneous manifestation of dermatomyositis. *Br J Dermatol* 1997; 136: 768–771.
24. Tsao H, Busam K, Barnhill RL, et al. Lesions resembling malignant atrophic papulosis in a patient with dermatomyositis. *J Am Acad Dermatol* 1997; 36: 317–319.
25. Shah M, lewis FM, Harrington CI. Scrotal pyoderma gangrenosum associated with dermatomyositis. *Clin Exp Dermatol* 1996; 21: 151–153.
26. Chen GY, Liu MF, Lee J, et al. Combination of massive mucinosis, dermatomyositis, pyoderma gangrenosum-like ulcer, bullae and fatal intestinal vasculopathy in young female. *Eur J Dermatol* 2005; 15: 396–400.
27. Yoo WH, Moon SK, Park TS, et al. A case of Sweet's syndrome in patient with dermatomyositis. *Korean J Intern Med* 1999; 14: 78–81.
28. Sasaki T, Nishizawa H, Sugita Y. Chondrodermatitis nodularis helices in childhood dermatomyositis. *Br J Dermatol* 1999; 141: 363–365.
29. Lupton JR, Figueroa P, Berberian BJ, et al. An unusual presentation of dermatomyositis: The type Wong variant revised. *J Am Acad Dermatol* 2000; 43: 908–912.
30. Narbutt J, Torzecka JD, Sysa-Jedrzejowska A, et al. Pemphigus foliaceus in an 11-year-old boy with dermatomyositis: simple coincidence or familial immunological background? *Br J Dermatol* 2003; 148: 823–842.
31. Lipton JH, McLeod BD, Brownell AK. Dermatomyositis and granulomatous myopathy associated with sarcoidosis. *Can J Neurol Sci* 1988; 15: 426–429.
32. Ito A, Kazama T, Ito M. A unique case of sarcoidosis: coexistence of sarcoidal granuloma and histological changes consistent with dermatomyositis. *Br J Dermatol* 2003; 149: 430–432.
33. Bedlow AJ, Vittay G, Stephenson J, et al. Deep cutaneous infection with *Mycobacterium avium-intracellulare* complex in an immunosuppressed patient with dermatomyositis. *Br J Dermatol* 1998; 139: 920–922.
34. Durmischew A, Lasarowa A, Krasrewa M, et al. Dermatomyositis und Tuberculosis miliaris (Fallbeobachtung mit exitus letalis). *Z Hautkrh* 1988; 63(1): 42–43.
35. Leung YY, Choi KW, Ho KM, et al. Disseminated cutaneous infection with *Mycobacterium chelonae* mimicking panniculitis in a patient with dermatomyositis. *Hong Kong Med J* 2005; 11(6): 515–519.
36. Batz R, Sofka CM, Adler RS, et al. Dermatomyositis and calcific myonecrosis in the leg: ultrasound as an aid in management. *Skeletal Radiol* 2006; 35(2): 113–116.
37. Dalakas M. Polymyositis, dermatomyositis and inclusion body myositis. *N Engl J Med* 1991; 325(21): 1487–1498.
38. Marie I, Hatron PY, Hachulla E, et al. Pulmonary involvement in polymyositis and in dermatomyositis. *J Rheumatol* 1998; 25: 1336–1343.
39. Caro I. Dermatomyositis as a systemic disease. *Med Clin North Am* 1989; 73: 1181–1192.
40. Targoff IN, Reichlin M. The association between Mi-2 antibodies and dermatomyositis. *Arthritis Rheum* 1985; 28: 796–803.
41. Mierau R, Dick T, Genth E, et al. An update on HLA association of Mi-2 autoantibodies: the association with a tryptophan at position 9 of the HLA-DRbeta chain is strong but not absolute. *Arthritis Rheum* 1999; 42(7): 1552–1553.
42. Love LA, Leff RL, Fraser DD, et al. A new approach to the classification of idiopathic inflammatory myopathy: myositis-specific autoantibodies define useful homogeneous patient groups. *Medicine* 1991; 70: 360–374.

43. Gurely RC, Love LA, Targoff IN, et al. Associations among myositis-specific autoantibodies (MSA) and HLA-DQA1 aleles [abstract]. *Arthritis Rheum* 1991; 34: S137.
44. Miller FW. Myositis-specific autoantibodies: touchstones for understanding the inflammatory myopathies. *JAMA* 1993; 270: 1846–1849.
45. Nilasena DS, Trieu EP, Targoff IN. Analysis of the MI-2 autoantigen of dermatomyositis. *Arthritis Rheum* 1995; 38: 123–128.
46. Yasuda S, Tsutsumi A, Nakabayashi T, et al. Haemophagocytic syndrome in a patient with ermatomyositis. *Br J Rheumatol* 1998; 37: 1357–1358.
47. Madaule S, Porte L, Couret B, et al. Fatal haemophagocytic syndrome in the course of dermatomyositis with anti-Mi2 antibody. *Rheumatology* 2000; 39: 11–57–58.
48. Rider LG, Miller FW, Targoff IN, et al. A broadened spectrum of juvenile myositis. Myositis-specific autoantibodies in children. *Arthritis Rheum* 1994; 37: 1534–1538.
49. Targoff IN. Immune mechanisms in myositis. *Curr Opin Rheumatol* 1990; 2: 882–888.
50. Brouwer R, Hengstman GJ, Vree Egberts W, et al. Autoantibody profiles in the sera of European patients with myositis. *Ann Rheum Dis*. 2001; 60(2): 116–123.
51. Sherer Y, Livenh A, Levy Y, et al. Dermatomyositis and polymyositis associated with the antiphospholipid syndrome — a novel overlap syndrome. *Lupus* 2000; 9: 42–45.
52. Rencic A, Laman S, Nousari HC. Peripheral T-cell lymphoma presenting as dermatomyositis-like eruption. *J Cutan Med Surg* 2002; 6(3): 218–220.
53. Chandesris MO, Crétel-Durand E, Jean R, et al. Dermatomyositis associated with hepatosplenic gamma delta T-cell lymphoma. *Rev Med Interne* 2007; 28(8): 552–555 [French].
54. Mazabrey D, Bonafé JL, Viraben R, et al. Association of dermatomyositis, toxoplasmosis and tuberculosis. *Ann Dermatol Venereol* 1982; 109(3): 277–280 [French].
55. Cooper C, Fairris G, Cotton DK, et al. Dermatomyositis associated with idiopathic thrombocytopenia. *Dermatologica* 1986; 172: 173–176.
56. Hardman CM, Garioch JJ, Leonard JN, et al. Autoimmune haemolytic anaemia associated with dermatomyositis. *Clin ExpDermatol* 1996; 21: 437–439.
57. Hay EM, Makris M, Winfield J, et al. Evans' syndrome associated with dermatomyositis. *Ann Rheum Dis* 1990; 49: 793–794.
58. Chang DK, Yoo DH, Kim TH, et al. Induction of remission with intravenous immunoglobulin and cyclophosphamide in steroid-resistant Evans' syndrome associated with dermatomyositis. *Clin Rheumatol* 2001; 20: 63–66.

Juvenile Dermatomyositis 20

In 1918 Amedeo Modigliani painted a portrait of an 8- to 9-year-old girl ("fillette en bleu") with purple–red cheeks, thickened fingers with rough skin and pure red knuckles, reminiscent of features of juvenile DM [1]. Could Modigliani have depicted signs of disease on his little sitter?

Dermatomyositis, as with most diseases in children, is other than in adults and is manifested differently in each patient. There is variation in the onset, symptoms, physical findings, laboratory data, associated problems, response to therapy, and prognosis [2]. Despite these variations, the similarity of findings is significant enough to establish a real entity [3]. Juvenile DM represents approximately 5% of annual visits to pediatric rheumatology reference centers [4].

The diagnosis of juvenile DM is based at least in part upon the original Bohan and Peter criteria. Both childhood and adult forms of DM adhere to the same diagnostic criteria, but juvenile DM has unique features of vasculitis and calcinosis [5]. A clinicopathological, as well a serological, classification of juvenile IIMs was suggested in line with the classification for adult myositis [6]. Changes in the nature of these criteria have been based on clinical practice observations and advances in investigations [7] (Table 20.1). This reflects a growing trend not to use EMG and/or biopsies to establish the diagnosis, particularly in childhood, especially where the classical rash is present with obvious proximal muscle weakness and muscle enzyme elevation [7]. Magnetic resonance imaging or high-frequency ultrasound of affected muscles have increasingly been used to support diagnosis and monitor disease progression [8]. According to the published criteria, the majority of cases would have to be classified as possible or probable juvenile DM, when in practice there is no doubt about the diagnosis [7]. Suggested modifications to the criteria include the use of such imaging, and newly described MSAs.

DM in children usually starts before the age of 10 years with a severe, persistent, "sunburn" eruption, often initiated after an outdoor exposure, and mild nonspecific constitutional symptoms (tiredness, crankiness, fever). The disease has a bimodal age distribution with peaks at 5 and 9 and 10–14 years of age [9].

The most common onset age of juvenile DM is 6 years for boys and for girls there are two peaks at 6 and 10 years. The overall average age of disease onset is 7 years [4]. The

L.A. Dourmishev and A.L. Dourmishev, *Dermatomyositis: Advances in Recognition, Understanding and Management,*

20

Table 20.1 Criteria for diagnosis of juvenile DM [7]

1. Typical skin rash
– Heliotrope eyelid rash
– Gottron's papules/sign
2. Symmetrical proximal muscle weakness
3. Elevation of serum skeletal muscle enzymes
4. Specific EMG changes
5. Specific muscle biopsy abnormalities
6. MSAs (antisynthetase, Mi2, SRP)
7. MRI or ultrasound evidence of active myositis/fasciitis

Definite JDM: criterion 1. plus at least three of the other six criteria (2–7)
Probable JDM: criterion 1. plus two of the other six criteria (2–7)

clinical presentation in children is more frequently insidious, and may be dominated by constitutional symptoms of fatigue, malaise, fever, anorexia, and weight loss. Low-grade fever and general malaise are the initial and most common symptoms occurring in the majority of children with DM [10–12]. There is often a tiredness, lethargy, and a change in attitude to being difficult with frequent emotional outbursts [3]. The parents often misinterpret these findings, and consider them as a normal phase of childhood that will pass.

The onset of juvenile DM can be more insidious, and initial cutaneous signs are often nonspecific, causing delays in diagnosis. Some children develop quite marked cutaneous findings, while in others they are insignificant. Children may manifest all of the features of classic DM in adults. The cutaneous findings are characteristic in both their distribution and morphology. It involves the face in a sunburn configuration, with the added sign of eyelid involvement; but also involved are pressure points of the elbows, knees, and buttocks over the ischeal tuberosity. The morphology of the skin lesions is distinctive. They have a bluish red color (known as heliotrope) which is accentuated in the face and especially in the upper eyelids. In some patients it may be more extensive and even desquamative, and in others a photosensitive distribution may be seen, with widespread facial and shoulder involvement. The eyelids may also show some edema. The blood vessels in the lids of white children can be easy observed through the thin skin. The bulbar conjunctiva show areas with dilated vessels and areas that look white and avascular [13].

The classical pattern of skin involvement in juvenile DM is the erythematous, often scaling papular rash on the tops of the knuckles (Gottron's papules) over the hands, but this is seen only rarely on the toes [3]. They present as elevated area of skin a few millimeters in diameter over the knuckle of the fingers. Usually several papules are grouped over the joints and form small plaques (similar to psoriasis). Lister et al. [14] reported two Vietnamese children (boy and girl, respectively 7 and 8 years old) with DM, in whom the initial manifestations were follicular, papular, and pustular lesions on the extensor surface of elbows and knees clinically different from typical Gottron's papules. The authors suggest that the Oriental patients were predisposed to this type of eruption. Histology of a specimen showed a dilated follicular infundibulum plugged with keratin and a surrounding inflammatory cell infiltrate. A less common, but more troublesome finding is white patches (Gottron's sign) anywhere from a few millimeters to several centimeters in size [3]. They are somewhat vitiliginous in appearance but seem more atrophic, and are areas of compromised perfusion leading to difficult-healing ulcerations [3, 4]. In one study of 35 patients with juvenile DM, cutaneous ulcers were found in four patients (11.42%) (including one of the two fatal cases); calcinosis was present in five (14.28%) and systemic involvement in nine patients (27.71%) [4]. All cases presented alterations in the serum levels of muscle enzymes. In another retrospective study it was concluded that the most common initial physical examination findings were an extremity rash (94%) and periungual erythema (75%) [15].

Another common finding is noted in the proximal nailfolds of the fingers [16, 17]. Periungual skin changes are typical, and can be severe and scarring. Capillary microscopy identifies vessel changes, thromboses, and hemorrhage, and correlation of morphologic nailfold capillary bed vasculature with clinical course [17]. The skin in these areas appears atrophic, and dilated vessels can be seen separated by areas of avascularity. Cutaneous involvement in juvenile DM often begins with an extremity rash and persistent periungual erythema and nailfold telangiectasias [15].

Some patients present with marked edema of the subcutaneous tissues, which is often prominent with periorbital distribution [18], but may be widespread [19, 20] and severe (anasarca) [21]. If it is severe, it is usually associated with a more resistant disease [19, 21].

Vasculopathic lesions are more common in juvenile DM, and portend a more severe course with a poorer functional outcome [22, 23]. These lesions are associated with vascular occlusion [24], resulting in cutaneous necrosis with ulceration and calcinosis at the site of inflammation. Cutaneous ulcers have been mentioned as occurring in 6% to 30% of cases in various studies [4, 15, 25, 26]. Additionally, children have more often a multisystem vasculitis, which may involve the skin, gastrointestinal mucosa, heart, and retina. In the most severe forms of the skin disease in juvenile DM, large areas of infarction and skin ulceration occur [3, 4]. The infarction leads to necrosis formation. The ulcered areas develop crusting. True skin ulceration is a feature in up to 25% of pediatric cases, and may be relatively minor in some (e.g., periorbitally, near the inner canthus or behind the ear), or severe, full-thickness ulcers on the limbs or trunk, associated with life-threatening disease in others [7].

Some authorities have subdivided childhood DM into the Brunsting-Perry and Banker variants [27]. Approximately one half of the patients have the Banker type, characterized by rapid onset and progressive muscular weakness, fever, anorexia, and clinical and histologic widespread vasculitis in striated muscles and in the gastrointestinal tract, in addition to classic cutaneous and muscle abnormalities [5]. The rest of children with juvenile DM have the Brunsting-Perry type, characterized by protracted course, more subacute presentation with gradual progression of muscle weakness and subsequent calcinosis, which hardly responds to systemic administrated corticosteroids [27].

Rider et al. [28] and European Working Group for juvenile DM have suggested a proposed subclassification of childhood DM [7] (Table 20.2).

Table 20.2 Clinical variants of juvenile DM

Variant	Features
I. Classic JDM	Presents with typical rash and proximal muscle weakness and few associated other clinical features. It is responsive to steroids and disease-modifying NSAIDs.
II. Vasculopathic/ulcerative JDM	Associates with severe and widespread skin vascular changes, often with severe periungual capillary alterations and livedo reticularis. The patients are at high risk of early skin and gastrointestinal ulcers, and calcinosis. Muscle and skin biopsies reveal evidence of major abnormalities of the microvasculature. It is relatively resistant to standard therapies.
III. Overlap JDM	Presents with typical rash and muscle weakness; early prominent polyarthritis and features of "dry synovitis." Facial scleroderma-type skin changes and distal extremities may occur.
IV. JDM sine myositis	Refers to a group of patients with classic skin changes but no clinical evidence of muscle involvement; laboratory mild muscle enzyme elevation may be seen.

Recently, gingival telangiectases in five patients of juvenile DM have been reported [29] and are proposed as an important diagnostic marker of disease. The development of telangiectatic blood vessels scattered over the trunk had been described also in late stages of juvenile DM [3].

A new uncovered association of juvenile DM included pruritus in about 38% of patients and scalp scaly dermatosis in 25% of reported cases [15]. Peculiarities of juvenile DM are the frequent association with cutaneous and muscle calcinosis in 30%–70% of patients, resulting in flexural contractures [30]. Cutaneous calcinosis is frequently located on the elbows, knees and other acral parts, and can cause significant disability with severe pain, joint contracture, skin ulcers and muscle atrophy [31, 32]. Calcium deposit in the deeper tissues presents as hard, large size subcutaneous plaques [33, 34]. The calcification in juvenile DM is thought to develop through a dystrophic mechanism.

Lipodystrophy is also more commonly seen in juvenile DM [35, 36], with loss of subcutaneous fat over the masseter and on the upper and lower extremities, allowing clear definition of muscle groups [37]. In one series of 20 patients with juvenile DM, it was indicated that 25% of them had evidence of lipodystrophy, whereas 50% showed hypertriglyceridemia and insulin resistance [35]. Because the diagnosis of lipodystrophy in all studies has been based on a subjective clinical evaluation, it is possible that the prevalence rates in juvenile DM might be higher [26, 38]. Lipodystrophy can be associated with hirsutism, acanthosis nigricans, insulin-dependent diabetes mellitus, and hypertriglyceridemia [35]. Partial profound lipodystrophy/atrophy has been seen in some patients [38–40], sometimes with an associated insulin-resistant type of diabetes mellitus [35].

The vasculopathy, calcinosis, and lipodystrophy seen in juvenile DM are more prevalent in children carrying the TNF-α-308A allele [41].

Uncommon skin manifestations in juvenile DM include panniculitis [29, 42], partial lipoatrophy [39, 40], generalized [43, 44] or localized hypertrichosis [45], angiokeratomas [46], chondrodermatitis nodularis helices [47], and others.

Only three case reports of panniculitis in juvenile DM have been published [29, 39, 42]. A 3-year-old girl developed clinical paniculitis concurrently with her DM [42], while a 10-year-old boy [39] and a 14-year-old girl [29] have presented with symptoms of panniculitis 1 and 4 years respectively after the initiation of the juvenile DM.

Hypertrichosis in DM patients is described as the excessive growth of thick vellus hairs on any part of body without signs of virilization [43]. Generalized hypertrichosis has been rarely reported as a cutaneous manifestation of juvenile DM [43, 44]. Turner [48] reported the first case of localized acquired hypertrichosis in a 9-year-old girl with juvenile DM who had an abundance of thick pigmented hair on the forearms. In 1948 Reich and Reinchard [49] described a 9-year-old boy with thick black hairs on the forehead, femoral regions, elbows, and infrapatellar areas. Piantanila et al. [50] reported a 5-year-old African-American girl with classic clinical signs of juvenile DM and infrapatellar hypertrichosis.

There are few reports in the literature on the adverse cutaneous reaction of drugs used for treatment of juvenile DM. Narbut et al. [51] reported an 11-year-old boy who had a 2-year history of juvenile DM, and who after 9 months therapy with methotrexate 7.5 mg weekly, and enalapril 5 mg daily developed pemphigus foliaceus. Bloom et al. [52] reported case in which the hydroxychloroquine therapy aggravated the rash of juvenile DM.

Muscle disease usually manifests itself as a combination of muscle pain and weakness [7]. Usually the weakness manifests as difficulty in arising from a chair, climbing up stairs, reaching for objects, riding a bicycle, etc. Gower's sign is seen in juvenile DM and reflects truncal weakness [3, 53]. Sometime muscle weakness may have sudden onset and could be severe. A number of younger children do not complain of pain but might be miserable. At the time of DM onset, muscle involvement in children is generally mild. The muscles are usually tender, especially early in the course, and may be indurated or edematous (or the overlying subcutaneous tissue may become edematous). The proximal muscle groups, namely the shoulder, hip, and neck muscle, are more noticeably involved. The more distal muscles are also involved, but their affection is usually not recognized. With progression or severity, difficulty walking and getting out of bed, and exertion-induced dyspnea or dyspnea at rest may be noticeable due to respiratory muscle weakness [7]. The strength of muscles could be graded according to their ability to act against pressure and resistance offered by an examiner, as proposed by the well-known MRC grading system [54]. However, such a system has the disadvantage of being rather subjective, depending on the examiner's impression. Clinical muscle strength improvement in juvenile DM usually lags behind decreasing CK values [11]. Muscle involvement causes weakness but later leads to contractures [3]. Perifascicular atrophy has been observed as early as 1 month from

20

the onset of symptoms, and has persisted for at least 64 months of the active disease. The inflammatory infiltration seems to be more evident in the first 6 months of the disease. After 1 year, even if untreated, there is apparently a decrease in the inflammatory alterations [4].

Noncutaneous manifestations of juvenile DM include arthritis and lung and intestinal involvement, as observed in adults. Symmetric arthritis of both large and small joints is common, with joint contractures developing secondary to persistent inflammation and lack of physical therapy [9]. Joint contractures of the knees, elbows, wrists, and ankles are a common complication of juvenile DM, and can be seen early in the disease course, mainly in cases with prolonged immobility. In part, the contractures are caused by musculo-tendinous structure scarring; however, in some cases the joint disorder is due to associated inflammatory arthritis [12, 55].

Lungs are affected in juvenile DM, primarily or through complications of muscle weakness. Clinically apparent ILD is rare in juvenile DM, but is usually associated with significant morbidity and mortality [56, 57]. It usually presents insidiously with gradual onset of dyspnea and cough, whilst other aspects of disease may appear relatively stable [7]. Recurrent apparent chest infections or possible aspiration pneumonia could be diagnosed initially but fail to clear with appropriate therapy. In a study of 35 juvenile DM patients, aspirative pneumonia was found in two and ILD in three patients [4]. Much more common is respiratory muscle weakness, which may appear infrequently, as many of the patients have become rather immobile, and is only obvious with attempted physical activity [7]. Elevated respiratory rate (especially when resting in bed or at night) and accessory muscle use are seen in some patients. The pathological mechanisms of ILD remain unknown. There is evidence that both cell-mediated and humoral immunity play a role in the pathogenesis of this lesions. More recently, the role of the anti-Jo-I antibody has been highlighted in association with pulmonary interstitial disease [58, 59]. However, in the study by Sallum et al., the anti-Jo-I antibody was negative in all 35 patients with juvenile DM, even in those patients with interstitial disease [4], which corroborates previous reports describing the rarity of its presence in childhood.

Abnormal esophageal motor function is a complication of the disease, and esophageal symptoms such as esophageal reflux, dysphagia, and upper digestive tract bleeding are frequently present [4]. Abnormal esophageal motor function is a complication of the disease, and esophageal symptoms are seen in 6–41% of patients [15, 25].

Juvenile DM associates with motor dysfunction of the entire gastrointestinal tract. Gastrointestinal subclinical or mild involvement is probably quite common, as measured by occult or visible blood in the feces and/or episodes of abdominal pain and dysmotility [7]. Rare but often life-threatening gastrointestinal complications of juvenile DM include bleeding, ulceration and perforation, and associated peritonitis or mediastinitis [11, 60, 61]. Small- and large-bowel involvement has also been reported in literature [62]. Thromboses of the bowel blood vessels are part of the pathology of gastrointestinal ulcerations in juvenile DM [60, 63]. Large-bowel infarction secondary to vasculopathy has occurred in juvenile patients with myositis. Apparent colitis or subacute bowel obstruction and other disorders are reported [62] as a forerunner of actual perforation. Increased gastrointestinal involvement in children often manifests as decreased absorption of nutrients, perforation, and pneumatosis interstitialis [64].

Pancreatitis is relatively rare in children. There have only been four reports of pancreatitis in juvenile DM [65–68]. Baar and Wolff [65] reported a 2-year-old boy with juvenile DM who developed abdominal pain and who subsequently died. The postmortem showed necrosis of the pancreas and peripancreatic fatty tissue. Petrou et al. [66] published a case of a 11-year-old girl with juvenile DM with recurrent pancreatitis, and Heckmatt et al. [67] reported two out of 14 children with juvenile DM entering a trial of cyclosporin A who had previously developed pancreatitis. See et al. [68] reported two boys with juvenile DM complicated by pancreatitis. One of them had hepatitis and mild bowel vasculitis, while the other developed a catastrophic bowel vasculitis with multiple perforations.

There are few reports in the literature on cardiac involvement in juvenile DM. A few patients had cardiac murmurs or pericardial friction rubs and a high proportion showed ECG changes [69]. Electrocardiogarphic abnormalities are seen in half of cases, manifesting as asymptomatic conduction abnormalities or right bundle branch block, and subclinical, decreased ventilatory capacity is evident in the majority of patients [9, 70]. In one study, three of 35 patients (8.5%) with juvenile DM presented tachicardia with hyperkinetic circulatory state by ECG [4].

Clinically apparent involvement of the kidney is rare in juvenile DM. Despite the glomerulonephropathy and low-grade proteinuria seen in some patients, the major impairment of renal function is uncommon [71]. Central nervous system involvement has been reported in a few cases, with seizures or organic brain disorder, reflecting the underlying vasculopathy prominent in this disorder [72].

The association of DM/PM with malignancy in children is rare [73, 74] (see Chapter 18). The scattered reports of malignancies in children with juvenile DM include lymphoid tumors [75], neuroblastoma [76], nasopharyngeal carcinoma [77], three cases of lymphoproliferative disorders [73], acute lymphoblastic leukemia, and hepatocarcinoma [74].

Juvenile DM is a condition in which the predisposition to calcinosis and permanent disabling due to limb contractures are the most severe complications [7].

The routine laboratory findings in juvenile DM such as the elevations of ESR, LDH, and ASAT are indistinguishable of those in classic DM [15].

Although the clinical manifestations resemble those of the adult form of DM, juvenile DM has been considered to be a distinct clinical entity because of several reasons [78–83]:

(i) Pathological examination usually reveal that selective atrophy and/or necrosis of perifascicular fibers is much more common in juvenile DM than in adult DM or PM patients.

(ii) The results of tests for ANA are positive in about 60% of patients with juvenile DM, but MSAs are much less frequently found in children (10%) than in adult patients [12]. It is noteworthy that the juvenile patients with positive MSA share similar clinical characteristics with adult patients with identical autoantibody profiles [6].

(iii) About 50% of children with juvenile DM have circulating evidences of endothelial cell damage (increased von Willebrand factor Ag), whereas others have different indicators of disease activity, such as elevated neopterin [12, 52] or increased circulating B cells with peripheral lymphopenia [12].

(iv) In peripheral blood of juvenile DM patients, there is simultaneous increase of B cells and decrease of CD8 + T cells during the acute phase of disease [84–87], strongly suggesting autoimmune mechanism involvement in the pathogenesis of this childhood illness. However, the cause of the immune abnormality has not been clarified yet.

Predictive parameters to guide the correct therapeutical approach, and for prognosis, are still lacking in juvenile DM. Most studies do not recommend routine clinical testing for anti-Mi-2, since the yield is likely to be low. Moreover, it seems not to be a prognostic factor of the disease activity [58].

The prognosis for a normal life span is favorable. Once remission is achieved, children appear to return to normal muscle strength and function more frequently than adults with DM [4]. Children with juvenile DM experience decreased mortality and improved outcome in comparison to the patients with "classic" DM in adults [25].

References

1. Bitsori M, Galanakis E. Modigliani's "fillette en bleu": a case of juvenile dermatomyositis? *Int J Dermatol* 2003; 42: 327–329.
2. Spencer CH, Hanson V, Singsen BH, et al. Course of treated juvenile dermatomyositis. *J Pediatr* 1986; 105: 339–408.
3. Norins AL. Juvenile dermatomyositis. *Med Clin North Am* 1989; 73: 1193–1209.
4. Sallum AM, Kiss MH, Sachetti S, et al. Juvenile dermatomyositis: clinical, laboratorial, histological, therapeutical and evolutive parameters of 35 patients. *Arq Neuro-Psiquiatr São Paulo* 2002; 60(4): 1–14.
5. Miller OF, Newman ED. Dermatomyositis and Polymyositis. In: *Cutaneous Medicine and Surgery*, Arndt KA, Leboit PC, Robinson JK, et al. (eds), W.B. Saunders, Philadelphia, 1996; 283–290.
6. Rider LG, Miller FW, Targoff IN, et al. A broadened spectrum of juvenile myositis. Myositis-specific autoantibodies in children. *Arthritis Rheum* 1994; 37: 1534–1538.
7. Murray KJ. Juvenile dermatomyositis: advances in understanding and management. *APLAR J Rheumatol* 2003; 6: 50–63.
8. Medsger TA Jr, Oddis CV. Classification and diagnostic criteria for polymyositis and dermatomyositis. *J Rheumatol* 1995; 22: 581–585.
9. Kovacs SO, Kovacs SC. Dermatomyositis. *J Am Acad Dermatol* 1998; 39: 899–920.
10. Sullivan DB, Cassidy JT, Petty RE, et al. Prognosis in childhood dermatomyositis. *J Pediatr* 1972; 80: 555–563.
11. Sullivan DB, Cassidy JT, Petty RE, et al. Dermatomyositis in the pediatric patient. *Arthritis Rheum* 1977; 20: 327–331.
12. Pachman LM. Juvenile dermatomyositis. *Pediatr Clin North Am* 1995; 42: 1071–1098.
13. Van Nouhuys CE, Sengers RC. Bilateral avascular zones of the conjunctiva in a patient with juvenile dermatomyositis. *Am J Ophtalmol* 1987; 104: 440–442.
14. Lister RK, Cooper ES, Paige DG. Papules and pustules of the elbows and knees: An uncommon clinical sign of dermatomyositis in Oriental children. *Pediatr Dermatol* 2000; 17: 37–40.
15. Peloro TM, Miller OF III, Hahn TF, et al. Juvenile dermatomyositis: a retrospective review of a 30-year experience. *J Am Acad Dermatol* 2001; 45: 28–34.

16. Spencer-Green G, Crowe WE, Levinson JE. Nailfold capillary abnormalities and clinical dermatomyositis. *Arthritis Rheum* 1982; 25: 954–958.
17. Silver RM, Maricq HR. Childhood dermatomyositis: serial microvascular studies. *Pediatrics* 1989; 83: 278–283.
18. Sevigny GM, Mathes BM. Periorbital edema as the presenting sign of juvenile dermatomyositis. *PediatrDermatol* 1999; 16: 43–45.
19. Maillard SM, Cleary G, Davidson JE, et al. Widespread oedema as a presenting feature of severe juvenile dermatomyositis. *Ann Rheum Dis* 2002; 61: S144.
20. Karabiber H, Aslan M, Alkan A, et al. A rare complication of generalized edema in juvenile dermatomyositis: a report of one case. *Brain Dev* 2004; 26: 269–272.
21. Mitchell JP, Dennis GJ, Rider LG. Juvenile dermatomyositis presenting with anasarca: a possible indicator of severe disease activity. *J Pediatr* 2001; 138: 942–945.
22. Bowyer SL, Clark RA, Ragsdale CG, et al. Juvenile dermatomyositis: histological findings and pathogenic hypothesis for the associated skin changes. *J Rheumatol* 1986; 13: 753–758.
23. Fisler RE, Liang MG, Fuhlbrigge RC, et al. Aggressive management of juvenile dermatomyositis results in improved outcome and decreased incidence of calcinosis. *J Am Acad Dermatol* 2002; 47(4): 505–511.
24. Lutz J, Huwiler KG, Fedczyna T, et al. Increased plasma thrombospondin-1 (TSP-1) levels are associated with the TNF alpha-308A allele in children with juvenile dermatomyositis. *Clin Immunol* 2002; 103: 260–263.
25. Ramanan AV, Feldman BM. Clinical outcomes in juvenile dermatomyositis. *Curr Opin Rheumatol* 2002; 14: 658–662.
26. Singh S, Bansal A. Twelve years experience of juvenile dermatomyositis in North India. *Rheumatol Int* 2006; 26(6): 510–515.
27. Ackerman AB. Dermatomyositis. In: *Diagnosis of Inflammatory Skin Diseases. An Algorithmic Method Based on Pattern Analysis*. Williams & Wilkins, Baltimore, MD, 1997; 289–293.
28. Rider LG, Miller FW. Idiopathic inflammatory muscle disease: clinical aspects. *Baillieres Best Pract Res Clin Rheumatol* 2000; 14(1): 37–54.
29. Ghali FE, Stein LD, Fine JD, et al. Gingival telangiectases: an underappreciated physical sign of juvenile dermatomyositis. *Arch Dermatol* 1999; 135: 1370–1374.
30. Wananukul S, Pongprasit P, Wattanakrai P. Calcinosis cutis presenting years before other clinical manifestations of juvenile dermatomyositis: report of two cases. *Australas J Dermatol* 1997; 38: 202–205.
31. Halbert AR. Juvenile dermatomyositis. *Australas J Dermatol* 1996; 37: 106–108.
32. Eddy MC, Leelawattana R, McAlister WH, et al. Calcinosis universalis complicating juvenile dermatomyositis: resolution during probenecid therapy. *J Clin Endocrinol Metabol* 1997; 82: 3536–3542.
33. Blane CE, White SJ, Braunstein EM, et al. Patterns of calcification in childhood dermatomyositis. *AJR Am J Roentgenol* 1984; 142: 397–400.
34. Ichiki Y, Akiyama T, Shimozawa N, et al. An extremely severe case of cutaneous calcinosis with juvenile dermatomyositis, and successful treatment with diltiazem. *Br J Dermatol* 2001; 144: 894–897.
35. Huemer C, Kitson H, Malleson PN, et al. Lipodystrophy in patients with juvenile dermatomyositis: evaluation of clinical and metabolic abnormalities. *J Rheumatol* 2001; 28: 610–615.
36. Rider L, Ruiz-Hidalgo M, Labora J, et al. Lipodystrophy in juvenile dermatomyositis is associated with calcinosis, but not with hepatocyte differentiation factor DLK levels [abstract]. *Arthritis Rheum* 2001; 44: S264.

37. Santmyire-Rosenberger B, Dugan EM. Skin involvement in dermatomyositis. *Curr Opin Rheumatol* 2003; 15(6): 714–722.
38. Quecedo E, Febrer I, Serrano G, et al. Partial lipodystrophy associated with juvenile dermatomyositis: report of two cases. *Pediatr Dermatol* 1996; 13: 477–482.
39. Commens C, O'Neill P, Walker G. Dermatomyositis associated with multifocal lipoatrophy. *J Am Acad Dermatol* 1990; 22: 966–969.
40. Kavanagh GM, Colaco CB, Kennedy CT. Juvenile dermatomyositis associated with partial lipoatrophy. *J Am Acad Dermatol* 1993; 28: 348–351.
41. Pachman LM. Juvenile dermatomyositis: immunogenetics, pathophysiology, and disease expression. *Rheum Dis Clin North Am* 2002; 28: 579–602.
42. Naidenbach PJ, Sahn EE, Helton J. Panniculitis in juvenile dermatomyositis. *J Am Acad Dermatol* 1995; 33: 305–307.
43. Pope DN, Strimling RB, Mallory SB. Hypertrichosis in juvenile dermatomyositis. *J Am Acad Dermatol* 1994; 31: 383–387.
44. Faure Fontanela MA. Severe hypertrichosis as an uncommon feature of juvenile dermatomyositis. *J Am Acad Dermatol* 1995; 33: 691.
45. Piantanida NA, Person DA, Piantanida EW. Infrapatellar hypertrichosis: An unusual cutaneous manifestation of juvenile dermatomyositis. *Pediatr Dermatol* 2002; 19: 135–137.
46. Shannon PL, Ford MJ. Angiokeratomas in juvenile dermatomyositis. *Pediatr Dermatol* 1999; 16: 448–452.
47. Sasaki T, Nishizawa H, Sugita Y. Chondrodermatitis nodularis helices in childhood dermatomyositis. *Br J Dermatol* 1999; 141: 363–365.
48. Turner JC. Dermatomyositis: a study of 3 cases. *N Engl J Med* 1937; 216: 158–161.
49. Reich NE, Reinchard JB. Dermatomyositis associated with hypertrichosis. *Arch Dermatol Syphilol* 1948; 57: 725–732.
50. Piantanida NA, Person DA, Piantanida EW. Infrapatellar hypertrichosis: an unusual cutaneous manifestation of juvenile dermatomyositis. *Pediatr Dermatol* 2002; 19(2): 132–135.
51. Narbutt J, Torzecka JD, Sysa-Jedrzejowska A, et al. Pemphigus foliaceus in an 11-year-old boy with dermatomyositis: simple coincidence or familial immunological background? *Br J Dermatol* 2003; 148(4): 838–839.
52. Bloom BJ, Tucker LB, Klein-Gitelman M, et al. Worsening of the rash of juvenile dermatomyositis with hydroxychloroquine thearpy. *J Rheumatol* 1994; 21: 2171–2172.
53. Jacobs JC. *Pediatric Rheumatology for the Practioners*. Spinger-Verlag, New York, 1993; 6.
54. Miller LC, Michael AF, Baxter TL. Quantitative muscle testing in childhood dermatomyositis. *Arch Phys Med Rehabil* 1988; 69: 610–613.
55. Tse S, Lubelsky S, Gordon M, et al. The arthritis of inflammatory childhood myositis syndromes. *J Rheumatol* 2001; 2: 192–197.
56. Trapani S, Camiciottoli G, Vierucci A, et al. Pulmonary involvement in juvenile dermatomyositis: a two-year longitudinal study. *Rheumatology* 2001; 40: 216–220.
57. Al-Mayouf SM, Al-Eid W, Bahabri S, et al. Interstitial pneumonitis and air leakage in juvenile dermatomyositis. *Rheumatology* 2001; 40: 588–590.
58. Feldman BM, Reichlin M, Laxer RM, et al. Clinical significance of specific autoantibodies in juvenile dermatomyositis. *J Rheumatol* 1996; 23: 1794–1797.
59. Marie I, Hatron PY, Hachulla E, et al. Pulmonary involvement in polymyositis and in dermatomyositis. *J Rheumatol* 1998; 25: 1336–1343.
60. Michailov G, Vlasov V. Upon visceral changes in dermatomyositis: case report. *Savr Med* 1974; 12: 47–50 [Bulgarian].
61. Magil HL, Hixon SD, Whitington G, et al. Duodenal perforation in childhood dermatomyositis. *Pediatr Radiol* 1984; 14: 28–30.

62. Laskin BL, Choyke P, Keenan GF, et al. Novel gastrointestinal tract manifestations in juvenile dermatomyositis. *J Pediatr* 1999; 135: 371–374.
63. Banker BQ, Victor M. Dermatomyositis (systemic angiopathy) of childhood. *Medicine* 1966; 45: 261–289.
64. Braunstein EM, White SJ. Pneumatosis intestinalis in dermatomyositis. *Br J Radiol* 1980; 53: 1011–1012.
65. Barr HS, Wolff OH. Pancreatic necrosis in cortisone treated children. *Lancet* 1957; 272 (6973): 812–815.
66. Petrou P, Balagh Z, Rosdy B, et al. Recurrent pancreatitis in Juvenile Dermatomyositis. *Orv Hetil* 1989; 180: 1937–1939.
67. Heckmatt J, Saunders C, Peters AM, et al. Cyclosporin in juvenile dermatomyositis. *Lancet* 1989; 13: 1063–1066.
68. See Y, Martin K, Roony M, et al. Severe juvenile dermatomyositis complicated by pancreatitis. *Br J Rheumatol* 1997; 36: 912–916.
69. Dubowitz V. Inflammatory myopathies. In: *Muscle Disorders in Childhood*, Dubowitz V (ed.), 2nd ed. W.B. Saunders, Philadelphia, 1995; 422–456.
70. Pachman LM. Polymyositis and dermatomyositis in children. In: *Oxford Texbook of Rheumatology*, Maddison PJ, Isenberg DA, Woo P, et al. (eds), Oxford University Press, Oxford, 1993; 821–828.
71. Picco P, Gattorno M, Barbano GC, et al. Mesangial glomerulonephritis and transient SLE manifestations in an adolescent with dermatomyositis. *Lupus* 1997; 6: 72–73.
72. Ramanan AV, Sawhney S, Murray KJ. Central nervous system complications in two cases of juvenile onset dermatomyositis. *Rheumatology* 2001; 40: 1293–1298.
73. Falcini F, Taccetti G, Trapani S, et al. Acute lymphoblastic leukemia associated with dermatomyositis in a child. *Pediatr Dermatol* 1993; 10: 199–200.
74. Leaute-Labreze C, Perel Y, Taieb A. Childhood dermatomyositis associated with hepatocarcinoma. *N Engl J Med* 1995; 333: 1083.
75. Taieb A, Guichard C, Salamon R, et al. Prognosis in juvenile dermato polymyositis: a cooperative retrospective study of 70 cases. *Pediatr Dermatol* 1985; 2: 275–281.
76. Kalmanti M, Athanasiou A. Neuroblastoma occurring in a child with dermatomyositis. *Am J Pediatr Hematol Oncol* 1985; 7: 387–388.
77. De Bersques J. Deux cas de dermatomyosite chez des adolescentes. *Nouv Dermatol* 1987; 6: 499.
78. Comola M, Johnson MA, Howel D, et al. Spatial distribution of muscle necrosis in biopsies from patients with inflammatory muscle disorders. *J Neurol Sci* 1987; 82: 229–244.
79. Iannone F, Cauli A, Yanni G, et al. T-lymphocyte immunophenotyping in polymyositis and dermatomyositis. *Br J Rheumatol* 1996; 35: 839–845.
80. Pachman LM. Juvenile dermatomyositis. *Pediatr Clin North Am* 1986; 33: 1097–1117.
81. Pachman LM. Juvenile dermatomyositis (JDM): new clues to diagnosis and pathogenesis. *Clin Exp Rheumatol* 1994; 12: 69–73.
82. Pachman LM, Hayford JR, Chung A, et al. Juvenile dermatomyositis at diagnosis: clinical characteristics of 79 children. *J Rheumatol* 1998; 25: 1198–1204.
83. Mizuno K, Yachie A, Nagaoki S, et al. Oligoclonal expansion of circulating and tissue-infiltrating CD8 + T cells with killer/effector phenotypes in juvenile dermatomyositis syndrome. *Clin Exp Immunol* 2004; 137: 187–194.
84. Mantegazza R, Bernasconi P. Cellular aspects of myositis. *Curr Opin Rheumatol* 1994; 6: 568–574.
85. Eisenstein DM, O'Gorman MR, Pachman LM. Correlations between change in disease activity and changes in peripheral blood lymphocyte subsets in patients with juvenile dermatomyositis. *J Rheumatol* 1997; 24: 1830–1832.

86. O'Gorman MR, Bianchi L, Zaas D, et al. Decreased levels of CD54 (ICAM-1) — positive lymphocytes in the peripheral blood in untreated patients with active juvenile dermatomyositis. *Clin Diagn Lab Immunol* 2000; 7: 693–697.
87. Kikuchi Y, Koarada S, Tada Y, et al. Difference in B cell activation between dermatomyositis and polymyositis: analysis of the expression of RP105 on peripheral blood B cells. *Ann Rheum Dis* 2001; 60: 1137–1140.

Amyopathic Dermatomyositis

21

In 1991 Euwer and Sontheimer [1] proposed a revision of Bohan and Peter's [2] original classification system of DM/PM, and included amyopathic DM as a sixth clinical type. Thereafter, the nomenclature of amyopathic DM is controversial. Some authors continue to use the historical term "DM sine myositis" [3, 4], others prefer the term "amyopathic DM" [5], a third group use the designations "premyopathic DM" [6] or "hypomyopathic DM" [5], but a few workers still prefer to use the terms "DM with normal muscle enzymes" [7, 8] or "DM without muscle weakness" [9, 10].

Amyopathic DM refers to a condition in which the typical cutaneous eruption of DM is present but muscle disease is lacking [1, 3, 5, 7]. This clinical variant of DM is the opposite of PM, in which muscle disease is present but cutaneous disease is lacking. The category of amyopathic DM is controversial, since according to the strict Bohan and Peter criteria patients with this presentation only fulfill one criterion and may have a suspected DM [11]. The clinical entity amyopathic DM includes patients with either cutaneous disease alone [7], or patients with cutaneous disease and minimal muscle involvement [12, 13]. However, the former definition lacks the criteria of Bohan and Peter for possible DM, and due to the low specificity of the skin lesions, it might be difficult to distinguish cases of amyopathic DM from those with other early connective tissue diseases such as lupus erythematosus [3, 14].

In 1975 when Bohan and Peter [1] published their five diagnostic criteria defining PM and DM, Krain [15] described the first six patients with "DM sine myositis," four of whom were adults, who presented with typical DM skin lesions and lack of muscle disease; later on, all of them developed overt myositis at an interval of between 3 months and 10.5 years. In Krain's series, one patient presented initially with cutaneous rash and weakness, which spontaneously remitted, and then presented again with only skin disease, but without muscle disease for 6 years. Another two patients who started with skin eruption and muscle weakness had normal muscle enzymes, demonstrated by EMG and a biopsy specimen. Muscle biopsy and EMG were performed, however, in only three patients with initial evolution of disease. Later on, Pearson [16] noted three cases of juvenile DM with "very mild muscular weakness and more prominent cutaneous features, but relatively stable course over a 6-month to 3-year period." Bohan et al. [17] reported that, in their series, at the initiation of DM the muscle strength was normal in

48 of 173 patients (31%); there were three patients (~2%) who failed to develop significant muscle weakness but met other diagnostic criteria (e.g., abnormal enzyme, EMG, or muscle biopsy), and one women with rash alone but without overt myositis who had cancer of the uterus. The term "amyopathic dermatomyositis" was introduced by Pearson in 1979 [12] for patients who had typical cutaneous findings of DM, but did not have any clinical or laboratory signs of muscle disease at least 2 years after the onset of the skin pathology. He reported five women with only cutaneous manifestations of DM, and six other patients (four women and two men) in whom the skin lesions were florid, whereas weakness and EMG changes were minimal [12]. Rockerbie et al. [9] described 28 of 50 patients (56%) who had DM with skin rash preceding muscle weakness, at intervals varying from 1 month to more than 4 years. Six patients (12%) only had cutaneous lesions more than 21 months before the onset of muscle weakness. Euwer and Sontheimer [1] described six patients who did not develop evidence of myositis for at least 2 years after the onset of cutaneous rash and defined cutaneous manifestation of amyopathic DM ("DM sine myositis"). However, EMG and muscle biopsy were not performed in any of these patients. Because five of these six cases were treated with moderate doses of prednisone and none of them developed overt myositis, Euwer and Sontheimer suggested that a "more aggressive approach to treating the skin disease may prevent the development of muscle disease in cases who initially have only cutaneous involvement." Euwer and Sontheimer [13] divided patients with amyopathic DM into three groups: (i) Type 1 represents pure amyopathic DM patients who have only cutaneous manifestations, (ii) Type 2 are patients with skin lesions who have subjective myalgias and weakness, but without laboratory evidence of muscle disease (as seen in Krain's series), and (iii) Type 3 are patients with eruptions, without features of muscle disease, but having evidence of abnormal laboratory tests at some time during their course. In 1993, Stonecipher et al. [7] reported 13 patients with typical DM rash and normal serum enzyme levels. The patients were separated into three groups: (i) four patients with only cutaneous changes without muscle involvement after 4–11 years follow-up (i.e., amyopathic DM), (ii) seven patients with cutaneous changes at baseline and subsequent development of myosits, and (iii) two patients with cutaneous changes and normal muscle enzymes in whom, however, the diagnostic evaluation showed subclinical evidence of muscle involvement demonstrated by EMG and/or muscle biopsy. This classification approach has been utilized by others [18]. Stonecipher et al. [7] have suggested the avoidance of therapy with systemic corticosteroids or other immunosuppressive drugs in patients with lack of overt muscle disease. In a retrospective study of 12 patients with typical DM rash but without reported weakness (i.e., with amyopathic DM) in France, Cosnes et al. [10] found eight cases with an increased enzyme levels, seven patients had myopathic finding on EMG and nine patients had abnormal muscle biopsy, of whom five had histopathologically confirmed myositis. After approximately 5 years follow-up, no patient developed overt muscle disease, and cutaneous manifestations improved in nine of all 12 patients [10]. Hydoxychloroquine sulfat was the first line therapeutic agent in all patients. None of the patients in this group received systemic corticosteroid treatment. Some clinically amyopathic DM patients have been observed to exhibit continuing skin disease activity for more than 20 years without ever developing clinically evident muscle weakness or other systemic features of DM [19].

As with classic DM in adults, amyopathic DM is more common in women [20]. In Sontheimer's 2004 study, 80% of patients with amyopathic DM were female, and the mean age was found to be 43 years [19]. The large majority of these patients experienced the onset of DM skin disease as adults. Amyopathic DM is more common in adults, but is observed also in children [18, 21–24]. In the USA and Europe, it has been estimated to occur with approximately 10–11% of the incidence of classic DM [5, 20], whereas in Asia it is more common and varies between 14% and 46% [25, 26]. Among children, in Pachman's study amyopathic DM occurs from 3% to 5% of patients [24] but in other studies the frequency is higher, up to 12% [27].

The cutaneous findings which are diagnostic for amyopathic DM include [1]:

(i) Violaceous discoloration of interfalangeal joints (Gottron's sign) and/or Gottrons' papules
(ii) Periungual erythema and/or telangiectasia
(iii) Violaceous discoloration of the face and upper trunk

Macular violaceous erythema overlying the extensor aspect of the upper extremities with or without Gottron's papules is present more frequently in both classic DM and amyopathic DM than periorbital heliotrope rush [1, 5, 18, 26, 27] (Table 21.1).

These cutaneous findings are diagnostic for amyopathic DM when the skin biopsy specimen is consistent with DM. Suggested diagnostic criteria for cutaneous manifestation of DM by Euwer and Sontheimer [1], were accepted by the American Academy of Dermatology [28]. Sontheimer [5] proposed a provisional minimal set of hallmark cutaneous manifestations of DM for the purpose of defining amyopathic DM. Most authors agree that there is no difference in skin findings in classic DM and amyopathic DM (Table 21.2). However, a recent study indicated that patients with amyopathic DM were more likely to have lesions in acral areas than on the face or trunk [18]. Cutaneous changes previously seen only in classic DM patients, and later on recognized in amyopathic DM, are: pruritic scaling scalp lesions associated with nonscarring alopecia in 25% of patients [27],

Table 21.1 Cutaneous manifestation of DM [1]

Pathognomonic	1. Gottron's papules 2. Gottron's sign – symmetric macular violaceous erythema with or without edema overlying the dorsal aspect of the unterfalangeal joints of the hands, olecranon processus, patellas, and medial malleoli
Characteristic	1. Periorbital violaceous eruthema with associated edema of eyelids and periorbital tissue (heliotrope) 2. Periungual telangiectasia with associated dystrophic cuticles 3. Macular violaceous erythema overlying the dorsal aspect of hands, extensor forearms and arms, deltoids, posterior shoulders, nape of neck, V-area of neck, upper chest, and forehead
Compatible	1. Poikiloderma atrophicans vasculare (poikilo-dermatomyositis) 2. Subepidermal bullous lesions and superficial erosions

Amyopathic dermatomyositis
One or two pathognomic signs in association with one or more characteristic signs and a compatible skin biopsy specimen (hematoxilin–eosin stain)

21

Table 21.2 Hallmark cutaneous manifestation of DM[a] [5]

Major cutaneous criteria	***Heliotrope rash***
	Gottron's papules
	Gottron's sign
Minor cutaneous criteria	***Macular violaceous erythema***
	Scalp or anterior hairline
	Malar eminences of face, or forehead, or chin
	V-area of neck or upper chest (open colar area, V-sign)
	Nape of the neck or posterior aspect of shoulders (shawl sign)
	Extensor surface of the arms or forearms
	Linear streaking overlying extensor tendons on the dorsal hands
	Periungual areas
	Lateral surface of the thighs or hips (holster sign)
	Medial malleoli (involvement of each above anatomical region qualifies as a single minor criterion)
	Periungual nailfold telangiectasia or cuticular hemorrhage-infarct with or without dystrophic cuticules
	Poikiloderma
	Mechanic's hand lesions
	Cutaneous calcinosis
	Cutaneous ulcers
	Pruritus

[a]The presence of two major criteria or one major and two minor criteria and biopsy on the skin lesion shows changes consistent with cutaneous DM

vesiculo-bullous lesions and oral ulcers [29], pathologic calcifications [22], or calcinosis universalis [30], mechanic's hands without arthritis, Raynaud's phenomenon, interstitial pneumonia, or MSAs [5]. Dystrophic calcification seems to be quite uncommon in both adult [18, 20] and juvenile-onset amyopathic DM [23]. The diagnosis of amyopathic DM is confirmed by clinical–pathological correlation. The pattern of the skin disease is relatively characteristic and when an interface dermatitis is demonstrated on skin biopsy the diagnosis may be relatively firm [31].

Clinical evidence of muscle weakness in amyopathic DM is controversial [10, 15, 21]. In one retrospective analysis of all 746 DM patients seen at the Mayo Clinic, 32 (4%) had had amyopathic DM; five of these had subjective muscle weakness without demonstrable muscle abnormalities [18]. Of 19 patients with amyopathic DM who were followed up, ten patients (67%) did not developed muscle weakness after 2–10 years, four patients (25%) had muscle affection within 1 year, two (11%) cases developed weakness within 5 years, and three patients showed evidence of muscle weakness 8–17 years after diagnosis amyopathic DM.

Fatigue and myalgia without evidence of muscle inflammation have been reported in a number of amyopathic DM patients [5]. The symptoms of fatigue, muscle pain, and muscle tenderness associated with fibromyalgia have also been observed [32].

Recently, a 50-year-old woman with typical cutaneous manifestations of DM and fasciitis has been reported [33]. The patient had no clinically evident muscle weakness, and the serum muscle enzymes were within the normal range. Magnetic resonance imaging (MRI) and muscle biopsy showed inflammation of the fascia and mild myopathic changes. The term "dermato-fasciitis" had been suggested. Steroid therapy was efficacious against the skin eruptions and fasciitis seen on T2-weighted MRI [33].

Arthritis has been observed in some cases of juvenile-onset amyopathic DM [34]. In one study of five cases with juvenile amyopathic DM for a period of 5 years, three patients (60%) were determined to have arthritis [34].

Although by definition amyopathic DM lacks muscle involvement, complications may arise from other forms of systemic involvement. Recently, several authors have reported amyopathic DM associated with ILD, and absence of other findings of an antisynthetase syndrome [18, 35]. Interstitial pneumonitis and pulmonary fibrosis that complicate amyopathic DM have been observed [36–39]. Since 1979, when the first DM patient without apparent myositis complicated by fibrosing alveolitis was published, [40] up to 2002 34 cases of amyopathic DM with symptomatic ILD had been reported [5]. Interstitial lung disease, a potentially fatal complication of classic DM, was reported to have occurred in only 4% of the 336 published cases of clinically amyopathic DM [19]. In a study at the Mayo Clinic, radiologic evidence of pulmonary fibrosis and the absence of clinical manifestation of lung disease was determined in five patients with amyopathic DM [18]. The prevalence of interstitial pneumonitis in amyiopathic DM has not yet been determined, but according to Sontheimer [5] it may approach between 5% and 10% of published cases. Higher incidence of amyopathic DM patients with ILD has been reported in Japan, probably because in this country interstitial pneumonitis is a common complication of classic DM in adults. In addition, the acute pattern of pulmonary disease presenting with rapidly progressive dyspnea, hypoxemia, therapeutic resistance, and fatal outcome has been observed in a high percentage of patients with amyopathic DM [5, 35, 36]. Amyopathic DM complicated by ILD and pneumomediastinum has also been reported [38]. Interstitial lung disease with autoantibody against aminoacyl-tRNA synthetase and absence of clinically apparent myositis [41], and autoantibody to 140-kD proteins in Japanese patients with adult-onset amyopathic DM having interstitial pneumonia, have been determined [42].

Dermatomyositis sine myositis may also present as a paraneoplastic syndrome [3, 18, 43–45]. Amyopathic DM, like its classical counterpart, also shows an association with malignancy. Some authors consider the risk of malignancy is the same as in classical DM in adults, while others suggest that the risk is lower. The occurrence of internal malignancy was reported in 12% of all 336 cases published by Sontheimer in 2004 [19]. Stonecipher et al. [7] were the first to report the possible association of malignancy in patients with amyopathic DM. In their series, two female patients of 13 reported cases were diagnosed to have adenocarcinoma of the breast [7]. Whitmor et al. [3] found three women and one man with associated malignancy among 12 patients with amyopathic DM. Two female

21

patients had papillary serous ovarian cancer; one was detected 8 months after the initial presentation of amyopathic DM. In another patient, the cancer was detected 31 months after the initial symptoms of amyopatic dermatomyositis. One female patient had two malignant diseases, an ovarian cancer and supraglottic squamous carcinoma, detected 26 and 16 months respectively arter cutaneous manifestation appearance. The male patient had squamous cell carcinoma, detected 24 months after the onset of cutaneous eruption [3]. Nasopharyngeal carcinoma is the most commonly associated malignancy in classic DM in adults, as well as in amyopathic DM patients of Chinese origin, particularly those from Southern China, as reported in cohorts from Singapore [25, 46], Hong Kong [47], Guangzhou in Southern China [48], and Taiwan [49] in which nasopharyngeal carcinoma comprises 40–80% of the associated malignancies. Although nasopharyngeal carcinoma is a relatively common malignancy seen in Chinese, it is disproportionately represented among the malignancies associated with DM, both classical and amyopathic forms [50]. Current knowledge supports the idea that adult patients with classic DM and amyopathic DM have an increased risk of harboring a malignancy, which increases with age.

Certain drugs can induce DM-like cutaneous eruptions indistinguishable from amyopathic DM (i.e., drug-induced amyopathic DM) [51]. Some authors, however, have considered that drugs do not participate in the initiation of DM [52, 53]. Dermatomyositis-like eruption is a rather stereotypical cutaneous adverse reaction to hydroxyurea, which appears on the dorsa of the interfalangeal and metacarpophalageal joints as Gottron's papules or Gottron's signs, associated with atrophic and telangiectatic changes, or poikilodermatous plaques and prominent nailfold telangiectasia [54–59]. Cutaneous eruption is clinically and histopathologically similar to specific skin lesions in idiopathic DM [59, 60]. This cutaneous syndrome usually occurs after 2–10 years discontinuous hydroxyurea therapy. In most patients, clinical manifestations improve following the discontinuation of hydtroxyurea treatment. According to Rocamora et al. [59], DM sine myositis is clinically indistinguishable from this drug reaction. Recently, Ruiz-Genao et al. [61] reported three patients on a 19-month chemotherapeutic treatment with hydroxyurea followed by cyclophosphamide and high doses of etoposide, who developed the hallmark cutaneous manifestations of DM. These lesions disappeared in all cases in a few days without any treatment after drug removal, and patients did not show relapse of the cutaneous lesions during the follow-up time.

Magnetic resonance imaging (MRI) and P-31 magnetic resonance spectroscopy (MRS) are methods of choice for diagnosing minimal muscle involvement in myositis patients, and in amyopathic DM [8, 62, 63]. Two studies have demonstrated that MRI and muscle biopsy went on to manifest muscular involvement in nine of 13 patients without muscle enzyme elevation for up to 11 years follow-up, and in three of five patients with normal findings of muscle enzyme levels and EMG [7, 8]. Functional metabolic changes in muscles have been indentified in some amyopathic DM patients [62]. Park and Olsen [62] have proposed dividing amyopathic DM into three subsets: (i) pure amyopathic DM — with skin disease only, (ii) skin disease with subjective myalgias, and (iii) skin disease with normal muscle strength but with some laboratory abnormalities.

ANA are positive in most of the published cases with amyopathic DM [5]. Positive ANA assays were reported in 79% of the 336 cases with amyopathic DM published in literature [19]. Patients with amyopathic DM do not seem to produce MSAs or MAAs. In a preliminary study, Targoff et al. identified the presence of a unique pair of new autoantibodies that react with a 155 kDa autoantigen and/or the Se autoantigen by immunoprecipitation/immunoblotting in 16 of 19 (84%) North American clinically amyopathic DM patients [64]. These autoantibodies, which are associated with RNA might serve as serologic markers of amyopathic DM [64, 65]. In five Japanese patients with adult-onset amyopathic DM and interstitial pneumonia, antibodies reactive with a 140-kD polypeptide have been reported [42]. More recently, the presence of an autoantibody to a 140 kDa autoantigen designated as the "US" autoantigen was reported in eight of 15 Japanese patients with amyopathic DM (53%) [66].

The debate about the possibility of juvenile-onset amyopathic DM patients developing clinically significant myositis is not resolved, since some authors report a relatively low risk [23] while other investigators have found a relatively high risk [22].

Those involved in the management of such patients with amyopathic DM should consider the following facts:

(i) Some or more of patients with amyopathic DM develop symptomatic myositis 2 years after disease onset.
(ii) Classic DM has a refractory nature and resistance to treatment.
(iii) Patients with amyopathic DM are potentially at risk for developing ILD (the risk is greater in some ethnic groups such as Japanese).
(iv) Individuals with amyopathic DM may have a statistically significant increased risk of internal malignancy.
(v) Children with amyopathic DM who are not aggressively treated frequently develop calcifications [22].
(vi) Topical therapy with broad-spectrum sunscreens, anti-inflammatories, and antipruritics is useful [5].
(vii) Some amyopathic DM could be induced by drugs [51].

References

1. Euwer RL, Sontheimer RD. Amyopathic dermatomyositis (dermatomyositis sine myositis). Presentation of six new cases and review of the literature. *J Am Acad Dermatol* 1991; 24: 959–966.
2. Bohan A, Peter JB. Polymyositis and dermatomyositis. *N Engl J Med* 1975; 292: 344–347.
3. Whitmore E, Watson R, Rosenshein NB, et al. Dermatomyositis sine myositis: association with malignancy. *J Rheumatol* 1996; 23: 101–106.
4. Olhoffer IH, Carrol C, Watsky K. Dermatomyositis sine myositis presenting with calcinosis universalis. *Br J Dermatol* 1999; 141: 365–366.
5. Sontheimer RD. Dermatomyositis: an overview of recent progress with emphasasis on dermatologic aspects. *Dermatol Clin* 2002; 20: 387–408.
6. Trautmann C, Badawy Abdel-Nasar MB, Soehnchen R, et al. Prämyopathische versus amyopathische Dermatomyositis. *Hautarzt* 1995; 46: 47–52.
7. Stonecipher MR, Jorizzo JL, White WL, et al. Cutaneous changes of dermatomyositis in patients with normal muscle enzyme concentrations: Dermatomyositis sine myositis? *J Am Acad Dermatol* 1993; 28: 951–956.

21

8. Stonecipher MR, Jorizzo JL, Monu J, et al. Dermatomyositis with normal muscle enzyme concentrations. A single-blind study of the diagnostic value of magnetic resonance imaging and ultrasound. *Arch Dermatol* 1994; 130: 1294–1299.
9. Rockerbie NR, Woo TY, Callen JP, et al. Cutaneous changes of dermatomyositis without muscle weakness. *J Am Acad Dermatol* 1989; 24: 959–966.
10. Cosnes A, Amaudric F, Gherardi R, et al. Dermatomyositis without muscle weakness. Long-term follow-up of 12 patients without systemic corticosteroids. *Arch Dermatol* 1995; 131: 1381–1385.
11. Kovacs SO, Kovacs SC. Dermatomyositis. *J Am Acad Dermatol* 1998; 39: 899–920.
12. Pearson CM. Polymyositis and dermatomyositis. In: *Arthritis (and Allied Conditions)*, Mc Carty DJ (ed.), 9th ed. Lea & Febiger, Philadelphia, 1979; 742.
13. Euwer RL Sontheimer RD. Amyopathic dermatomyositis: a review. *J Invest Dermatol* 1993; 100(Suppl): S124–127.
14. Smith CA, Pinals RS. Periorbital edema in systemic lupus erythematosus. *Arch Intern Med* 1982; 142: 1711–1712.
15. Krain LS. Dermatomyositis in six patients without initial muscle involvement. *Arch Dermatol* 1975; 111: 241–246.
16. Pearson CM. Patterns of polymyositis and their response to treatment. *Ann Intern Med* 1976; 59: 827–838.
17. Bohan A, Peter JB, Bowman RL, et al. A computer-assisted analysis of 153 patients with polymyositis and dermatomyositis. *Medicine* 1977; 56: 255–286.
18. el-Azhary R, Pakzad SY. Amyopathic dermatomyositis: retrospective review of 37 cases. *J Am Acad Dermatol* 2002; 46: 560–565.
19. Sontheimer RD. Skin manifestations of systemic autoimmune connective tissue disease: diagnostics and therapeutics. *Best Pract Res Clin Rheumatol* 2004; 18(3): 429–462.
20. Caproni M, Cardinali C, Parodi A, et al. Amyopathic dermatomyositis, a review by the Italian Group of Immunodermatology. *Arch Dermatol* 2002; 138: 23–27.
21. Schmid MH, Trüeb RM. Juvenile amyopathic dermatomyositis. *Br J Dermatol* 1997; 136: 431–433.
22. Eisenstein DM, Paller AS, Pachman LM. Juvenile dermatomyositis presenting with rash alone. *Pediatrics* 1997; 100: 391–392.
23. Plamondon S, Dent PB. Juvenile amyopathic dermatomyositis: results of a case finding descriptive survey. *J Rheumatol* 2000; 27: 2031–2034.
24. Pachman LM. Juvenile dermatomyositis: immunogenetics, pathophysiology, and disease expression. *Rheum Dis Clin North Am* 2002; 28: 579–602.
25. Ang P, Sugeng MW, Chau SH. Classic and amyopathic dermatomyositis seen at the National Skin Centere of Singapore: a 3-year retrospective review of their clinical characteristics and association with malignancy. *Ann Acad Med Singapore* 2000; 20: 219–223.
26. Chen YJ, Wu CY, Shen JL. Predicting factors of malignancy in dermatomyositis and polymyositis: a case control study. *Br J Dermatol* 2001; 144: 825–831.
27. Peloro TM, Miller OF, Hahn TF, et al. Juvenile dermatomyositis: a retrospective review of a 30-year experience. *J Am Acad Dermatol* 2001; 45: 28–34.
28. Drake L, Dinehart SM, Farmer ER, et al. Guidelines of care for dermatomyositis. *J Am Acad Dermatol* 1996; 34: 824–829.
29. Seno A, Tokuda M, Yamasaki H, et al. A case of amyopathic dermatomyositis presenting blister and oral ulcer. *Ryumachi* 1999; 39: 836–840 [Japanese].
30. Olhoffer IH, Carroll C, Watsky K. Dermatomyositis sine myositis presenting with calcinosis universalis. *Br J Dermatol* 1999; 141(2): 365–366.

31. Callen JP. Relation between dermatomyositis and polymyositis and cancer. *Lancet* 2001; 357(9250): 85–86.
32. Thune P. The coexistence of amyopathic dermatomyositis and fibromyalgia. *Acta Derm Venereol* 2000; 80: 453–454.
33. Tsuruta Y, Ikezoe K, Nakagaki H, et al. A case of dermato-fasciitis: amyopathic dermatomyositis associated with fasciitis. *Clin Rheumatol* 2004; 23: 160–162.
34. Tse S, Lubelsky S, Gordon M, et al. The arthritis of inflammatory childhood myositis syndromes. *J Rheumatol* 2001; 28: 192–197.
35. Sontheimer RD, Miyagawa S. Potentially fatal interstitial lung disease can occur in clinically amyopathic dermatomyositis. *J Am Acad Dermatol* 2003; 48: 797–798.
36. Tokiyama K, Tagawa H, Yokota E, et al. Two cases of amyopathic dermatomyositis with fatal rapidly progressive intestinal pneumonitis. *Ryumachi* 1990; 30: 204–209.
37. Mihailovic B, Karadaglic D, Dostanic I, et al. Amyopathic dermatomyositis with interstitial lung disease. *Vajnosanit Pregl* 1997; 54: 260–271.
38. Santiago MB, Chalhoub M, Pereira ST. Amyopathic dermatomyositis complicated by interstitial pulmonary disease and pneumomediastinum. *J Rheumatol* 1998; 25: 2042–2043.
39. Chow SK, Yeap SS. Amyopathic dermatomyositis and pulmonary fibrosis. *Clin Rheumatol* 2000; 19: 484–485.
40. Fernandes L, Goodwill CJ. Dermatomyositis without apparent myositis, complicated by fibrosing alveolitis. *J R Soc Med* 1979; 72: 777–779.
41. Friedman AW, Targoff IN, Arnet FC. Interstitial lung disease with autoantibody against aminoacyl-tRNA synthetase in the absence of clinically apparent myositis. *Semin Arthritis Rheum* 1996; 26: 459–467.
42. Satoh S, Hirakata M, Suwa A, et al. Antibodies to 140 kDa proteins in Japanase patients with amyopathic dermatomyositis [abstract]. *Arthritis Rheum* 2001; 44: S205.
43. Goyal S, Nousari HC. Paraneoplastic amyopathic dermatomyositis associated with breast cancer recurrence. *J Am Acad Dermatol* 1999; 41: 874–875.
44. Russ BW, English JC, King DH, et al. Amyopathic dermatomyositis associated with transitional cell carcinoma of the bladder. *Cutis* 1999; 63: 73–76.
45. Celebi S, Gul A, Kamali S, et al. Amyopathic dermatomyositis associated with cervical cancer. *Clin Rheumatol* 2001; 20: 438–440.
46. Leow YH, Goh CL. Malignancy in adult dermatomyositis. *Int J Dermatol* 1997; 36: 904–907.
47. Fung WK, Chan HL, Lam WM. Amyopathic dermatomyositis in Hong Kong — association with nasopharyngeal carcinoma. *Int J Dermatol* 1998; 37: 659–663.
48. Hu WH. Nasopharyngeal carcinoma with dermatomyositis — an analysis of 30 cases. *Chung Hua Chung Liu Tsa Chih* 1986; 8: 133–135 [Chinese].
49. Peng JC, Sheen TS, Hsu MM. Nasopharyngeal carcinoma with dermatomyositis. Analysis of 12 cases. *Acta Otolaryngol Head Neck Surg* 1995; 121: 1298–1301.
50. Ee HL, Ng PP, Tan SH. Exacerbation of amyopathic dermatomyositis in Orientals: a high alert for nasopharyngeal carcinoma. *Australas J Dermatol* 2004; 45(1): 77–78.
51. Dourmishev A, Dourmishev L. Dermatomyositis and drugs. *Adv Exp Med Biol* 1999; 455: 187–191.
52. Erel A, Toros P, Tokcear AB, et al. Amyopathic dermatomyositis. *Int J Dermatol* 2000; 39: 771–773.
53. Price CJ, Frankel JP, Hammans SR. Palatal palsy in dermatomyositis (Letter). *Eur J Neurol* 2001; 8: 197–198.
54. Richard M, Trucheter F, Friedel J, et al. Skin lesions simulating chronic dermatomyositis during long-term hydroxyurea therapy. *J Am Acad Dermatol* 1989; 21: 797–799.

55. Senet P, Aractingi S, Porneuf M, et al. Hydroxyurea-induced dermatomyositis-like eruption. *Br J Dermatol* 1995; 133: 455–459.
56. Bahadoran P, Castanet J, Lacour JP, et al. Pseudo-dermatomyositis induced by long-term hydroxyurea therapy: report of two cases. *Br J Dermatol* 1996; 134: 1161–1163.
57. Velez A, Lopez-Rubio F, Moreno JC. Chronic hydroxyurea-induced dermatomyositis-like eruption with severe dermal elastosis. *Clin Exp Dermatol* 1998; 23: 94–95.
58. Varma S, Lanigan SW. Dermatomyositis-like eruption and leg ulceration caused by hydroxyurea in a patient with psoriasis. *Clin Exp Dermatol* 1999; 24: 164–166.
59. Rocamora V, Puig L, Alomar A. Dermatomyositis-like eruption following hydroxyurea therapy. *J Eur Acad Dermatol Venereol* 2000; 14: 227–228.
60. Marie I, Joly P, Levesque H, et al. Pseudo-dermatomositis as a complication of hydroxyurea therapy. *Clin Exp Rheumatol* 2000; 18: 536–537.
61. Ruiz-Genao DP, Sanz-Sánchez T, Bartolomé-González B, et al. Dermatomyositis-like reaction induced by chemotherapeutical agents. *Int J Dermatol* 2002; 41: 885–887.
62. Park JH, Olsen NJ, King LE, et al. Use of magnetic resonance imaging and P-31 magnetic resonance spectroscopy to detect and quantify muscle dysfunction in the amyopathic and myopathic variants of dermatomyositis. *Arthritis Rheum* 1995; 38: 68–77.
63. Park JH, Olsen NJ. Utility of magnetic resonance imaging in the evolution of patients with inflammatory myopathies. *Curr Rheumatol Rep* 2001; 3: 334–345.
64. Targoff IN, Trieu EP, Sontheimer RD. Autoantibodies to 155kD and Se antigens in patients with clinically amyopathic dermatomyositis [abstract]. *Arthritis Rheum* 2000; 43(Suppl 9): S194.
65. Sontheimer RD, Targoff I, Trieu E, et al. Autoantibodies to 155kD and Se antigens in a patients with clinically amyopathic dermatomyositis. *J Invest Dermatol* 2001; 117: 466.
66. Sato S, Suwa A, Kuwana M, et al. Clinical and immunological associations of autoantibodies to the 140kDa polypeptide (the US autoantigen) in patients with clinically amyopathic dermatomyositis. *Arthritis Rheum* 2003; 48: S102.

Paraneoplastic Dermatomyositis 22

Retrospective investigations show the variation in frequency of this clinical form of DM between 4.4% and 60% [1–6]. The malignancy can precede, occur concurrently with, or follow the appearance of DM. From their Scandinavian epidemiological population-based study on 618 cases, Hill et al. [7] found the coincidence of neoplasia in 32% of patients with DM in adults. Moreover, DM and PM associates with specific cancer types, most frequently ovarian, lung, and pancreatic carcinomas as well as non-Hodgkin's lymphoma (NHL) for DM, and NHL, lung, and bladder cancer for PM [7]. Burnouf et al. [8] reported 26 adults presenting with DM, hospitalized in Bichat–Claude Bernard Hospital Paris between 1993 and 2000, and found cancers in eight (31%) of them and five patients (62.5%) with cutaneous necrosis. In one study of 788 patients, the death rate was higher in those with DM owing to the presence of malignancy [3]. In women, ovarian cancer is the most frequent, which makes mandatory the screening for ovarian malignancy of all women with DM [4]. Physical examination and imaging techniques, however, may not succeed in detecting it early enough for a favorable prognosis.

Only a few papers with relatively small populations have reported with regard to the predictive signs of malignancies in DM/PM [1, 5, 9, 10]. Advanced age of onset and male gender have been proposed as indicating a greater risk for developing cancers [1, 5], but without significant differences in multivariate analysis. Sparsa et al. [11] did not find any association between malignancy and increasing age, in contrary to many other studies [10, 12–17]. Cutaneous necrosis [1, 5, 9] and an elevated ESR [1] have also been proposed as predictive signs of malignancies (Table 22.1). The evaluation of ESR above 40 mm in the first hour, a predictive criteria retained by Basset-Seguin et al. [1], was not confirmed in Burnouf's 2003 trial [8], nor in the preceding 1996 study [9]. In an univariate analysis Chen et al. [10] did not remain ESR as a factor predictive of cancer during the multivariate analysis. The study by Burnouf et al. [8] provides identical results by including the various muscle enzymes and the presence of cutaneous necroses in the same model. Only the presence of necroses remained significantly associated with the presence of cancer.

Several predictive factors of cancer other than patient's age and male gender have been proposed, such as the presence of cutaneous necroses, increased erythrocyte sedimentation rate (ESR), and increase or normality of creatine kinase (CK) [1, 5, 9, 10, 18]. Patients with primary idiopathic DM, with an older age of onset, higher serum CK levels and male

22

Table 22.1 Predictive value of the paraneoplastic nature of cutaneous necroses [8][a]

		DM with cancer		DM without cancer	
	P	*N*	With necrosis (%)	*N*	With necrosis (%)
Basset-Seguin [1]	0.05	13	4 (30.7%)	19	1 (5.2%)
Gallais [12]	0.002	9	6 (64.4%)	23	2 (8.7%)
Mautner [13]		6	0	5	0
Burnouf [15]	0.01	8	5 (62.5%)	18	2 (11.1%)
Total = 101		36	15 (41.7%)	65	5 (7.7%)

[a]Among 101 studied cases of DM, 36 were associated with a neoplasia (35.6%). The positive predictive value of cutaneous necrosis for an associated cancer is 81%, with sensitivity of 58.3%, and specificity of 92.3%.

gender, had more risk to develop concomitant malignancies [10]. An increased risk of cancer has been reported among male DM patients older than 50 years [19].

According to Sparsa et al. [11], factors associated with malignancy in DM patients are a rapid onset of disease, a presence of constitutional symptoms, lack of Raynaud's phenomenon, and elevated ESR and CK levels. In Fudman and Schnitzer's trial [18], however, the increased risk of cancer correlates with normal levels of CK. Moreover, Montagna et al. [20] have found that 5 of 17 patients with elevated CK had malignancy, compared with three of nine cases with normal CK. The number of patients in these studies is too small to firmly conclude that normal CK is a marker of malignancy in patients with DM.

The increased levels of CK, although reported to be associated with an increased risk of cancer in the study by Chen et al. [10] in univariate analysis, did not remain a cancer-predictive factor in the multivariate analysis, and if they coincided with DM complications, especially ILD, had a lower risk for association with neoplasia.

Cutaneous necrosis may be similarly linked [5], as may be resistance to therapy, combined with an elevated ESR, elevated C-reactive protein, and advanced age [1]. Cutaneous necrosis occurs in between 7% and 55% of those with malignancy-associated DM [1, 11, 21, 22]. Necrotic skin lesions have been suggested as predictive of concomitant neoplasia [5, 9, 10, 23], as well as advanced age greater than 55 years and persistent pruritus [9]. A patient with metastatic hepatocellular carcinoma with two of these risk factors, cutaneous necroses and advanced age, has been reported [23]. Hunger et al. [24] also proposed that leukocytoclastic vasculitis was associated with malignancy in DM.

The presence of cutaneous vasculitis may also be a predictive sign of malignancy [25]. Feldman et al. [25] found clinical evidence of vasculitis manifested as dermal or subcutaneous nodules, periungual infarcts, or digital ulceration in seven of 76 patients. Two of these patients had cancer, compared with four of those without vasculitis. In addition, the vasculitic lesions occurred primarily in patients with DM (six of seven patients). It has been reported that DM patients with recurrent ulcers and vasculitis had a poor prognosis [26]. Recently, Hunger et al. [24] have reported the greater prevalence of neoplasia when histopathological evidence of vasculitis was found in skin biopsy. Four of their five patients with vasculitis had cancer, compared with three of 18 patients without vasculitis ($p < 0.05$).

Table 22.2 Predictive factors for malignancy in DM patients

Predictive factors	Comments
I. Cutaneous features	
(a) Cutaneous necroses	
(b) Vasculitis	Subcutaneous nodules, periungual infarcts
(c) Ulcers	
(d) Vesicule and bulla	Ovarian and gastric cancer
(e) Poikiloderma	
(f) Pruritus	
II. Laboratory features (data)	
(a) Elevated ESR	
(b) Elevated C-reactive protein	
(c) CK level	Normal or high serum CK levels
III. Demographic data	
(a) Advanced age	>40, >50, >55 years
(b) Male gender	
IV. Evolution of disease	
(a) Rapid onset	
(b) Severe constitutional symptoms	

Vesicle and bulla formation in DM may strongly correlate with ovarian [2] and gastric cancer [27], while these subepidermal lesions are not associated with immunoglobulin deposition [2].

Cases with generalized hyperkeratotic follicular papules, hyperkeratotic papules on the palms and soles, and nonscarring alopecia are frequently associated with internal malignancy [28].

Dourmishev [29] characterized the differences between classic and paraneoplastic DM. Paraneoplastic DM is more often associated with poikiloderma, ulcerations, and an increased ESR than classic DM in adults (Table 22.2).

DM and acquired ichthyosis are both considered as paraneoplastic dermatoses. Acquired ichthyosis was recently reported as concomitantly occurring with the onset of DM in a patient found to have hepatocellular carcinoma [30].

Pruritus in DM has also been implicated as potentially indicative of underlying malignancy [9]. However, pruritus is well known for its potential association with malignancy, especially lymphomas and leukemias. Unexplained, persistent pruritus should always prompt a search for underlying malignancy, especially when appearing in older patients.

The amyopathic nature of DM also does not appear to be predictive of the absence of concomitant neoplasia. Single case reports and some small case series of this cohort have described an association of amyopathic DM with malignancy [31, 32]. Even though this association appears rare [10], observations of paraneoplastic amyopathic DM have been reported [33–35].

DM in childhood associated with cancer, although very rare, has been also reported [36, 37] (see also Chapter 18).

For years, the value of an extensive search for occult malignancy in patients with DM has been discussed. Some form of screening for malignancy should be made in every patient

22

with DM, and should be planned individually, taking into consideration the patient's age, sex, and ethnicity. Every DM patient should be investigated for underlying malignancy during the first 3–5 years of disease onset.

References

1. Basset-Seguin N, Roujeau J-C, Gherardi R, et al. Prognostic factors and predictive signs of malignancy in adult dermatomyositis. A study of 32 cases. *Arch Dermatol* 1990; 126: 633–637.
2. Kubo M, Sato S, Kitahara H, et al. Vesicle formation in dermatomyositis associated with gynecologic malignancies. *J Am Acad Dermatol* 1996; 34: 391–394.
3. Sigurgeirsson B, Lindelof B, Edhag O, et al. Risk of cancer in patients with dermatomyositis or polymyositis. *N Engl J Med* 1992; 326: 363–367.
4. Davis MD, Ahmed I. Ovarian malignancy in patients with dermatomyositis and polymyositis: a retrospective analysis of fourteen cases. *J Am Acad Dermatol* 1997; 37: 730–733.
5. Mautner GH, Grossman ME, Silvers DN, et al. Epidermal necrosis as a predictive sign of malignancy in adult dermatomyositis. *Cutis* 1998; 61: 190–194.
6. Goyal S, Nousari HC. Paraneoplastic amyopathic dermatomyositis associated with breast cancer recurrence. *J Am Acad Dermatol* 1999; 41: 874–875.
7. Hill CL, Zhang Y, Sigurgeirsson B, et al. Frequency of specific cancer types in dermatomyositis and polymyositis: a population-based study. *Lancet* 2001; 357: 96–100.
8. Burnouf M, Mahe E, Verpillat P, et al. Cutaneous necrosis is predictive of cancer in adult dermatomyositis. *Ann Dermatol Venereol* 2003; 130: 313–316.
9. Gallais V, Crickx B, Belaich S. Facteurs pronostiques et signes prédictifs de cancer au cours de la dermatomyosite de l'adulte. *Ann Dermatol Venereol* 1996; 123: 722–726.
10. Chen YJ, Wu CY, Shen JL. Predicting factors of malignancy in dermatomyositis and polymyositis: a case-control study. *Br J Dermatol* 2001; 144: 825–831.
11. Sparsa A, Fiazon E, Hertman F, et al. Routine vs extensive malignancy search for adult dermatomyositis and polymyositis. A study of 40 patients. *Arch Dermatol* 2002; 138: 885–890.
12. Manchul LA, Jin A, Pritchard KI, et al. The frequency of malignant neoplasms in patients with polymyositis–dermatomyositis. A controlled study. *Arch Intern Med* 1985; 145(10): 1835–1839.
13. Benthassal J, Gelel D, Parhoil K, et al. Prognostic factors in polymyositis/dermatomyositis: a computer-assisted analysis of ninety-two cases. *Arthritis Rheum* 1985; 28: 249–256.
14. Tymms KE, Webb J. Dermatomyositis and other connective tissue diseases: a review of 105 cases. *J Rheumatol* 1985; 12: 1140–1148.
15. Bonnetblanc JM, Bernard P, Fayol J. Dermatomyositis and malignancy. *Dermatologica* 1990; 180: 212–216.
16. Marie I, Hatron PY, Levesque H, et al. Influence of age on characteristics of polymyositis and dermatomyositis in adults. *Medicine* 1999; 78: 139–147.
17. Pautas E, Cherin P, Pielte DC, et al. Features of polymyositis and dermatomyositis in the elderly: a case control study. *Clin Exp Rheumatol* 2000; 18: 241–244.
18. Fudman EJ, Schnitzer TJ. Dermatomyositis without creatine kinase elevation: poor prognosis sign. *Am J Med* 1986; 80: 329–332.
19. Wakata N, Kurihara T, Saito E, et al. Polymyositis and dermatomyositis associated with malignancy: a 30-year retrospective study. *Intern J Dermatol* 2002; 41: 729–734.
20. Montagna GL, Manzo C, Califanc E, et al. Absence of elevated creatine kinase in dermatomyositis does not exclude malignancy. *Scand J Rheumatol* 1988; 17: 73–74.

21. Parodi A, Caproni M, Marzano AV, et al. Dermatomyositis in 132 patients with different clinical subtypes: cutaneous signs, constitutional symptoms and circulating antibodies. *Acta Derm Venereol* 2002; 82(1): 48–51.
22. Mahe E, Descamps V, Burnouf M, et al. A helpful clinical sign predictive of cancer in adult dermatomyositis: cutaneous necrosis. *Arch Dermatol* 2003; 139: 539.
23. Maruani A, Armingaud P, Nseir A, et al. Erythroderma and cutaneous necrosis in patient with dermatomyositis. *Ann Dermatol Venereol* 2003; 150: 353–356.
24. Hunger RE, Durr D, Brand CU. Cutaneous leukocytoclastic vasculitis in dermatomyositis suggests malignancy. *Dermatology* 2001; 202: 123–126.
25. Feldman D, Hochberg MC, Zizic TM, et al. Cutaneous vasculitis in adult polymyositis/dermatomyositis. *J Rheumatol* 1983; 10: 85–89.
26. Yamamoto T, Ohkubo H, Katayama I, et al. Dermatomyositis with multiple skin ulcers showing vasculitis and membrano-cystic lesion. *J Dermatol* 1994; 21: 687–689.
27. Fujimoto M, Murakami T, Murata S, et al. Acute onset vesiculo-bullous dermatomyositis associated with massive mucosal necrosis of the intestines. *Clin Exp Dermatol* 2002; 27: 714–722.
28. Wong KO. Dermatomyositis: a clinical investigation of 23 cases in Hong Kong. *Br J Dermatol* 1969; 81: 544–547.
29. Dourmishev LA. Dermatomyositis associated with malignancy. 12 case reports. *Adv Exp Med Biol* 1999; 455: 193–199.
30. Inuzuka M, Tomita K, Tokura Y, et al. Acquired ichthyosis associated with dermatomyositis in a patient with hepatocellular carcinoma. *Br J Dermatol* 2001; 144: 415–448.
31. Caproni M, Cardinali C, Parodi A, et al. Amyopathic dermatomyositis, a review by the Italian group of immunodermatology. *Arch Dermatol* 2002; 138: 23–27.
32. el-Azhary RA, Pakzad SY. Amyopathic dermatomyositis: retrospective review of 37 cases. *J Am Acad Dermatol* 2002; 46: 560–565.
33. Russ BW, English JC, King DH, et al. Amyopathic dermatomyositis associated with transitional cell carcinoma of the bladder. *Cutis* 1999; 63: 73–76.
34. Goyal S, Nousari HC. Paraneoplastic amyopathic dermatomyositis associated with breast cancer recurrence. *J Am Acad Dermatol* 1999; 41: 874–875.
35. Celebi S, Gul A, Kamali S, et al. Amyopathic dermatomyositis associated with cervical cancer. *Clin Rheumatol* 2001; 20: 438–440.
36. Falcini F, Taccetti G, Trapani S, et al. Acute lymphocytic leukemia with dermatomyositis-like onset in childhood. *J Rheumatol* 1993; 20(7): 1260–1262.
37. Léaute-Labrèze C, Perel Y, Taïeb A. Childhood dermatomyositis associated with hepatocarcinoma. *N Engl J Med* 1995; 333(16): 1083.

Overlap Syndromes 23

Overlap syndromes (OS) are a spectrum of disorders with clinical features of two or more classical connective tissue diseases (CTD). Patients with PM/DM may have evidence of another CTD, such as systemic sclerosis, systemic LE, rheumatoid arthritis, or Sjögren's syndrome. Systemic sclerosis is the most common associated disease (36%), compared with systemic LE (28%), rheumatoid arthritis (13%), and Sjögren's syndrome (9%). In Bohan et al.'s study [1], 21% of patients were classified as a PM or DM associated with a CTD. Overlap syndromes often confuse the diagnostic process, since inflammatory myopathies mimicking DM and PM may appear in patients with SSc, systemic LE, and Sjögren's syndrome [1]. The most common is overlap of SSc with systemic LE and myositis, termed "mixed connective tissue disease" (MCTD) [2].

Only DM but not PM truly overlaps with SSc and MCTD [3–5]. Specific signs of SSc or MCTD, such as sclerotic thickening of the dermis, contractures, esophageal hypomotility, microangiopathy, and calcinosis are present in DM, but not PM, whereas signs of systemic LE, rheumatoid arthritis, or Sjögren's syndrome are very rare in DM [3, 4]. Fever, fatigue, weight loss, Raynaud's phenomenon, and nondeforming arthritis frequently occur in OS [1, 3, 6].

Advances in immunology allowed the identification of specific biologic markers of overlap syndrome, such as anti-Ku and PM-Scl antibodies, that are the main markers for Japanese and Caucasian patients [5, 7, 8]. Numerous autoantibodies such as anti-nuclear protein complex (anti-PM-Scl), anti-U1RNP, anti-U2RNP (both anti-RNP antibodies), and anti-Ku have been described in PM/DM overlap syndrome [8]. Anti-Ku antibody is found in a wide spectrum of CTD, including overlap syndromes with SS and DM [9]. In some cases, antibodies to Ku antigen might contribute to the complication of multiple autoimmune diseases [5, 9].

DM associated with features of SSc is one of the most common and heterogeneous overlap syndrome variants, and is termed *sclerodermatomyositis* (SDM) or *scleromyositis* (SM) [5, 7, 10]. The term sclerodermatomyositis was introduced by Corson in 1967 [10]. Scleromyositis is scleroderma/myositis OS, combining clinical features of DM and SS with a chronic and relatively benign course and an association with anti-PM-Scl antibodies [7, 11]. It is a clinical variant separate from both MCTD and the concomitant occurrence of SSc and DM [11]. The syndrome is not uncommon in children [7]. Sclerodermatomyositis associated with the anti-PM-Scl antibody is probably the best characterized entity among OS [7, 12], and seems to be the most frequent systemic CTD of childhood [7].

Anti-PM-Scl scleromyositis has been described mainly in adults [13], and only occasional pediatric cases in one series of 14 children have been reported [7]. Anti-PM-Scl-associated childhood scleromyositis usually starts insidiously, before the age of 12, with arthralgia or arthritis [7, 14]. Exceptionally, the onset can be sudden, with fever, severe myalgia, arthritis, or Raynaud's phenomenon. Cutaneous features of both DM (periorbital erythema, Gottron's sign) and SSc (scleroderma-like changes of the face and hands) develop slowly within the first years of the illness, and are variably pronounced in its course. The symptoms of myositis are clinically indistinguishable from those of primary PM or DM. In the study by Jablonska et al. (1999), EMG showed shortening of mean duration of motor unit action potentials and polyphasic potentials in over 80% of cases [15]. In another study, the sympathetic skin response was abnormal in the vast majority of patients [16]. However, the myalgia may be severe, although the muscle enzyme levels are normal or slightly elevated. The cutaneous and muscle features of DM are usually transient and may regress spontaneously, whereas those of scleroderma tend to persist. Other common features that have usually appeared later in the disease course include arthritis, transient Raynaud's phenomenon or calcinosis. Visceral involvement is often mild or absent, although other immunogenetic associations have been reported [5, 7, 12, 13, 17]. Pulmonary involvement presented as ILD and fibrosis varies between 34% and 78% of cases [12, 15]. A strong correlation has been found between scleromyositis and elevated titers of ANA with homogeneous fluorescence pattern, which mainly correspond to anti-PM-Scl-antibody. This antibody is detectable in more than 50% of adults and in all children with sclerodermatomyositis [5, 11, 18]. Between 43% and 76% of patients with anti-PM-Scl-antibody show features of PM/DM and SSc overlap, although this antibody has been also detected in patients with myositis (8%) and SSc (3%) [8, 11, 13]. Certain HLA genotypes are typical of scleromyositis. The PM-Scl autoantibodies verify with great probability the presence of the HLA DQA1 in about 100% and DRD1 antigens in 90% of cases. These data demonstrate that scleromyositis with PM-Scl autoantibodies should be regarded as a separate immunogenetic entity [19, 20]. All Polish patients with PM-Scl antibodies have HLA-DQA1*0501 and 94% HLA-DRB1*0301 suballeles [21]. Systemic scleroderma in children often displays features of other CTDs [7], including a mild, noninflammatory myopathy with normal serum enzyme levels [13]. Sclerodermatomyositis differs from systemic sclerosis by the absence of hallmark cutaneous features as the induration of face and trunk, thinning of the lips, perioral furrowing, prominent telangiectasia, contracture of the fingers, digital pits and ulcers, as well as the lack of acro-osteolysis, avascular areas of capillaroscopy, and severe visceral involvement [7, 18]. It is distinguished from MCTD by variously pronounced manifestations of DM and lack of SLE symptoms, and by serological associations such as the presence of highly characteristic but not disease-specific PM-Scl antibodies, in contrast to U1-RNP antibodies in MCTD.

Several case reports noted the presence of "mechanic's hands" as a clinical feature of scleromyositis. Garcia-Patos et al. [14] reported a 16-year-old boy with overlap manifestations of SSc and DM (sclerodermatomyositis), with Gottron's papules, mechanic's hands and calcinosis, ANA with a homogeneous nucleolar fluorescence pattern and anti-PM-Scl antibody demonstrated by immunoblotting in sera. Török et al. [22] reported a 56-year-old woman presenting PM-Scl autoantibody-positive scleromyositis, concomitant interstitial lung fibrosis, and mechanic's hands.

The PM-Scl autoantibody-positive SSc–PM overlap syndrome is a chronic disease with a benign course, and remission is achieved with low- or medium-dose steroid therapy. Involution of symptoms, however, is accompanied by the persistence of the serologic markers [15]. A patient with SSc-PM overlap syndrome accompanied by autoimmune hepatitis and mediastinal sarcoidosis, who was positive for ANA, anti-Ku, ASMA (anti-smooth muscle antibodies), rheumatoid factor and anticardiolipine antibodies was reported [23].

Within the overlap syndromes, a combination of DM/PM and localized scleroderma has been observed [24]. However, cases of concurrent DM/PM and morphoea have been rarely documented [24, 25]. Park et al. [26] reported a 35-year-old woman who presented with DM determined both clinically and in the laboratory over 3 years and with circumscribed multiple sclerotic plaques with central depressions (profound morphoea). Clinically, DM/PM and morphoea OS appears as indurated plaques or nodules that remain stable or enlarge progressively, and often heal with subcutaneous atrophy and residual hyperpigmentation [27]. Histology of cutaneous lesions shows characteristic hyaline sclerosis and thickening of collagen bundles mainly within the lower dermis and septae between adipous lobules in subcutis, without notable changes in the epidermis or upper dermis. These findings are the most helpful feature in differentiating the disorder from localized scleroderma and lupus panniculitis [27, 28]. Overlap syndrome has been reported in a 66-year-old woman with disseminated scleroderma and Hashimoto thyroiditis who developed clinical manifestations of PM after initiation of d-penicillamine therapy [29].

While the overlap syndrome of DM and PM with anti-PM-Scl positive SSc is frequently reported, inclusion body myositis (IBM) has only once previously been described in association with anti-PM-Scl-positive systemic sclerosis [30]. Recently, a 72-year-old patient with a 10-year history of anti-PM-Scl-positive SS and "mechanic's hands" associated with IBM has been reported [31].

There is controversy concerning MCTD as a separate entity due to heterogeneity of the clinical manifestations, the infrequent transformation into definite CTD and the variation of classification criteria [15]. Many studies have shown that only DM, but not PM, truly overlaps in up to 20% of patients with other CTD, and only with SSc and MCTD [1, 3, 32]. In MCTD women are found to be affected 6–9 times more often than men, whereas in DM the female to male ratio is 3:1.

Clinical manifestations of MCTD (Sharp's syndrome) include:

1. The presence of edema of hands
2. Raynaud's phenomenon (with typical capillaroscopy)
3. Puffy, sausage-shaped fingers or sclerodactyly (acrosclerosis)
4. Myositis or myalgia
5. Synovitis
6. Esophageal hypomotility
7. Higher titers of U1-RNP antibodies to 70 kD polypeptide (≥320) in sera; in single cases antibodies may disappear if patient is in clinical remission
8. Variable association with HLA – HLA-DR2, DR4, and DRB1*0405
9. Chronic, relatively mild course; in children (about 30% of cases) there could be a more severe course with generalized vasculopathy, glomerulonephritis, and pulmonary complications
10. Response to small or moderate doses of corticosteroids [15, 33–36]

23

The set shows high specificity (85.7%) and sensitivity (76.5%) [35].

Patients with MCTD and DM overlap syndrome rarely develop internal neoplasms.

Adults with myositis associated with other CTD may have prominent weakness. However, in contradistinction to DM and PM patients, muscle enzyme abnormalities are generally much less prominent. In a study of 177 patients, 19 patients with PM and two DM patients showed the overlap with other CTD [13].

Polymyositis/antisynthetase overlap syndrome observed in 29 patients has been reported by Jablonska et al. [15]. This syndrome is characterized by myositis, ILD, arthritis, and Raynaud's phenomenon, in association with anti-aminoacyl transfer RNA synthetase antibodies, mainly with anti-histidyl-tRNA synthetase (anti-Jo-1). In over 85% of cases, genetic association with DQA1*0501 alleles was found. Cutaneous scleroderma-like changes of the face and hands were more frequent and prominent (65.4%) that those of DM type (42.3%), which include Gottron's papules or sign and periorbital heliotrope rash. The onset of disease is usually acute, with fever. The disease course is moderate or severe.

In addition, clinical features of myositis have been recognized in approximately 5% patients with anti-Ro (SS-A) antibody-positive Sjögren's syndrome. Histology from affected muscles in those patients reveals perivascular mononuclear inflammatory infiltrates. Schmidt et al. [37] reported 18 patients with anti-Jo-1 syndrome, one of whom had clinical features of Sjögren's syndrome and anti-Ro- and La-antibodies in sera. In a study of 34 patients with PM/DM, 11% of cases had features of Sjögren's syndrome/ overlap, presenting with subjective xerostomia, signs of salivary hypofunction, fibrosis of the minor salivary glands, and periductal lymphocytic infiltration, but only one of them showed the characteristic for Sjögren's syndrome positive focus score [38].

Overlap syndrome of SLE associated with DM has been reported in a 22-year-old man with arthritis, fever, diffuse myalgia, and periorbital skin heliotrope rash [39]. EMG and muscular biopsy were suggestive of DM. The patient developed nephrotic syndrome in relation with diffuse proliferative glomerulonephritis. Antibodies against native ds DNA were positive, and DIF of normal skin biopsy showed immune complex deposit on the dermo–epidermal junction, suggestive of SLE [39].

References

1. Bohan A, Peter JB, Bowman RL, et al. Computer-assisted analysis of 153 patients with polymyositis and dermatomyositis. *Medicine* 1977; 56: 255–286.
2. Sharp GC, Irvin WS, Tan EM, et al. Mixed connective tissue disease: an apparently distinct rheumatic disease syndrome associated with a specific antibody to an extractable nuclear antigen (ENA). *Am J Med* 1972; 52: 148–159.
3. Dalakas M. Polymyositis, dermatomyositis and inclusion body myositis. *N Engl J Med* 1991; 325(21): 1487–1498.
4. Tymms KE, Webb J. Dermatomyositis and other connective tissue diseases: a review of 105 cases. *J Rheumatol* 1985; 12: 1140–1148.
5. Mimori T. Scleroderma–polymyositis overlap syndrome. *Int J Dermatol* 1987; 26: 419–425.
6. Hochberg MC, Feldman D, Stevens MB. Adult onset polymyositis – dermatomyositis: an analysis of clinical and laboratory factors and survival in 76 patients with a review of the literature. *Semin Arthritis Rheum* 1986; 15: 168–191.

7. Blaszczyk M, Jablonska S, Szymanska-Jagiello W, et al. Childhood scleromyositis: an overlap syndrome associated with PM-Scl antibody. *Pediatr Dermatol* 1991; 8: 1–8.
8. Targoff IN. Humoral immunity in polymyositis/dermatomyositis. *J Invest Dermatol* 1993; 100: 116S–125S.
9. Kamei N, Yamane K, Yamashita Y, et al. Anti-Ku antibody-positive scleroderma–dermatomyositis overlap syndrome developing Graves' disease and immune thrombocytopenic purpura. *Int Med* 2002; 41: 1199–1203.
10. Corson JK. Slerodermatomyositis. *Arch Dermatol* 1967; 96: 596–597.
11. Jablonska S, Chorselski TP, Blaszczyk M, et al. Scleroderma/polymyositis overlap syndromes and their immunologic markers. *Clin Dermatol* 1992; 10: 457–472.
12. Marguerie C, Brunn CC, Copier J, et al. The clinical and immunologic features of patients with autoantibodies to the nuclear antigen PM-Scl. *Medicine (Baltimore)* 1992; 71: 327–336.
13. Oddis CV, Okano Y, Rudert WA, et al. Serum antibody to the nuclear antigen PM-Scl. *Arthritis Rheum* 1992; 35: 1211–1217.
14. Garcia-Patos P, Bartlarot R, Fonollosa V, et al. Childhood sclerodermatomyositis: report of a case with the anti-PM/Scl antibody and mechanic's hands. *Br J Dermatol* 1996; 135: 613–616.
15. Jablonska S, Blaszcyk M. Scleroderma overlap syndromes. *Adv Exp Med Biol* 1999; 455: 85–92.
16. Hausmanowa-Petrusewicz I, Blaszcyk M, Kowalska-Oledzka, et al. Neuromuscular studies in scleromyositis. *Acta Cardiomiologica* 1994; 6: 99–110.
17. Genth E, Mierau R, Genetzky P, et al. Immunogenetic associations of scleroderma-related antinuclear autoantibodies. *Arthritis Rheum* 1990; 33: 657–665.
18. Blaszczyk M, Jarzabek-Chorzelska M, Jablonska S, et al. Autoantibodies to nuclear antigens in systemic scleroderma: clinical correlations. *Br J Dermatol* 1990; 123: 421–430.
19. Jablonska S, Blaszcyk M. Scleromyositis: a scleroderma/polymyositis overlap syndrome. *Clin Rheumatol* 1998; 17: 465–467.
20. Genth E, Mireau R, Geneczky P, et al. Immunogenetic associations of scleroderma- related antinuclear antibodies. *Arthritis Rheum* 1999; 33: 657–665.
21. Hausmanowa-Petrusewicz I, Kowalska-Oledzka E, Miller FW, et al. Clinical, serological and immunogenetic features in Polish patients with idiopathic inflammatory myopathies. *Arthritis Rheum* 1997; 40: 1257–1266.
22. Török L, Dankó K, Cserni G, et al. PM-SCL autoantibody positive scleroderma with polymyositis (mechanic's hand: clinical aid in the diagnosis). *JEADV* 2004; 18: 356–359.
23. Lis-Swety A, Brzezinska-Wcislo L, Pierszchala E, et al. Systemic-sclerosis–polymyositis overlap syndrome accompanied by immune hepatitis and sarcoidosis of mediastinal lymphonodes. *J Eur Acad Dermatol Venereol* 2006; 20: 107–108.
24. Venables PJ. Polymyositis-associated overlap syndromes. *Br J Rheumatol* 1996; 35: 305–306.
25. Al Attia HM, Ezzeddin H, Khader T, et al. A localised morphoea/idiopathic polymyositis overlap. *Clin Rheumatol* 1996; 15(3): 307–309.
26. Park JH, Lee CW. Concurrent development of dermatomyositis and morphoea profunda. *Clin Exp Dermatol* 2002; 27: 324–327.
27. Requena L, Yus ES. Panniculitis. Part I. Mostly septal panniculitis. *J Am Acad Dermatol* 2001; 45: 163–183.
28. Stork J, Vosmik F. Lupus erythematosus panniculitis with morphea-like lesions. *Clin Exp Dermatol* 1994; 19: 79–82.
29. Dourmishev LA, Stomonjakova SR, Dourmishev AL. D-Penicillamine induced polymyositis and morphea dissemination in woman with Hashimoto thyroiditis. *J Eur Acad Dermatol Venereol* 2002; 16: 538–539.
30. Selva-O'Callaghan A, Mijares-Boeckh-Behrens T, Labrador-Horillos M, et al. Anti-PMScl antibodies in a patient with inclusion body myositis. *Rheumatology (Oxford)* 2003; 42: 1016–1018.

31. Kim S, Genth E, Krieg T, et al. PM-Scl antibody positive systemic sclerosis associated with inclusion body myositis. *Z Rheumatol* 2005; 64: 499–502.
32. Uthman I, Vazques-Abad D, Senecal JL. Distinctive features of idiopathic inflammatory myopathies in French Canadians. *Semin Arthritis Rheum* 1996; 26: 447–458.
33. Alarcon-Segovia D, Cardiel MM. Comparison between three diagnostic criteria for mixed connective tissue disease. Study of 593 patients. *J Rheumatol* 1989; 16: 328–334.
34. Hoffman RW, Sharp GC, Deutscher SL. Analysis of anti-U1 RNP antibodies in patients with connective tissue diseases: association with HLA and clinical manifestations of disease. *Arthritis Rheum* 1995; 38: 1837–1844.
35. Amigues JM, Cantagrel A, Abbal M, et al. Evaluation of the classification criteria for mixed connective tissue disease [abstract]. *Arthritis Rheum* 1996; 39(9): S45.
36. Kuwana M, Okano Y, Kaburaki J, et al. Clinical correlation with HLA type in Japanese patients with connective tissue disease and anti-U1 small nuclear RNP antibodies. *Arthritis Rheum* 1996; 39: 986–996.
37. Schmidt WA, Wetzel W, Friedländer R, et al. Clinical and serological aspects of patients with anti-Jo-1 antibodies — an evolving spectrum of disease manifestations. *Clin Rheumatol* 2000; 19: 371–377.
38. Márton K, Hermann P, Dankó K, et al. Evaluation of oral manifestations and masticatory force in patients with polymyositis and dermatomyositis. *J Oral Pathol Med* 2005; 34(3): 164–169.
39. Kilani B, Amari L, Houmane H, et al. Association of systemic lupus erythematosus and dermato-polymyositis. *Tunis Med* 2005; 83: 230–232 [French].

Drug-Induced Dermatomyositis

24

Certain drugs seem to be capable of inducing both the cutaneous and muscle manifestations of DM. Beickert and Kühne are attributed as being the first to recognize that a drug might induce DM [1]. In 1960, they reported the case of a patient who developed DM after chlorpromazine treatment. Various medications have been reported that may cause muscle damage and skin lesions — **drug-induced dermatomyositis (DI-DM)** or syndromes that resemble DM (DM-like syndrome) [2]. During the last 45 years, more than 40 therapeutic substances have been reported that induce DM or PM as adverse reaction of their activity (Table 24.1). In recent years, both the number of observed cases of drug-induced DM and the list of the culprit medicines that provoke these clinical features have increased [3]. The association of drugs and DM/PM may present as follow:

(i) Induction of clinical features typical for classic DM
(ii) Occurrence of cutaneous DM-like lesions without muscle damage — i.e., amyopathic DM
(iii) Provocation of PM
(iv) Development of myalgia or muscle damage
(v) Induction of serum enzyme changes only [2]

Non-steroidal anti-inflammatory drugs (NSAIDs), lipid-lowering agents, anti-infectious, antineoplastic medicines, vaccines, radiotherapy, and other nonrelated drugs are of particular interest in induction of DM.

A NSAID-related medicine, disease-modifying drug d-penicillamine, is the most frequently reported agent that induced PM or DM. Forty-two cases with d-penicillamine-induced DM or PM have been published [3]. The drug can cause elevations in serum levels of sarcoplasmic enzymes, clinical features of PM, or DM, particularly in patients with associated immune disorders [3]. Treatment of rheumatoid arthritis with d-penicillamine is associated with the development of DM/PM in 0.2–1.2% of the cases, which occur 1.5–6 months after introduction of the drug [4]. Some authors do not share this observation, considering that d-penicillamine-induced DM/PM depends on neither the dose nor the duration of the treatment [5]. This complication is unpredictable in individual patients [3]. The condition is reversible once the treatment with drug is discontinued. Patients with

Table 24.1 Drugs which induce DM or similar syndromes

Drugs	ADM	DM	PM	M	E
Analgesics/antirheumatics/NSAIDs					
Acidum acetylsalicylicum	+				
Diclofenac	+				
Niflumic acid	+				
d-Penicillamine	+	+	+	+	+
Phenylbutazone		+			
Ibuprofen		+		+	
Anti-infectious					
Penicillins		+			
Sulfonamides		+	+		
Isonazide		+			
Zidovudine			+	+	+
Lipid-lowering agents					
Gemfibrozil			+		
Fenofibrate			+		
Atorvastatine		+			
Pravastatin		+		+	+
Lovastatin				+	+
Simvastatin		+		+	
Antineoplastic					
Hydroxyurea	+				
Tamoxifen		+			
Tegafur		+			
Cyclophosphamid	+				
Etopsid	+				
Nifumic acid (Nifuril®)	+	+			
Radiotherapy					
Others					
Chlorpromazine		+			
Antazoline		+			
Clemizole		+			
Mephenytoin		+			
Phenytoin		+			
Alfuzosin		+			
Interferon alpha		+			
Vaccines (BCG, polymyelitis, influenza)		+			

ADM =amyopathic DM; DM = dermatomyositis; PM = polymyositis; M = myopathia; E = serum enzyme changes (CPK, ASAT ALAT, …)

d-penicillamine-induced PM could promote insidious, but potentially life-threatening cardiac involvement such as complete heart block and must be carefully monitored [6, 7].

Other NSAIDs that induce DM/PM are diclofenac [8], ibuprofen [9], phenylbutazone [10], aspirin [11], and niflumic acid [8]. Periorbital infiltrated erythematous edema in association with inflammatory edema in lower extremities occurred abruptly in a 42-year-old female patient after 3 months therapy of oral diclofenac, 150 mg/day, for transient arthralgia [8]. DM-like syndrome regressed 1 week after the cession of treatment. Niflumic acid, 750 mg/day orally, was prescribed on day 8, for pain due to minor trauma. Two weeks later (day 21), erythematous nonpruriginous edema of face and lower extremities had reappeared. The patient complained of severe lassitude. Laboratory study showed ten times elevated CK, five times elevated LDH, and aldolase exceeding by seven times the normal range. EMG showed typical myopathic changes. Because muscle biopsy was performed late (day 47), only type II muscle fiber atrophy was determined. Photopatch tests with niflumic acid and diclofenac were negative. Niflumic acid was discontinued (day 24). The clinical features had disappeared and biological results had returned to normal values on the 55th day after the cessation of treatment. The patient was controlled for more than 12 months.

After 1-year treatment with alfuzosin, an alpha-adrenergic blocker used to treat benign prostatic hyperplasia in a 75-year-old man, the patient developed DM confirmed by EMG, muscle biopsy, and serum enzymes [12]. ANA in sera were slightly positive with spliced fluorescence pattern, while the anti-Jo-1 antibody, C3, C4, and ENA were negative. Diagnosis of DI-DM was confirmed by rapid improvement of clinical manifestation after discontinuing treatment with drug.

DI-DM has been linked to a variety of other drugs, although it appears that lipid-lowering agents are the most commonly reported [13–17]. With increasing usage of these drugs, more cases of toxic myopathy or rabdomyolysis have been described [18–20]. The effect is not specific to one class of compounds, almost all lipid-lowering agents have been implicated, including nicotinic acid and fibrates; however, the statins are the most frequently reported.

HMG-CoA (3-hydroxy-3-methylglutaryl coenzyme A) reductase inhibitors, known as statins, are used for the treatment of familial hypercholesterolaemia and for prevention of primary or secondary artherosclerosis. These medicaments are usually well-tolerated, but transient elevation of serum levels of skeletal muscle enzymes, especially CK, are common and cases of myopathy or rhabdomyolysis after therapy with these drugs have been reported [18–20]. Characteristic cutaneous lesions for DM or compatible with disease have been reported in patients treated with simvastatin [15], lovastatin [16], atorvastatin [17] pravastatin [21], and fluvastatin [22]. A report has been published on a patient treated with pravastatin presenting with erythematous and bullous skin lesions involving face, neck, shoulders, and chest who developed DM [13]. A 69-year-old woman with typical features of DM 2 years after the initiation of a treatment with pravastatin has also been reported; the statin therapy was discontinued and the patient slowly improved, with only a transient local corticosteroid treatment [21]. Eight other cases of DM after prolonged treatment with HMG-CoA reductase inhibitors are reported in the literature [23] as well as one unpublished case of a 82-year-old patient in whom myositis arose after combined atorvastatin and ezitimibine therapy of hyperlipidemia. All of them presented with classical features of DM. The discontinuation of the treatment was followed by spontaneous clinical and biological improvement in four of them. The other six cases received high doses of corticosteroids and improved, except one patient who died of respiratory failure due to pulmonary fibrosis despite the adjunction of oral cyclophosphamide. Cases of myositis with elevated CK levels, myalgia, and muscle weakness were observed as provoked by these drugs [13, 18, 24, 25]. It has been hypothesized that apoptosis of vascular smooth muscle cells induced by HMG-CoA reductase inhibitors is responsible for development of DM in patients treated with statins [26]. Some authors do not considered drug participation in initiated DM [27, 28]. Price et al. [28] reported a 68-year-old woman with past medical history of ischemic heart disease and essential hypertension who was on medication including aspirin, simvastatin, loratidine, and ramipril. She developed DM (confirmed by EMG and muscle biopsy) presenting with symptoms of limb muscle weakness, rash over the neck, face, and hands, and 70 times elevated CK in sera. The patient had Medical Research Council (MRC) grade 4 proximal upper limb and grade 3 proximal lower limb weakness. After 1 month, the patient developed nasal speech, nasal regurgitation of fluids, dysphagia, palatal palsy, and worsening of the facial rash. Fourteen months after initial symptoms, the patient presented with pathology revealing a diffuse large B-cell lymphoma, invading muscle. The authors did not, however, comment on the possibility of drug initiation of DM.

Drug-induced polymyositis has been reported in patients treated with fibrates as well as clofibrate [29], fenofibrate [30], and gemfibrocil [31].

Cutaneous lesions simulating chronic course DM have also been reported during long-term treatment with antineoplastic agents such as hydroxyurea [32], etoposide, cyclophosphamid [33], after tamoxifen-induced tumor regression [34], or triggered by tegafur [35], radiotherapy [36], or total body irradiation [33]. Most of reported patients with drug-induced DM from antineoplastic agents were treated with hydroxyurea [32, 37–42]. Hydroxyurea is considered the drug of choice in the treatment of myeloproliferative disorders such as chronic myeloid leukemia, polycythemia vera, and essential thrombocythemia, and is effective in the treatment of recalcitrant psoriasis. DM-like eruption is rather stereotypical cutaneous adverse reaction to hydroxyurea, which appears on the dorsa of the interfalangeal and metacarpophalageal joints as Gottron's papules or Gottron's signs, associated with atrophic or telangiectatic changes, and prominent nailfold telangiectasia [32, 33, 37–42]. Clinical manifestations of the acral lesions range from scaly, poikilodermatous plaques to atrophic erythema with violaceous papules. Eruption develops on the dorsa of the feet, elbows, palms, and soles. The face is involved with diffuse edema in some cases. The onset occurs usually from months to several years (2–10 years) after the initiation of hydroxyurea treatment. Clinical signs of muscle involvement and systemic symptoms have been never described. Elevated serum levels of sarcoplasmatic enzymes are not detected, and no ANA and circulating immune complex are reported in these patients. Painful leg ulcers are often seen in association with xerosis and cutaneous atrophy. Cutaneous eruption is clinical and histopathologically similar to idiopathic DM-specific skin disease [41, 43]. The course of eruption is benign [37], and in most patients the clinical manifestations improve after the discontinuation of hydroxyurea treatment. Such a clinical syndrome has been reported under different names, such as DM-like eruption [33, 37, 41, 44], lichenoid drug reaction [45], pseudo-dermatomyositis [43], poikiloderma, or hydroxyurea dermatopathy [39, 45, 46]. DM sine myositis could be clinically indistinguishable from this drug reaction [41]. Hydroxyurea DM-like eruption is a clinical manifestation example of drug-induced amyopathic DM. DM-like eruption from long-term use of hydroxyurea therapy has been reported in a woman with thrombocytopenia treated for 2 years [47]. Two years after discontinuation of the drug the patient developed multiple keratotic lesions, and 8 years later a metastasic neuroendocrine Merkel cell carcinoma located on the finger [47].

The mechanism for cutaneous lesions caused by long-term hydroxyurea therapy is related to a toxic effect of the drug due to inhibition of DNA synthesis and repair [48]. Hydroxyurea probably is responsible for vacuolar degeneration of the basal cells and colloidal bodies and epidermal atrophy seen in biopsy specimen of skin lesions in treated patients [32]. Ruiz-Genao et al. [33] reported three cases on chemotherapeutic treatment (the first patient with chronic myeloid leukemia treated with hydroxyurea for 19 months and cyclophosphamide, case two with follicular lymphoma treated with total body irradiation and cyclophosphamide, and the third case of a patient with acute lymphoblastic leukemia treated with high doses of etoposide) who developed the hallmark cutaneous manifestations of DM, such as periorbital erythema, erythema over the interphalangeal joints and on elbows, and periungual lesions. No muscular involvement, either clinical or biochemical, was present in any of the cases [33]. In all cases skin lesions disappeared in a few days after drug removal without any additional treatment, and patients did not show relapse during the follow-up time of up to 6 months. Autoantibody detection was performed only in case 2, and was negative. Subsequent long-term follow-up has shown a benign clinical course, with no further indication of evolving autoimmune disease. The cases described in the literature of DM-like reaction related to long-term hydroxyurea treatment present with exclusive cutaneous lesions resembling those of true amyopathic DM.

It is surprising that patients with DM or PM with a complex karyotype including monosomy 7, and trilineage dysplastic features treated with azatioprine, developed acute myeloid leukemia [49, 50]. Similar observations of the development of lymphomas associated with Epstein–Barr virus occurring during methotrexate therapy in DM patients have been reported [51–53] (Table 24.2). A patient with DM associated with uterine adenocarcinoma has been reported, who after removal of tumor and 18 months methotrexate therapy developed a second primary adenocarcinoma of the breast, [54]. Recently, a 48-year-old woman with

Table 24.2 Malignancy in DM patients after immunosuppressive treatment

Drug	DM preceding malignancy	Malignancy type	Author
Methotrexate	Yes	Breast cancer	Callen (1983)
		Lymphoma	Kamel et al. (1993)
		Hodgkin's lymphoma	Bittar and Rose (1995), Chai et al. (1999)
Azathioprine	Yes	Acute myeloid leukemia	Krishnan et al. (1994), Arnold et al. (1999)
Hydroxyurea	Yes	Neuroendocrine carcinoma	Bouldouyre et al. (2005)
Infliximab	Yes	Non-Hodgkin's lymphoma	Roddy et al. (2002)

refractory DM has been reported, who developed non-Hodgkin's lymphoma after treatment with human TNF-α monoclonal antibody infliximab (5 mg/kg) [55].

Anti-infectious drugs such as penicillins [56], sulfonamides [57], isoniazid [58], and zidovudine [59] have also been reported to induce DM or PM. HIV-positive patients receiving long-time antiviral zidovudine therapy can develop a toxic myopathy with elevated CK levels, myalgia, and weakness [59]. Histological and molecular biology studies indicate that zidovudine inhibiting the γ-DNA polymerase is responsible for abnormal production of muscle mitochondrial DNA [60]. A case series in 1987 [61] reported two patients with DM who developed muscular tuberculosis. Both patients developed a severe relapse, attributed to the initiation of rifampicin treatment. Despite an increase in steroid dose in both patients, there were relapses in myositis following rifampicin onset, requiring treatment with intravenous immunoglobulin.

There are many reports of induced DM by different types of vaccine — cholera, paratyphoid fever, poliomyelitis vaccine [62], BCG [63], and single communications of other drugs such as chlorpromazine [1], antazoline [64], clemizole, mephenytoin [65], phenytoin [66], interferon alpha [67], and leflunomide [68].

Recently, Lee and Werth [69] have reported a patient with newly diagnosed DM shortly after starting a herbal supplement containing the algae *Spirulina platensis* and *Aphanizomenon flos-aquae*. The skin symptoms remained stable when she discontinued the supplement, and worsened upon rechallenge. The skin biopsy showed interface dermatitis and ANA titer was 1:160. Over the next 6 months, additional features of DM developed, including muscle weakness accompanied by elevated CK and aldolase levels. The patient proved to be heterozygous for a TNF-α promoter polymorphism, manifested by a phenotype of increase TNF-α production.

Herbal supplements such as *S. platensis* manifest a range of immunostimulatory functions [69], including enhanced production of IL-1, IL-6, and TNF-α [70], augmented interferon production and increased phagocytic activity of macrophages, and enhanced NK cell activity [71]; the alga *Aflos aquae* increases expression of TNF-α in vitro [72].

It is almost impossible to rule out primary idiopathic DM in these patients, because removal of the drug alone has not always caused the clinical manifestations to cease, and most patients have undergone a long corticosteroid course to control the disease [73].

It is well-known that antihistone antibodies are detected in sera of more than 90% of patients with drug-induced lupus erythematosus, and these antibodies are fairly specific for drug-induced lupus [74, 75]. Anti-histone antibodies have been detected also in patients with various autommune diseases. Recently, anti-histone antibodies in sera have been found by ELISA in 17% of patients with PM/DM [76]. No significant correlation between anti-histone antibodies and clinical and laboratory findings in the patients with PM/DM were found. Moreover, serological studies showing an association between certain autoantibodies and drug-induced DM have not yet been reported. In one study, however, it was concluded that drug-induced DM is associated with HLA-B18, HLA-B35, and HLA-DR4 [77].

Recently, in one study the structural requirements for eliciting drug-induced DM and drug-induced PM have been determined [78]. The Common Reactivity Pattern (COREPA) approach is used to describe the structural requirements for eliciting side-effects of 20 drugs [78]. The specific atoms (atomic groups) defined to have characteristic ranges for their electronic properties (atomic charges), are found to be indicative for the possible

Table 24.3 Pharmacological activity in inducing of PM, DM, and amyopathic DM

Features	Polymyositis	Dermatomyositis	Amyopathic DM
1. Myositis	+	+	–
2. Cutaneous rash	–	+	+
3. Muscle enzymes	+	+	–
4. Pharmacological activity	Drugs containing oxygen atom from a carbonyl and hydroxyl group	Drugs containing reduced sulfur and nitrogen atom	Drugs containing nitrogen atom and additional condition for the nitrogen atoms participating in the structures

active centers responsible for eliciting the adverse reactions. The oxygen atoms of carbonyl and hydroxyl groups in the charge range of 0.350 < QO < −0.320 a.u. were found to induce PM side-effects [78]. (Table 24.3).

In another group of drugs, reduced sulfur in a charge range of $0.07 < Q_s < 0.450$ a.u. and a nitrogen atom (in a cyclical fragment and anticyclical in a sp3-hybridization) in a charge range of $-0.390 < Q_N < -0.140$ a.u were found to be active centers for DM side-effects [78].

In conclusion, clinical manifestations of drug-induced DM may be presented in three subgroups:

(i) With typical cutaneous and muscle features of classic DM
(ii) With only skin features of amyopathic DM
(iii) As paraneoplastic DM
    (a) In patients with cancers treated with chemotherapeutic agents who develop signs of DM, and vice versa
    (b) in DM patients treated with antineoplastic drugs (azathioprine, methotrexate) who develop malignancy (i.e., acute myelogenic leukemia, lymphomas)

References

1. Beickert A, Kühne W. Dermatomyositis mit Immunleucopenie, Phenothiazinschädigung. *Schweiz Med Wochenschr* 1960; 90: 132–135.
2. Dourmishev A, Dourmishev L. Dermatomyositis and drugs. *Adv Exp Med Biol* 1999; 455: 187–191.
3. Dourmishev LA, Stomonjakova SR, Dourmishev AL. D-penicillamine induced polymyositis and morphea dissemination in woman with Hashimoto thyreoiditis. *J Eur Acad Dermatol Venereol* 2002; 16: 538–539.
4. Kolosi R, Bahloul Z, Hachicha J, et al. Dermatomyositie induite par la d-pénicillamine au cours d'une polyarthrite rheumatoide. A propos d'un cas avec revue de la littérature. *Rev. Rheum Mal Osteo Articulaires* 1992; 59: 341–344.
5. Chapurlat R, Tebib JG, Noel E, et al. Dermatomyositis induite par la d-pénicillamine au cours d'une polyarthrite rheumatoide. *Rheumatologie* 1995; 47: 203–207.

24

6. Doyle DR, McCurely TL, Sergent JS. Fatal polymyositis in d-penicillamine-treated rheumatoid arthritis. *Ann Intern Med* 1983; 98: 327–330.
7. Wright GD, Wilson C, Bell AL. D-penicillamine induced polymyositis causing complete heart block. *Clin Rheumatol* 1994; 13: 80–82.
8. Grob JJ, Collet AM, Bonerandi JJ: Dermatomyositis-like syndrome induced by nonsteroid anti-inflammatory agents. *Dermatologica* 1989; 178: 178.
9. Ross NS, Hoppel CL. Partial muscle carnitine palmitoyltransferase-A deficiency. Rhabdomyolysis associated with transiently decreased muscle carnitine content after ibuprofen therapy. *JAMA* 1987; 257(1): 62–65.
10. Curran JJ, Jamieson TW. Dermatomyositis-like syndrome associated with phenylbutazone therapy. *J Rheumatol* 1987; 14(2): 397–398.
11. Shelly WB. Birch pollen and aspirin psoriasis. A study in salicylate hypersensitivity. *JAMA* 1964; 189: 985–958.
12. Vela-Casasempere P, Borras-Blasco J, Navarro-Ruiz A. Alfuzosin-Xatral®-associated dermatomyositis. *Br J Rheumatol* 1998; 37: 1135–1136.
13. Schalke BB, Schmidt B, Toyka K, et al. Pravastatin-associated inflammatory myopathy. *N Engl J Med* 1992; 111: 649–650.
14. Khattak FH, Morris IM, Branford WA. Simvastatin-associated dermatomyositis. *Br J Rheumatol* 1994; 32(2): 199.
15. Hill C, Zeitz C, Kirkham B. Dermatomyositis with lung involvement in a patient treated with simvastatin. *Aust NZ J Med* 1995; 25: 745–746.
16. Ridriguez-Gacia JI, Serrano Commino M. Lovastatin-associated dermatomyositis. *Postgrad Med J* 1996; 72: 694.
17. Noël B, Cerottini JP, Pires A, et al. Atorvastatine et dermatomyositis. *Ann Dermatol Venereol* 2000; 127: 4S77–227.
18. Pierce IR, Wysowski D, Gross TP. Myopathy and rhabdomyolysis, associated with lovastatin–gemfibrocil combination therapy. *JAMA* 1990; 264: 71–75.
19. Deslypere JP, Vermeulen A. Rhabdomyolysis with simvastatin. *Ann Intern Med* 1991; 114: 342.
20. Wallace CS, Mueller BA. Lovastatin-induced rhabdomyolysis in the absence of concomitant drugs. *Ann Pharmacol* 1992; 26: 190–192.
21. Zuech P, Pauwels C, Duthoit C, et al. Pravastatin-induced dermatomyositis. *Rev Med Interne* 2005; 26: 897–902 [French].
22. Thual N, Penven K, Chevallier JM, et al. Fluvastatin-induced dermatomyositis. *Ann Dermatol Venereol* 2005; 132(12): 996–999 [French].
23. Dourmishev LA, Dourmishev AL. Activity of certain drugs in inducing of inflammatory myopathies with cutaneous manifestations. *Exp Opin Drug Saf* 2008; 4: 421–433.
24. McDonagh J, Winocour P, Walker DJ. Musculoskeletal manifestations during simvastatin therapy. *Br J Rheumatol* 1992; 32: 647–648.
25. al-Jubouri M, Briston PG, Sinclair D, et al. Myxoedema revealed by simvastatin-induced myopathy. *Br Med J* 1994; 308: 588.
26. Guijaro C, Blanco-Colio LM, Ortego M, et al. 3-Hydroxy-3-methylglutaryl coenzyme A reductase and isoprenylation inhibitors induce apoptosis of vascular smooth muscle cells in culture. *Circ Res* 1998; 83: 490–500.
27. Erel A, Toros P, Tokcaer AB, et al. Amyopathic dermatomyositis. *Int J Dermatol* 2000; 39: 771–773.
28. Price CJ, Frankel JP, Hammans SR. Palatal palsy in dermatomyositis. *Eur J Neurol* 2001; 8(2): 197–198.
29. Mastaglia FL. Adverse effects of drugs on muscle. *Drugs* 1982; 24: 304–321.
30. Sauvaget F, Piette JC, Herson S, et al. Fenofibrate-induced polymyositis. *Rev Med Interne* 1991; 12(1): 52–54 [French].

31. Fusella J, Strosberg JM. Polymyositis exacerbated by gemfibrocil. *J Rheumatol* 1990; 17: 572.
32. Richard M, Truchetter F, Friedel J, et al. Skin lesions simulating chronic dermatomyositis during long-term hydroxyurea therapy. *J Am Acad Dermatol* 1989; 21: 797–799.
33. Ruiz-Genao DP, Sanz-Sánchez T, Bartolomé-González B, et al. Dermatomyositis-like reaction induced by chemotherapeutical agents. *Int J Dermatol* 2002; 41: 885–887.
34. Harris AL, Smith IE, Snaith M. Tamoxifen-induced tumor regression associated with dermatomyositis. *Br Med J* 1982; 284: 1674.
35. Akiyama C. Osada A, Sou K, et al. A case of dermatomyositis triggered by tegafur. *Acta Derm Venereol (Stockh)* 1997; 77: 490.
36. Monk BL, Pembroke AC. Dermatomyositis after radiotherapy. *Br J Dermatol* 1983; (Suppl 24): 103.
37. Senet P, Aractingi S, Porneuf M, et al. Hydroxyurea-induced dermatomyositis-like eruption. *Br J Dermatol* 1995; 133: 455–459.
38. Bahadoran P, Castanet J, Lacour JP, et al. Pseudo-dermatomyositis induced by long-term hydroxyurea therapy: report of two cases. *Br J Dermatol* 1996; 134: 1161–1163.
39. Suehiro M, Kishimoto S, Wakabayashi T, et al. Hydroxyurea dermatopathy with a dermatomyositis-like eruption and a large leg ulcer. *Br J Dermatol* 1998; 139: 748–749.
40. Velez A, Lopez-Rubio F, Moreno JC. Chronic hydroxyurea-induced dermatomyositis-like eruption with severe dermal elastosis. *Clin Exp Dermatol* 1998; 23: 94–95.
41. Rocamora V, Puig L, Alomar A. Dermatomyositis-like eruption following hydroxyurea therapy. *J Eur Acad Dermatol Venereol* 2000; 14: 227–228.
42. Oh ST, Lee DW, Lee JY, et al. Hydroxyurea-induced melanonychia concomitant with a dermatomyositis-like eruption. *J Am Acad Dermatol* 2003; 49(2): 339–341.
43. Marie I, Joly P, Levesque H, et al. Pseudo-dermatomyositis as a complication of hydroxyurea therapy. *Clin Exp Rheumatol* 2000; 18: 536–537.
44. Varma S, Lanigan SW. Dermatomyositis-like eruption and leg ulceration caused by hydroxyurea in a patient with psoriasis. *Clin Exp Dermatol* 1999; 24: 164–166.
45. Daoud MS, Gibson LE, Pittelkow MR. Hydroxyurea dermatopathy: a unique lichenoid eruption complicating long-term therapy with hydroxyurea. *J Am Acad Dermatol* 1997; 36: 178–182.
46. Kirby B, Rogers S. Hydroxyurea-induced dermatopathy: a unique lichenoid eruption complicating long-term therapy with hydroxyurea. *J Am Acad Dermatol* 1998; 38: 178–182.
47. Bouldouyre MA, Avril MF, Gaulier A, et al. Association of cutaneous side-effects of hydroxyurea and neuroendocrine carcinoma. *Eur J Dermatol* 2005; 15: 268–270.
48. Katou Y, Kanoh Y, Bando M, et al. S-phase checkpoint proteins Tof1 and Mrc1 form a stable replication-pausing complex. *Nature* 2003; 424(6952): 1078–1083.
49. Krishnan K, Adams P, Silveira S, et al. Therapy-related acute myeloid leukaemia following immunosuppression with azathioprine for polymyositis. *Clin Lab Haematol* 1994; 16: 285–289.
50. Arnold JA, Ranson SA, Abdalla SH. Azathioprine-associated acute myeloid leukaemia with trilineage dysplasia and complex karyotype: a case report and review of the literature. *Clin Lab Haem* 1999; 21: 289–292.
51. Kamel OW, van de Rijn M, Weiss LM, et al. Reversible lymphomas associated with Epstein–Barr virus occurring during methotrexate therapy for rheumatoid arthritis and dermatomyositis. *N Engl J Med* 1993; 328: 1317–1321.
52. Bittar B, Rose CD. Early development of Hodgkin's lymphoma in association with the use of methotrexate for the treatment of dermatomyositis. *Ann Rheum Dis* 1995; 54: 607–608.
53. Chai C, White WL, Shea CR, et al. Epstein–Barr virus-associated lymphoproliferative disorders primarily involving the skin. *J Cutan Pathol* 1999; 26: 242–247.
54. Callen JP. Dermatomyositis and multiple malignancies in a patient treated with methotrexate. *J Surg Oncol* 1983; 24: 113–116.

24

55. Roddy E, Couriney PA, Morrisw A. Non-Hodgkin's lymphoma in a patient with refractory dermatomyositis which had been treated with infliximab. *Rheumatology* 2002; 41: 1194–1195.
56. Parker CW. Drug allergy (in three parts). *N Engl J Med* 1975: 292(10): 511–514, 732–736, 957–960.
57. Mackie BS, Mackie LE. Systemic lupus erythematosus-dermatomyositis induced by sulphacetamide eye drops. *Australas J Dermatol* 1979; 20(1): 49–50.
58. Fayolle J, Vallon C, Claudy E, et al. Dermatomyositis induite par l'isoniazide. *Lyon Med* 1975; 223: 135.
59. Bessen LJ, Green GB, Louie E, et al. Severe polymyositis-like syndrome associated with zidovudine therapy of AIDS and ARC. *New Engl J Med* 1988; 318: 708.
60. Dalakas MC, Illa I, Pezeshkpour GH, et al. Mitochondrial myopathy caused by long-term zidovudine therapy. *N Engl J Med* 1990; 332: 1098–1105.
61. Camus JP, Koeger AC, Nahoul K, et al. Isolated muscular tuberculosis treated with corticosteroids. Developing outbreak of dermatomyositis under rifampicin treatment. 2 cases. *Ann Med Interne* (Paris) 1987; 138: 524–526 [French].
62. Cotterill JA, Shapiro H. Dermatomyositis after immunization. *Lancet* 1978; 2(8100): 1158–1159.
63. Kass F, Straume S, Mellbaye OJ, et al. Dermatomyositis associated with BCG vaccination. *Scand J Rheumatol* 1979; 8: 187–191.
64. Mackie B. Dermatomyositis induced by drugs. *Aust J Dermatol* 1966; 8: 249.
65. Zangemeister WH, Weisner B. A progressive systemic sclerosis-like disease due to anticonvulsive therapy? *Fortschr Neurol Psychiatr Grenzgeb* 1977; 45(9): 501–507 [German].
66. Dimachkie MM, Vriesendorp FJ, Heck KA. Phenytoin-induced dermatomyositis: case report and literature review. *J Child Neurol* 1998; 13: 577–580.
67. Dietrich LL, Bridges AJ, Albertini MR. Dermatomyositis after interferon alpha treatment. *Med Oncol* 2000; 17: 64–69.
68. Gomez Rodriguez N, Zulaica Garate A. Development of dermatomyositis in a woman with rheumatoid arthritis treated with leflunomide. *An Med Interna* 2005; 22: 300–301 [Spanish].
69. Lee AN, Werth VP. Activation of autoimmunity following use of immunostimulatory herbal supplements. *Arch Dermatol* 2004; 140: 723–727.
70. Burger RA, Torres AR, Warren RP, et al. Echinacea-induced cytokine production by human macrophages. *Int J Immunopharmacol* 1997; 19: 371–379.
71. Hirahashi T, Matsumoto M, Hazeki K, et al. Activation of the human innate immune system by *Spirulina*: augmentation of interferon production and NK cytotoxicity by oral administration of hot water extract of *Spirulina platensis. Int Immunopharmacol* 2002; 2: 423–434.
72. Pugh N, Pasco DS. Characterization of human monocyte activation by a water soluble preparation of *Aphanizomenon flos-aquae. Phytomedicine* 2001; 8: 445–453.
73. Kovacs SO, Kovacs SC. Dermatomyositis. *J Am Acad Dermatol* 1998; 39(6): 899–920.
74. Hess E. Drug-related lupus. *N Engl J Med* 1988; 318: 1460–1462.
75. Price EJ, Venables PT. Drug-induced lupus. *Drug Safety* 1995; 12: 283–290.
76. Kubo M, Ihn H, Yazawa Y, et al. Prevalence and antigen specificity of anti-histone antibodies in patients with polymyositis/dermatomyositis. *J Invest Dermatol* 1999; 112: 711–715.
77. Wilson CL, Bradlow A, Wonjarowska F. Cutaneous problems with drug therapy in rheumatoid arthritis. *Int J Dermatol* 1991; 30: 148–149.
78. Kamenska V, Dourmishev L, Dourmishev A, et al. Quantitative structure–activity relationship modeling of dermatomyositis activity of drug chemicals. *Arzneimittelforschung* 2006; 56(12): 856–865.

Other Idiopathic Inflammatory Myopathies

Polymyositis

25

PM is a disease complex comprising heterogeneous groups of acquired muscle disorders. They are collectively defined as IIMs due to the presence of major clinical symptoms (muscle weakness, pain, and tenderness) and histologic signs of skeletal muscle inflammation.

PM can viewed as a syndrome of different causes that may occur separately or in association with systemic autoimmune or CTD and certain known viral or bacterial infections. Muscle inflammation may have a definite (i.e., viral, bacterial, or parasitic) or indefinite (i.e., idiopathic) etiology [1]. Certain bacteria, such as *Borrelia burgdorferi*, which cause Lyme disease [2] and *Legionella pneumophila*, which causes Legionnaire's disease [3] have been reported to induce PM. In the tropics, a bacterial pyogenic myositis known as tropical PM was reported, induced by *Staphylococcus aureus*, *Yersinia*, *Streptococcus*, or other anaerobes [4]. PM is found in patients with the acquired immunodeficiency syndrome (AIDS) [5], and it has been associated with other viral infectious agents such as influenza A or B [6–9], coxsackie B [10, 11], and hepatitis B virus [12]. Clinical symptoms such as myalgia and elevation of serum CK values in these patients were limited to a few days. Since specific regions of the viral RNA, a possible epitope of VPI shell protein synthesis of encephalomyocarditis virus, show significant sequence homology to the myositis-specific antigens (Jo-1 antigen or histidyl-tRNA synthetase) and myosin heavy and light chains, the picornaviruses are thought to be possible causative agents of myositis [13–16]. The most evidential connection of a viral induction of PM is found in retroviruses [17]. At least six different retroviruses have been associated with PM and IBM [18–23]. Monkeys infected with simian HIV [18], and human beings infected with HIV and HTLV-I, [19, 21] develop PM either as an isolated clinical entity or concurrently with other manifestations of AIDS or HTLV-1 infection [19, 21–24]. HIV seroconversion may coincide with myoglobulinuria and acute myalgia, suggesting that myotropism for HIV can be symptomatic early in the infection. The retroviruses are found only in occasional endomysial macrophages [21–24], and do not replicate within the muscle fibers or cause persistent infection [22–24].

Several animal parasites, such as *Trichinae*, *Trypanosoma cruzi*, *Shistosoma*, *Cysticerca*, and *Toxoplasma gondii* have been reported that can give symptoms similar to those of PM and produce a focal or diffuse inflammatory myopathy termed as parasitic PM [25].

Some drugs, such as d-penicillamine indicated for the treatment of rheumatoid arthritis [26] and zidovudine prescribed in AIDS patients [27], have been reported to induce a

L.A. Dourmishev and A.L. Dourmishev, *Dermatomyositis: Advances in Recognition, Understanding and Management,* © Springer-Verlag Berlin Heidelberg 2009

myopathy with endomysial inflammation. Other drugs, such as cocaine, heroin, emetine, ipecac, alcohol, chloroquine, steroids, and interferons can cause a toxic, noninflammatory myopathy that is histologically different from PM [16].

In patients with idiopathic PM, there are no skin lesions, family history of neuromuscular disease, history of contacts with myotoxic drugs or toxins, endocrinopathy, diseases of the nervous system or dysphonia, history of eye and facial muscle involvement, or decrease in muscle enzymes. The clinical hallmark of PM is the gradual onset over weeks to months of symmetrical proximal muscle weakness. Most of patients with PM have dysphagia due to the involvement of the oropharyngeal striated muscles and distal esophagus [28, 29]. Cardiac abnormalities such as tachyarrythmias, congestive heart failure, and myocarditis can be frequently seen in this patients [30, 31]. Half of PM patients have pulmonary involvement associated with antisynthetase autoantibodies [32, 33].

25.1 Autoantibody Defined Syndromes in PM/DM

25.1.1 Antisynthetase Syndrome [Anti-Jo-1 Antibody Syndrome]

The terms "antisynthetase syndrome" and "Jo-1 antibody syndrome" were introduced by Marguerie et al. [34] in 1990 and Ray et al. [35] in 1993 respectively. Antisynthetase syndrome is characterized by the presence of autoantibodies toward a subset of aminoacyl-tRNA synthetases, and a clinical syndrome consisting of myositis, symmetric nonerosive arthritis, interstitial lung disease, Raynaud's phenomenon, "mechanic's hands", unexplained low-grade fever, and other clinical features [33, 36, 37]. Patients with "antisynthetase syndrome" tend to have an acute onset of severe PM in spring, the HLA-DR3, HLA-DRw52, and HLA-DQA1*0501 haplotypes, an exacerbation of myositis with tapering of medications, moderate response to therapy, a 5-year survival rate of about 70%, and a fatal outcome in most cases from pulmonary complications [33, 36, 38–40]. Recently, in a study of 131 Caucasian patients with "antisynthetase syndrome" in the USA, it was reported that myositis onset peaked in March and April and that the disease predominates in male patients with PM [41].

Hyperkeratotic rhagadiform hand symptom (mechanic's hands) has been previously attributed only to antisynthetase syndrome with the incidence of 71%, and separately from PM and anti-Jo-1 antibodies syndrome [37]. The mechanic's hands skin lesion was originally reported to be a cutaneous marker for the antisynthetase syndrome [33]. Although not specific, mechanic's hands is a cutaneous marker of this syndrome in adults, signaling the potential for ILD. During the course of their Jo-1 syndrome, patients with autoantibodies to aminoacyl-tRNA synthetases express one or usually more characteristic signs of a spectrum of different organ manifestations, including myositis (PM/DM), ILD, arthritis (carpal tunnel syndrome, rheumatoid arthritis), features of connective tissue diseases (sclerodactyly, Sjögren's syndrome), calcinosis, mechanic's hands and capillary abnormalities (facial telangiectasia and Raynaud's phenomenon) [42]. The typical cutaneous lesions of DM were scarce and transient, mechanic hands however was constant. Anti-Jo-1 antibodies were detected in 75% of the cases. No malignancy was associated with this form of disease, except in one patient that presented melanoma 5 years later [37]. More recent observations, however, failed to support the specificity of this association [43]. Mechanic's hands can also be seen in cases of PM, classic DM, [43], amyopathic DM [44], and juvenile DM [45]. One reported patient with juvenile DM and antisynthetase antibodies presented with acral nonhealing cutaneous ulcers [45].

Schmidt et al. [42] investigated clinically and serologically 18 patients with Jo-1 syndrome, and compared them with those of 257 cases published in 15 case series and 30 case reports. Only three of their patients had the mechanic's hands sign (3/18, or 17%), compared to 21% of all reported patients. They concluded that there is a coincidence of mechanic's hands with anti-Jo-1 antibody in DM patients.

In one study in Barcelona, Spain, 25 of 124 patients (20%) with DM/PM had pulmonary involvement [37]. Interstitial lung disease is found in 50–70% of these patients [13, 32, 46] (see also Chapter 11). In fact, ILD in association with anti-Jo-1 (antihistidyl-tRNA synthetase) antibodies may occur in patients with minimal or no evidence of myositis. A polyarthritis occurs in approximately 70% of these patients, and Raynaud's phenomenon is common. The presence of characteristic nailfold changes and serum aspartate aminotransferase and ferritin levels were higher in patients with anti-Jo-1 antibody syndrome associated with ILD [47].

Recently, PM synthetase overlap syndrome observed in 29 patients has been reported [48]. This syndrome is characterized by myositis, ILD, arthritis, and Raynaud's phenomenon in association with anti-aminoacyl transfer RNA synthetase antibodies, mainly with antihistidyl-tRNA synthetase (anti-Jo-1). In over 85% of cases, a genetic association with DQA1*0501 alleles was found. Cutaneous scleroderma-like changes of the face and hands have been more frequently observed (65.4%) that those characteristics for DM type (42.3%) such as Gottron's papules, Gottron sign and periorbital heliotrope rash. The onset of disease is usually acute with fever, and the course moderate or severe. A 58-year-old man with occupational PM chronically exposed to vinyl chloride with availability of antihistidyl-t-RNA-synthetase antibody has been reported [49].

The muscle biopsy findings in patients with Jo-1 antibody syndrome have differed from pathological patterns in DM, PM, and IBM [50]. The myopathology in 11 patients with Jo-1 antibody syndrome consistently included regions of fragmented, rarefied perimysial connective tissue with macrophage-predominant inflammation [50]. Perifascicular myopathic changes, including atrophy, regenerating muscle fibers, and some muscle fiber necrosis, were most common in regions near the connective tissue pathology, and were most prominent in patients with more severe weakness. The pathology in perimysial connective tissue in patients with Jo-1 antibody syndrome is similar to that seen in patients with fasciitis. Alkaline phosphatase staining of the perimisium was frequently positive (91%). Unlike many other inflammatory myopathies, inflammation in endomysial and perivascular regions in Jo-1 syndrome was uncommon [50], and in contrast with DM the capillary density was normal.

25.1.2
Anti-Signal Recognition Particle Syndrome [Anti-SRP Syndrome]

Patients with anti-signal recognition particle syndrome, often black women, have an acute onset of severe PM with myalgias and cardiac involvement with palpitations. They are

25

frequently HLA-DR5, HLA-DRw52, and HLA-DQA1*0301 genotype carriers and have a poor response to standard corticosteroid therapy, show frequent exacerbation and have a 5-year survival rate of only 25% due to cardiac complications [15, 33, 39, 40, 51]. A milder illness has recently been described in some patients [52]. The peak of the disease onset in patients with anti-SRP-positive myositis is between September and February [51]. In contrast to previous findings, patients with anti-SRP autoantibodies in the USA do not have significant seasonal variations in disease onset [41]. Association between cardiac involvement and anti-signal recognition particle (SRP) antibodies has been reported, largely based on two studies in the past decade that included a total of 20 patients with those antibodies [15, 33]. Of these patients, only one was diagnosed with a true cardiomyopathy. Most patients had associated cardiac palpitations by report with no further investigative studies. More recent evidence suggests that anti-SRP antibodies are not quite specific for PM, and may not contribute to cardiac involvement to the degree that was suspected [52, 53]. In a recent study of 23 patients with autoantibodies directed against SRP, three patients were diagnosed with dermatomyositis, whereas all others had polymyositis [54]. Muscle involvement included marked muscle weakness in 22 of 23 patients, and dyspnoea on exertion was present in half of the patients, whereas palpitations, or symptoms of heart failure and chest pain were found in less than 20% of patients. None of the patients with anti-SRP autoantibodies had capillary abnormalities in muscle biopsies, nor did they show capillary deposition of complement deposits, suggesting that the myopathy could be secondary to multifocal ischemia [54].

The presence of novel anti-7SL RNA autoantibodies appeared to be associated with DM and finger swelling with PM patients [55]. The seasonal onset of the disease for Japanese PM/DM patients was different in those with anti-7SL RNA antibodies, who developed the illness between October and January from that of patients without these antibodies, who developed it between June and August [55].

References

1. Krajac I. Dermatomyositis: diagnosis and evolution of dermatomyositis, polymyositis and inclusion-body myositis. *Adv Exp Med Biol* 1999; 455: 181–186.
2. Atlas E, Novak SN, Duray RD, et al. Lyme myositis: muscle invasion by *Borrelia burgdorferi*. *Ann Intern Med* 1988; 109: 245–256.
3. Warner CL, Fayad PB, Heffner RR Jr. Legionella myositis. *Neurology* 1991; 41: 750–752.
4. Shepherd JJ. Tropical myositis: is it an entity and what is its cause? *Lancet* 1983; 2: 1240–1242.
5. Gaut P, Wong PK, Myer RD. Polymyositis in a patient with the acquired immunodeficiency syndrome. *Arch Intern Med* 1988; 148: 1608–1610.
6. Middleton PJ, Alexander RM, Szymanski MT. Severe myositis during recovery from influenza. *Lancet* 1970; 2: 533–535.
7. Mejlszenkier JD, Safran AP, Healy JJ, et al. The myositis of influenza. *Arch Neurol* 1973; 29: 441–443.
8. Koch M, Brody JA, Nemo GJ, et al. Antibody levels to parainfluenza, rubella, measles, and influenza A virus in children with polymyositis. *Arthritis Rheum* 1975; 18: 353–355.
9. Dietzman DE, Schaller AP, Ray CG, et al. Acute myositis associated with influenza B infection. *Pediatrics* 1976; 57: 255–258.

10. Schiraldi O, Iandolo E. Polymyositis accompanying coxsackie virus B2 infection. *Infection* 1978; 6: 32–34.
11. Gyorkey F, Cabral GA, Gyorkey PK, et al. Coxsackie aggregates in muscle cells of a polymyositis patient. *Intervirology* 1978; 10: 69–77.
12. Mihas AA, Kirby D, Kent SP. Hepatitis B antigen and polymyositis. *JAMA* 1978; 239: 221–222.
13. Walker EJ, Jeffrey PD. Sequence homology between encephalomyocarditis virus protein VPI and histidyl-tRNA synthetase supports a hypothesis of molecular mimicry in polymyositis. *Med Hypotheses* 1988; 25: 21–26.
14. Targoff IN. Immunologic aspects of myositis. *Curr Opin Rheumatol* 1989; 1: 432–442.
15. Targoff IN. Immune mechanisms in myositis. *Curr Opin Rheumatol* 1990; 2: 882–888.
16. Dalakas M. Polymyositis, dermatomyositis and inclusion body myositis. *N Engl J Med* 1991; 325(21): 1487–1498.
17. Dalakas MC, Hohfeld R. Polymyositis and dermatomyositis. *Lancet* 2003; 362: 971–982.
18. Dalakas MC, London WT, Gravell M, et al. Polymyositis in an immunodeficiency disease in monkeys induced by a type D retrovirus. *Neurology* 1986; 36: 569–572.
19. Dalakas MC, Pezeshkpour GH, Gravell M, et al. Polymyositis in patients with AIDS. *JAMA* 1986; 256: 2381–2383.
20. Dalakas MC, Pezeshkpour GH. Neuromuscular diseases associated with human immunodeficiency virus infection. *Ann Neurol* 1988; 23 (Suppl): 38–48.
21. Morgan OS, Rodgers-Johnson P, Mora C, et al. HTLV-1 and polymyositis in Jamaica. *Lancet* 1989; 2: 1184–1187.
22. Leon-Monzon M, Illa I, Dalakas MC. Polymyositis in patients infected with HTLV-I: the role of the virus in the cause of the disease. *Ann Neurol* 1994; 36: 643–649.
23. Cupler EJ, Leon-Monzon M, Miller J, et al. Inclusion body myositis in HIV-I and HTLV-I infected patients. *Brain* 1996; 119: 1887–1893.
24. Illa I, Nath A, Dalakas MC. Immunocytochemical and virological characteristics of HIV-associated inflammatory myopathies: similarities with seronegative polymyositis. *Ann Neurol* 1991; 29: 474–481.
25. Banker BQ. Parasitic myositis and other inflammatory myopathies. In: *Myology*, Engel AG, Banker BQ (eds), McGraw–Hill, New York, 1986; 1467–1524.
26. Doyle DR, McCurely TL, Sergent JS. Fatal polymyositis in d-penicillamine-treated rheumatoid arthritis. *Ann Intern Med* 1983; 98: 327–330.
27. Dalakas MC, Illa I, Pezeshkpour GH, et al. Mitochondrial myopathy caused by long-term zidovudine therapy. *N Engl J Med* 1990; 332: 1098–1105.
28. Dietz F, Logeman JA, Sahgal V, et al. Cricopharyngeal muscle dysfunction in the differential diagnosis of dysphagia in polymyositis. *Arthritis Rheum* 1980; 23: 491–495.
29. DeMerieus P, Verity MA, Clements PJ, et al. Esophageal abnormalities and dysphagia in polymyositis and dermatomyositis: clinical, radiographic and pathologic features. *Arthritis Rheum* 1983; 26: 961–968.
30. Taylor AJ, Worthman DC, Burge JR, et al. The heart in polymyositis: a prospective evolution of 26 patients. *Clin Cardiol* 1993; 16: 802–806.
31. Anders HJ, Wanders A, Rihl M, et al. Myocardial fibrosis in polymyositis. *J Rheumatol* 1999; 26: 1840–1842.
32. Bernstein RM, Morgan SH, Chapman J, et al. Anti-Jo-1 antibody: a marker for myositis with interstitial lung disease. *Br Med J (Clin Res Ed)* 1984; 289(6438): 151–152.
33. Love LA, Leff RL, Fraser DD, et al. A new approach to the classification of idiopathic inflammatory myopathy: myositis-specific autoantibodies define useful homogeneous patient groups. *Medicine* 1991; 70: 360–374.

34. Marguerie C, Bunn CC, Beynon HL, et al. Polymyositis, pulmonary fibrosis and autoantibodies to aminoacyl-tRNA synthetase enzymes. *Q J Med* 1990; 282: 1019–1038.
35. Ray DW, Bridger J, Hawnaur J, et al. Transverse myelitis as the presentation of Jo-1 antibody syndrome (myositis and fibrosing alveolitis) in long-standing ulcerative colitis. *Br J Rheumatol* 1993; 32: 1105–1108.
36. Targoff IN. Humoral immunity in polymyositis/dermatomyositis. *J Invest Dermatol* 1993; 100(1): 116S–123S.
37. Herrero C, Grau JM, Lecha M. Anti-synthetase syndrome. *J Eur Acad Dermatol Venereol* 2000; 14(Suppl 1): 17.
38. Arnett F, Hirsch T, Bias W, et al. The Jo-1 antibody system in myositis: relationships to clinical features and HLA. *J Rheumatol* 1981; 8: 925–930.
39. Gurely RC, Love LA, Targoff IN, et al. Associations among myositis-specific autoantibodies (MSA) and HLA-DQA1 alleles. *Arthritis Rheum* 1991; 34(Suppl): S137.
40. Miller F. Myositis-specific autoantibodies. Touchstones for understanding the inflammatory myopathies. *J Am Med Assoc* 1993; 270: 1846–1849.
41. Sarkar K, Weinberg CR, Oddis CV, et al. Seasonal influence on the onset of idiopathic inflammatory myopathies in serologically defined groups. *Arthritis Rheum.* 2005; 52: 2433–2438.
42. Schmidt WA, Wetzel W, Friedländer R, et al. Clinical and serological aspects of patients with anti-Jo-1 antibodies — an evolving spectrum of disease manifestations. *Clin Rheumatol* 2000; 19: 371–377.
43. Watanabe C, Okubo Y, Ohi T, et al. A case of dermatomyositis associated with mechanic's hand. *J Dermatol* 2000, 27: 711–716.
44. Sontheimer RD. Dermatomyositis: an overview of recent progress with emphasis on dermatologic aspects. *Dermatol Clin* 2002; 20(3): 387–408.
45. Rider LG, Miller FW, Targoff IN, et al. A broadened spectrum of juvenile myositis. Myositis-specific autoantibodies in children. *Arthritis Rheum* 1994; 37(10): 1534–1538.
46. Yoshida S, Akizuki M, Mimori T, et al. The precipitating antibody to an acidic nuclear antigen protein, the Jo-1, in connective tissue diseases: a marker for a subset of polymyositis with interstitial pulmonary fibrosis. *Arthritis Rheum* 1983; 26: 604–611.
47. Marie I, Hatron PY, Levesque H, et al. Influence of age on characteristics of polymyositis and dermatomyositis in adults. *Medicine* 1999; 78: 139–147.
48. Jablonska S, Blaszcyk M. Scleroderma overlap syndromes. *Adv Exp Med Biol* 1999; 455: 85–92.
49. Serratrice J, Granel B, Pache X, et al. A case of polymyositis with anti-histidyl-t-RNA synthetase (Jo-1) antibody syndrome following extensive vinyl chloride exposure. *Clin Rheumatol* 2001; 20: 379–382.
50. Mozaffar T, Pestronk A. Myopathy with anti-Jo-1 antibodies: pathology in perimyium and neighbouring muscle fibres. *J Neurol Neurosurg Psychiatry* 2000; 68: 472–478.
51. Leff RL, Burgess SH, Miller FW, et al. Distinct seasonal patterns in the onset of adult idiopathic inflammatory myopathy in patients with anti-Jo-1 and anti-signal recognition particle autoantibodies. *Arthritis Rheum* 1991; 34(11): 1391–1396.
52. Hengstman GJ, van Engelen BG, Vree Egberts WT, et al. Myositis-specific autoantibodies: overview and recent developments. *Curr Opin Rheumatol* 2001; 13: 476–482.
53. Kao AH, Lacomis D, Lucas M, et al. Anti-signal recognition particle autoantibody in patients with and patients without idiopathic inflammatory myopathy. *Arthritis Rheum* 2004; 50(1): 209–215.
54. Hengstman GJ, ter Laak HJ, Vree Egberts WT, et al. Anti-signal recognition particle autoantibodies: marker of a necrotizing myopathy. *Ann Rheum Dis* 2006; 65(12): 1635–1638.
55. Satoh T, Okano T, Matsui T, et al. Novel autoantibodies against 7SL RNA in patients with polymyositis/dermatomyositis. *J Rheumatol* 2005; 32(9): 1727–1733.

"Inclusion Body" Myositis

26

Inclusion body myositis (IBM) belongs to the group of IIMs, but differs from PM and DM [1]. Since 1968, when Chou [2] originally described "myxovirus-like structures and accompanying nuclear changes in a patient with chronic PM", IBM has emerged as an apparently distinct and well-differentiated pathological entity among IIMs, with proposed diagnostic criteria [3] (Table 26.1). The term "inclusion body myositis" was coined by Yunis and Samaha [4] in describing a slowly progressive proximal myopathy affecting a young woman. The findings were similar to those reported 1 year earlier by Carpenter et al. [5], whose patient had both distal and proximal muscle weakness, and depressed or absent tendon reflexes. Subsequently, Carpenter et al. [6] reported six cases with a fairly homogeneous syndrome characterized by a protracted, painless disease involving distal as well as proximal muscles, loss of tendon reflexes, and predominantly affecting elderly men.

Population-based epidemiological data on IBM are scanty. An incidence of 2.2 cases/million population was reported from Sweden [7] and 4.9 patients/million inhabitants in the Netherlands [8]. When adjusted for age distribution, the prevalence was 16/million inhabitants aged over 50 years. The relative prevalence of disease in all IIMs was reported to vary between 16% and 28% in series from neuromuscular centers [9, 10]. Review of the reported cases revealed a considerable male predominance. The male to female ratio is 3:1 [3, 11]. The condition tends to affect the population over 50 years old; however, it may also occur in younger female, and a bimodal age–sex distribution has been suggested [12, 13]. Recent observations suggest the IBM differs from DM and PM since the epidemiology is more limited, the incidence and prevalence varies, clinic and histology present features of myopathy rather than myositis, as well as the fact that IBM responds only modestly or even not at all to immunosuppressive therapy [13]. Several groups with large number of patients with muscle disease have observed that IBM starts between 30 and 50 years [9, 14], but the most common cases of inflammatory myopathy were in patients over 50 years of age, due to slow development of weakness and difficulties in diagnosis [15]. Some argue that IBM should not be included among the IIMs since inflammation is often sparse and hence may play only a secondary role [16], and the response to anti-inflammatory therapy is recognized as at best modest.

IBM is sporadic, but diseases have been reported in twins [17], and cases with recessive or autosomal dominant inheritance [3, 18]. IBM has been observed in families

Table 26.1 Diagnostic criteria for inclusion body myositis (Adapted from [3])

Features	Criteria	Description
A. Clinical features	**1. Age at onset**	>30 years old Male predominance (male to female ratio is 3:1)
	2. Duration of illness	>6 months
	3. Proximal and distal muscle weakness of extremities including	(a) Finger flexor weakness
		(b) Wrist flexor > wrist extensor weakness
		(c) Quadriceps muscle weakness (equal to or less than grade 4 MRC) and/or atrophy
	4. Early loss of patellar and Achilles tendon reflexes	
	5. Therapeutic resistance	
B. Laboratory features	**1. Serum CK levels — normal or moderately raised**	
	2. Muscle biopsy	(a) Invasion of non-necrotic fibers by mononuclear cells
		(b) Vacuolated muscle fibers
		(c) Intracellular amyloid deposits or
		(d) 15–18 nm tubulofilaments by electron microscopy
	3. EMG	Features of inflammatory myopathy
C. Family history		

[19–21]. This condition is different from *hereditary inclusion body myopathy,* which is a rare autosomal dominant disease caused by mutations in the valosin-containing protein (VCP) gene [22]. The diagnosis of familial IBM requires specific histologic findings of the inflammatory component by muscle biopsy in addition to vacuolated muscle fibers, intracellular deposits of amyloid, and 15–18-nm tubulofilaments determined by electron microscopy. Familial cases have been reported in some ethnic groups [20] and cases with associated leucoencephalopathy [19].

Clinically, IBM presents with slowly progressive, sometimes asymmetrical painless weakness which predominantly affects the distal muscle groups, asymmetric muscle atrophy of the quadriceps, iliopsoas, triceps, and biceps muscles, early loss of patellar and Achilles tendon reflex and therapeutic resistance. IBM differs in its clinical presentation, as its hallmark is usually atrophy and weakness of the quadriceps and the wrist and finger flexors, producing predominantly distal rather than proximal weakness [13]. Fascial muscle weakness and dysphagia could be the early manifestations [23]. The involvement of distal muscles, especially foot extensors and finger flexors, is a early clue to clinical diagnosis in more than 50% of cases [1]. The distal weakness and the early loss of the patellar reflex resulting from severe weakness of the quadriceps muscle often raises suspicion of the presence of neurogenic disease [12].

In general, the serum muscle enzymes are within normal ranges, or only moderately elevated. EMG often reveals changes of denervation with fibrillations and large prolonged duration polyphasic potentials with late components on volitional activity [12].

Definitive diagnosis is confirmed by the histologic finding of endomysial inflammation with multiple membrane-lined basophilic acid phosphatase negative vacuoles, often containing basophilic masses, and occasionally eosinophilic inclusions. The typical "rimmed" vacuoles were observed in the muscle fibers, together with inflammatory infiltrates of mononuclear cells in the endomysium , atrophic fibers, sarcoplasmic, and intracellular filament inclusions [15]. The electron microscopic appearance in muscle biopsy is characteristic, and shows intracellular 15–18-nm tubofibrillar inclusion specimens as well as eosinophilic, cytoplasmic, and intracellular deposits of ectopic beta-amyloid, and ubiquitin [24, 25]. Immunocytochemical staining of biopsy muscle with SMI-31 monoclonal antibody, which recognizes the phosphorylated tau protein of paired helical filaments, also has a diagnostic value in sporadic IBM [26] The histopathological changes of IBM have also been reported in patients with DM [27, 28].

In only one population-based study of IIM including IBM, patients were reported to have an increased risk for the development of malignant disease after diagnosis, even if the first year after diagnosis was excluded (SIR = 2.7, 95% Cl = 2.3–8.1) [29]. Only 11 patients with neoplasms associated with IBM have been reported [30]. Cutaneous features of DM (erythema and periorbital edema, a "V"-shaped erythematous eruption on the upper chest) with normal levels of muscle enzymes, coupled with histology of IBM on muscle biopsy specimen and carcinoma of the urinary bladder, have been observed in one patient [28]. The authors suggest the diagnosis of possible IBM basis on the "rimmed vacuoles" in frozen muscle tissue but found no typical beta-amyloid deposition or filamentous inclusions in semithin or ultrathin sections [31].

In up to 15% of the cases, the IBM associates with systemic autoimmune or connective tissue diseases [19]. Similar cases with association of DM and IBM have been reported previously [9, 27], including some juvenile DM patients who later developed IBM [32]. Lane et al. reported a 53-year-old man with a prominent bluish/purple discoloration of the knuckles, thickening of the skin on the dorsum of the hands, and slight heliotrope facial rash. The facial muscles were slightly wasted and he had marked weakness and wasting of the sternomastoids, deltoids, spinati, biceps, and triceps muscles with relative preservation of distal muscles [27]. All upper limb reflexes were grossly diminished or absent. Muscle biopsies showed marked fibrosis with perivascular and endomysial lymphocytic infiltrations. Some of the fibers showed conspicuous vacuoles. The histologic criteria for classification as IBM were partial myophagia and the presence of "rimmed" vacuoles, along with additional fiber atrophy and endomysial fibrosis. Electron microscopic examination revealed the presence of both cytoplasmatic and intranuclear filament and numerous osmophilic membranous whorls [27].

In general, IBM excludes the presence of the anti-Jo-1 autoantibody in patient's sera [33]. However a 74-old man with IBM and anti-Jo-1 antibodies has recently been reported [34].

Three months after the initiation of treatment with prednisone (60 mg once daily) a marked improvement of muscle strength was found; serum CK normalized, the anti-Jo-1 autoantibody was no longer detectable and EMG demonstrated a significant improvement.

While the overlap syndrome of DM and PM with anti-PM-Scl-positive SSc is frequently reported, IBM has only once been described in association with anti-PM-Scl-positive SSc [35]. Recently, a 72-year-old patient with a 10-year history of anti-PM-Scl-positive SSc and "mechanic's hands" associated with IBM has been reported [36].

Proposed pathogenic mechanisms for the development of IBM of both the familial and the sporadic forms include:

(a) The concept of the increased transcription and accumulation of beta-amyloid precursor protein and its proteolytic fragments
(b) Abnormal accumulations of the components of lipid metabolism, including cholesterol, low-density lipoprotein receptor (LDLR), and very low-density lipoprotein receptor (VLDLR) immunoreactive inclusions; oxidative stress [37]
(c) Accumulations of Alzheimer's disease-related proteins [38]

Predisposing genetic factors such as the transthyretin Val122Ile mutation have also been proposed to contribute to the pathogenesis of IBM in select cases [39]. One variant of the apolipoprotein E gene, APO Eε4, was found increased in IBM patients compared with the general population [40]. Multiple mitochondrial DNA deletions in muscle fibers from IBM patients have been observed and a polymorphism, 1611C, in the coding region of mtDNA has been suggested as a potentially pathogenic role in IBM [40].

The most important step forward in the study of IBM in recent years was the identification of mutations in the UDP-*N*-acetylglucosamine 2-epimerase/*N*-acetylmannosamine kinase gene in the recessive familial quadriceps-sparing IBM first described in Iranian Jews but now more widely recognized [41].

At least retroviruses such as HIV-I and HTLV-I have been associated with IBM [42]. However, they are found only in occasional endomysial macrophages and do not replicate within the muscle fibers [42].

References

1. Dalakas M. Polymyositis, dermatomyositis and inclusion body myositis. *N Engl J Med* 1991; 325(21): 1487–1498.
2. Chou SM. Myxovirus-like structures and accompanying nuclear changes in a patient with chronic polymyositis. *Arch Pathol* 1968; 86: 649–658.
3. Griggs RC, Askanas V, DiMauro S, et al. Inclusion body myositis and myopathies. *Ann Neurol* 1995; 38: 705–713.
4. Yunis ET, Samaha FJ. Inclusion body myositis. *Lab Invest* 1971; 25: 240–248.
5. Carpenter S, Karpati G, Wolff L. Virus-like filaments and a phospholipid accumulation in skeletal muscle-study of a histochemically distinct chronic myopathy. *Neurology* 1970; 20: 889–903.
6. Carpenter S, Karpati G, Haller I, et al. Inclusion body myositis: a distinct variety of idiopathic inflammatory myopathy. *Neurology* 1978; 28: 8–17.

7. Lindberg C, Persson LI, Bjorkander J, et al. Inclusion body myositis: clinical, morphologic, physiological and laboratory findings in 18 cases. *Acta Neurol Scand* 1994; 89: 123–31.
8. Badrising UA, Maat-Schieman M, van Duinen SG, et al. Epidemiology of inclusion body myositis in the Netherlands: a nationwide study. *Neurology* 2000; 55: 1385–1387.
9. Lotz BP, Engel AG, Nishiono H, et al. Inclusion body myositis. Observation in 40 patients. *Brain* 1989; 112: 727–747.
10. Mhiri C, Gherardi R. Inclusion body myositis in French patients. A clinicopathological evaluation. *Neuropathol Appl Neurobiol* 1990; 16: 333–344.
11. Askanas V, Engel WK. New advances in the understanding of sporadic inclusion body myositis and hereditary inclusion body myopathies. *Curr Opin Rheumatol* 1995; 7: 486–496.
12. Eisen A, Berry K, Gibson G. Inclusion body myositis (IBM): myopathy or neuropathy? *Neurology (Cleveland)* 1983; 33: 1109–1114.
13. Christopher-Stine L, Plotz PH. Adult inflammatory myopathies. *Best Pract Res Clin Rheumatol* 2004; 18 (3): 331–344.
14. Dalakas MC, Sivakumar K. The immunopathologic and inflammatory differences between dermatomyositis, polymyositis and sporadic inclusion body myositis. *Curr Opin Neurol* 1996; 9(3): 235–239.
15. Petrov I, Kostov K, Ikonomov P. Inclusion body myositis: clinical and biopsy investigation. *Bulg Neurol* 2004; 4: 139–4143 [Bulgarian].
16. Plotz PH, Miller F, Hoffman E, et al. Workshop on inflammatory myopathy. Bethesda, 5–6 April 2000. *Neuromusc Disord* 2001; 11: 93–95.
17. Amato AA, Shedert RT. Inclusion body myositis in twins. *Neurology* 1998; 51: 598–600.
18. Neville HE, Baubach LL, Ringel SP, et al. Familial inclusion body myositis: evidence for autosomal dominant inheritance. *Neurology* 1992; 42: 897–902.
19. Cole AJ, Kuzniecky R, Karpati G, et al. Familial myopathy with changes resembling inclusion body myositis and periventricular leucoencephalopathy. *Brain* 1988; 111: 1025–1037.
20. Massa R, Weller B, Karpati G, et al. Familial inclusion body myositis among Kurdish-Iranian Jews. *Arch Neurol* 1991; 48: 519–522.
21. Mastaglia F, Price P, Walters S, et al. Familial inclusion body myositis in a mother and son with different ancestral MHC haplotypes. *Neuromuscul Disord* 2006; 16(11): 754–758.
22. Bersano A, Del Bo R, Lamperti C, et al. Inclusion body myopathy and frontotemporal dementia caused by a novel VCP mutation. *Neurobiol Aging* 2007 Sep 22 [Epub ahead of print].
23. Riminton DS, Chambers ST, Parkin PJ, et al. Inclusion body myositis presenting solely as dysphagia. *Neurology* 1993; 43: 1241–1243.
24. Prayson RA, Cohen ML. Ubiquitin immunostaining and inclusion body myositis: study of 30 patients with inclusion body myositis. *Hum Pathol* 1997; 28: 887–892.
25. Semino-Mora C, Amemiya K, Dalakas MC. Upregulation of IL-1b mRNA in inclusion body myositis (IBM) and coexpression with b-amyloid precursor protein: a mechanism for amyloid deposit. *Neurology* 1998; 50 (S4): A204.
26. Askanas V, Alvarez RB, Mirabella M, et al. Use of antineurofilament antibody to identify paired-helical filaments in inclusion-body myositis. *Ann Neurol* 1996; 39: 389–391.
27. Lane RJM, Fulthorpe JJ, Hudgson P. Inclusion body myositis: a case with associated collagen vascular disease responding to treatment. *J Neurol Neurosurg Psychiatry* 1985; 48: 270–273.
28. Talanin NY, Bushore D, Rasberry R, et al. Dermatomyositis with the features of inclusion body myositis associated with carcinoma of the bladder. *Br J Dermatol* 1999; 141: 926–930.
29. Buchbinder R, Forbes A, Hall S, et al. Incidence of malignant disease in biopsy-proven inflammatory myopathy. *Ann Intern Med* 2001; 134: 1087–1095.
30. Jensen ML, Wieting JM, Andary MT, et al. Inclusion body myositis and transitional cell carcinoma of the bladder: significant resolution of symptoms after tumour excision. *Arch Phys Med Rehabil* 1997; 78: 327–329.

31. Grau JM, Perea M. Dermatomyositis with the features of inclusion body myositis associated with carcinoma of the bladder: a true association? *Br J Dermatol* 2000; 143: 671.
32. Sivakumar K, Dalakas MC. Inclusion body myositis and myopathies. *Curr Opin Neurol* 1997; 10: 413–420.
33. Hengstman GJ, van-Engelen BG, Badrising U, et al. Presence of the anti-Jo-1 autoantibody in patient's sera excludes inclusion body myositis. *Ann Neurol* 1998; 44: 423.
34. Hengstman GJ, Terlak HJ, Van Engelen BG, et al. Anti-Jo-1 positive inclusion body myositis with marked and sustained clinical improvement after oral prednisone. *J Neurol Neurosurg Psychiatry* 2001; 70: 702–710.
35. Selva-O'Callaghan A, Mijares-Boeckh-Behrens T, Labrador-Horillos M, et al. Anti-PMScl antibodies in a patient with inclusion body myositis. *Rheumatology (Oxford)* 2003; 42: 1016–1018.
36. Kim S, Genth E, Krieg T, Hunzelmann N. PM-Scl antibody positive systemic sclerosis associated with inclusion body myositis. *Z Rheumatol* 2005; 64: 499–502.
37. Jaworska-Wilczynska M, Wilczynski GM, Engel WK, et al. Three lipoprotein receptors and cholesterol in inclusion body myositis muscle. *Neurology* 2002; 58: 438–445.
38. Askanas V, Engel WK. Unfolding story of inclusion body myositis and myopathies: role of misfolded proteins, amyloid-beta, cholesterol, and aging. *J Child Neurol* 2003; 18: 185–190.
39. Askanas V, Engel WK, McFerrin J, et al. Transthyretin Val122Ile, accumulated Abeta, and inclusion body myositis aspects in cultured muscle. *Neurology* 2003; 61: 257–260.
40. Oldorfs A, Fyhr IM. Inclusion body myositis: genetic factors, aberrant protein expression, and autoimmunity. *Curr Opin Rheum* 2001; 13: 469–475.
41. Eisenberg I, Avidan N, Potikha T, et al. The UDP-*N*-acetylglucosamine 2-epimerase/*N*-acetylmannosamine kinase gene is mutated in recessive hereditary inclusion body myopathy. *Nat Genet* 2001; 29: 83–87.
42. Cupler EJ, Leon-Monzon M, Miller J, et al. Inclusion body myositis in HIV-I and HTLV-I infected patients. *Brain* 1996; 119: 1887–1893.

Orbital Myositis

27

The rare involvement of the orbicularis oculi muscle in classic DM make the eyelids painful and tender [1]. Recently, several rare observed cases of orbital myositis in association with autoimmune rheumatic diseases have been reported [2–5]. Kokotis et al. [6], reported two patients with orbital myositis with orbital pain, proptosis, and exophthalmus in the course of previously undiagnosed DM, with red-purple edematous erythema on the upper palpebra and proximal muscle weakness and normal serum muscle enzymes. Orbital magnetic resonance imaging (MRI) was consistent with inflammatory myopathy of extrinsic ocular muscles. Marsani et al. [7] reported a 71-year-old woman who presented 10 years earlier a history of proptosis, initially unilateral but rapidly involving both eyes. She developed muscular fatigue and weakness of upper and lower limbs, and an inflammatory myopathy was diagnosed by muscle biopsy. Laboratory evaluation showed ANA with homogeneous pattern and titer 1:640; EMG of arm and leg muscles showed mild involvement confined to deltoid.

The clinical manifestation of ocular myositis should be distinguished from thyroid eye disease or Graves' ophthalmopathy, however, in ocular myositis; the inflammatory change is more diffuse and involves the whole muscle bellies and tendons [8]. Orbital myositis almost always leads to diplopia and/or ophthalmoplegia [9]. However, the absence of diplopia or ophthalmoplegia, an absence observed in 15% of the 52 patients with orbital myositis in Berkhoff et al.'s 1997 study, does not exclude the diagnosis [10]. Normal function of the affected muscles in 34 of 74 patients (45%) with idiopathic orbital myositis has also been observed [11].

There are three previously reported cases of idiopathic orbital myositis with giant cell myocarditis [12–14]. Three patients with bilateral periorbital erythema and edema, ophthalmoplegia, progressive heart failure, and endomyocardial biopsy-confirmed giant cell myocarditis have been reported [12]. Two patients died within days to months of the initial symptoms, but the third survived after cardiac transplantation. In 1989, Klein et al. [13] reported a 65-year-old woman with bilateral ophthalmoplegia. The extraocular muscles were thickened on CT. One month later, she developed a fatal cardiac arrhythmia. At autopsy, giant cell myocarditis was associated with a more diffuse extraocular and skeletal myositis without giant cells. The next year, Kattah et al. [14] reported a 37-year-old woman with bilateral painful periorbital swelling and ophthalmoplegia and extraocular muscles enlargement on CT. The patient improved subsequently with high-dose systemic

L.A. Dourmishev and A.L. Dourmishev, *Dermatomyositis: Advances in Recognition, Understanding and Management,*

27

corticosteroids, but after 18 months she developed fatal cardiac arrhythmia. Autopsy revealed giant cell myocarditis with an associated giant cell extraocular and skeletal myositis. In 1996, Stevens et al. [12] reported a 22-year-old white woman with bilateral periorbital edema and erythema, with proptosis and painful, limited extraocular movement. There was no ptosis and her vision, pupils, and fundi were normal. Vitiligo was present over the face, upper back, abdomen, and arms. Orbicular CT scan showed marked swelling of the extraocular muscles. The leukocyte count was $15 \times 10^9/l$, with 12% eosinophils, while ESR and CK levels were normal. An endomyocardial biopsy revealed findings of giant cell myocarditis. After failure to respond to a 7-day course of immunosuppressive therapy with cyclosporine, azathioprine, and high-dose corticosteroids, the patient underwent cardiac transplantation. Giant cell myocarditis is a rare idiopathic inflammatory heart disease characterized histologically by multinucleated giant cells and clinically by rapid, progressive heart failure, arrhythmias, or sudden death often within hours to days of initial symptoms [15]. Giant cell myocarditis should be monitored in the course of inflammatory orbital myopathy because of its life-threatening fulminant course.

References

1. Santmyire-Rosenberger B, Dugan EM. Skin involvement in dermatomyositis. *Curr Opin Rheumatol* 2003; 15(6): 714–722.
2. Billing K, Malhotra R, Selva D, et al. Orbital myositis in Churg–Strauss syndrome. *Acta Ophthalmol* 2004; 122: 393–396.
3. Younes M, Bejia I, Moussa A, et al. Oculomotor muscle involvement revealing dermatomyositis in a patient with rheumatoid arthritis. *Rev Med Interne* 2004; 25: 829–832.
4. Tsironi E, Eftaxias B, Karabatsas CH, et al. An unusually longstanding, strictly ocular, limited form of Wegener's granulomatosis. *Acta Ophthalmol* 2005; 83: 123–125.
5. Hattori H, Ohnishi S, Nakagawa Y, et al. An infant with idiopathic orbital myositis poorly responsive to steroid therapy: a case report. *Brain Dev* 2005; 27: 160–162.
6. Kokotis P, Theodossiadis P, Bouros C, et al. Bilateral ocular myositis as a late complication of dermatomyositis. *J Rheumatol* 2005; 32: 379–381.
7. Marasini B, Cossutta R, Massarotti M. Bilateral ocular myositis as a late complication of dermatomyositis. *J Rheumatol* 2005; 32(12): 2498–2499.
8. Liu DT, Chan AY. Bilateral ocular myositis as a late complication of dermatomyositis. *J Rheumatol* 2006; 33(3): 637.
9. Mannor GE, Rose GE, Moseley IF, et al. Outcome of orbital myositis: clinical features associated with recurrence. *Ophthalmology* 1997; 104: 409–414.
10. Berkhoff M, Sturzenegger M, Schroth G, et al. Ocular myositis. *Nervenartz* 1997; 68: 792–800.
11. Siatkowski RM, Capo H, Byrne SF, et al. Clinical and echographic findings in idiopathic orbital myositis. *Am J Ophthalmol* 1994; 118: 343–350.
12. Stevens AW, Grossman ME, Barr ML. Orbital myositis, vitiligo and giant cell myocarditis. *J Am Acad Dermatol* 1996; 35: 310–312.
13. Klein BR, Hedges TR, Dayal Y, et al. Orbital myositis and giant cell myocarditis. *Neurology* 1989; 39: 988–990.
14. Kattah JC, Zimmerman LE, Kolsky MP, et al. Bilateral orbital involvement in fatal giant cell polymyositis. *Ophthalmology* 1990; 97: 520–525.
15. Davis MJ, Pomerance A, Tear RD. Idiopathic giant cell myocarditis — a distinctive clinicopathological entity. *Br Heart J* 1975; 37: 192–195.

Eosinophilic Myositis/Perimyositis 28

Eosinophilic myositis/perimyositis (EM/P) is a diverse rare idiopathic inflammatory muscle disease, presenting with mass swelling, tenderness, pain and weakness, and associated with cutaneous lesions and peripheral and/or tissue eosinophilia [1]. EM is well described in the veterinary literature as it primarily affects the masticator muscles of dogs [2]; it has recently been discussed in the rheumatologic [3] and dermatologic literature [4, 5]. The spectrum of EM comprises a group of heterogeneous disorders affecting the muscles and their supporting connective tissue structures, with infiltration of mononuclear cells and/or eosinophils [5]. A clinical variant of EM have been termed "idiopathic eosinophilic myositis" [6], "subacute perimyositis" [7], or "relapsing eosinophilic perimyositis" [5, 8].

Relapsing eosinophilic perimyositis (REP) is a rare disease which appears as a part of the spectrum of eosinophilic myositis [5] and presents with an inflammation within perimysium and often epimysium without associated necrosis, in contrast with eosinophilic myositis, where a myonecrosis and inflammation of the endomysium appears. Only 12 patients with REP have been reported [3, 5, 8–10]. Trueb et al. (1995) described a 48-year-old Caucasian man with a 27-year history of relapsing febrile myopathy. The cutaneous manifestations included blotchy erythema overlying the swollen thigh muscles, Gottron's papules on the dorsa of the finger joints and erythematous papules on the palms. Laboratory findings showed peripheral blood eosinophilia $> 1.5 \times 10^9/l$ and histopathological features of eosinophilic perimysial inflammation [5].

Eosinophilic myositis/perimyositis [EM/P] encompasses a clinically and pathologically diverse group of rare, idiopathic, inflammatory muscle diseases associated with peripheral and tissue eosinophilia [3]. The term "eosinophilic perimyositis" was first coined by Serratrice et al. [8] in 1980. They described two patients with a benign relapsing myalgia involving the legs, with perimysial eosinophilic infiltrates, peripheral eosinophilia, normal CK levels, and no evidence of a systemic involvement. Later they claimed muscle involvement in eosinophilic fasciitis [10]. The cutaneous manifestations were, however, observed in only ten of 26 reported patients with EM/P [1]. The disease more frequently affects men, and the male to female ratio is 2.6:1. Skin manifestations such as cellulitis-like, deep subcutaneous indurations, erythema, angioedema, urticarial, and papular lesions are observed in 38% of patients [1]. Cutaneous biopsy specimens show a variable admixture of eosinophils, ranging from none to a widespread dermal infiltrate with eosinophilia

[1]. Elevated serum levels of CK, aldolase, eosinophilic cationic protein, and interleukin-5 are often detected [4]. Trueb et al. [4] reported a 39-year-old woman with a 2-year history of episodic swelling of the face, hands, arms, feet, and legs associated with pain and weakness of the proximal muscles of the arms and legs and joint pain of the hands and knees. The patient had elevated LDH and aldolase, and total eosinophil counts greater than 1.5×10^9/l. Muscle biopsy showed both perimysial and endomysial inflammatory infiltrates consisting of large number of eosinophils, but also of histiocytes and lymphocytes.

EM/P is a diagnosis of exclusion. The patients have to undergo a careful investigation for parasitic infestation or other eosinophilic disorders, such as l-tryptophan-associated eosinophilia–myalgia syndrome, eosinophilic fasciitis, drug-induced eosinophilic polymyositis from tranilast [11] or sulfisoxasol [12, 13], granulomatous eosinophilic polymyositis [14] or eosinophilic polymysitis [15]. Trueb et al. [4] reported a 44-year-old white woman with a 6-month history of recurrent pruritic urticarial skin lesions and plaques, with cutaneous swelling and erythema on the trunk and the extremities. The patient complained of a pronounced proximal muscle weakness of arms and legs. Laboratory studies revealed leukocytosis of (18.38×10^9/l), eosinophilia (32%), raised serum enzyme levels of CK and LDH, and elevated levels of soluble interleukin-2, IL-5, and GMCSF. Skin biopsy demonstrated a marked dermal infiltration predominantly with eosinophils forming a "flame figures" pattern. A muscle biopsy specimen showed eosinophilic infiltration in perimysial and endomysial areas. Of a total of 34 cases of idiopathic inflammatory muscle disease with eosinophilia hitherto published in literature,44% were classified as eosinophilic perimyositis, 35% as eosinophilic myositis and 21% as eosinophilic polymyositis [3, 5]. Among those with eosinophilic polymyositis, two had a poor outcome with cardiac and thromboembolic complications [14, 15].

Recently, a 9-year-old boy with eosinophilic PM has been reported [16]. Laboratory findings showed blood eosinophilia and raised serum transaminases and CK. Investigations for parasites were negative. His father, mother, and two siblings had normal results of laboratory tests. Muscle biopsy showed inflammatory myopathy with abundant eosinophils, no evidence of parasites, and no alteration of the membrane proteins dystrophin, sarcoglycan, and merosine. Corticosteroid treatment was not successful.

A case of eosinophilic gastroenteritis and PM occurring in the same patient is described by Sofat et al. in 2002 [17].

A 43-year-old man with an 8-year history of hypereosinophilia, persistent muscle pain, and mild weakness has been reported [18]. EMG and muscle enzymes were normal, but a needle muscle biopsy specimen revealed eosinophilic perimyositis. Treatment with methotrexate and corticosteroids was also ineffective.

A 51-year-old man with eosinophilic perimyositis and a monoclonal T-cell expansion has been reported [19]. The patient complained of exertional myalgias and muscle stiffness and mild proximal muscle weakness of the upper extremities and retraction of the digit flexors. Blood eosinophilia was present, but serum CK levels and an EMG study were normal. A skin–fascia–muscle biopsy of the calf revealed a macrophagic and CD4 + T-cell infiltration of the perimysium. T-cell expansion was observed in blood, bone marrow, and muscle. The patient showed a good clinical response to prednisone and azathioprine treatment.

Autopsy findings of EP in a 29-year-old woman have been reported [20]. Histological changes indicated tissue injuries, such as loss of muscle fibers, interstitial fibrosis, and infiltrates of lymphocytes in the skeletal muscles and heart but also in various visceral organs.

The etiology and pathogenesis of eosinophilic perimyositis remains elusive. It has been proposed that after an undefined triggering event such as an exposure to some unknown toxin, alcohol abuse, drugs, trauma, or other physical exertion, an increase in eosinophil production and activation, mediated by cytokines (GMCSF, IL-3, IL-5) appeared. This activation mechanism possesses an eosinophilopoietic activity and enhances eosinophilic cell survival and function, including leukotriene production [4].

As a rule, the outcome for most patients with EM is favorable and the overall prognosis is excellent. Moderate doses of corticosteroids are usually effective. The patients with eosinophilic PM with minimal manifestations limited only to one system other than the cardiovascular or nervous systems do not require specific therapy, but should be followed up at intervals of 3–6 months [4].

References

1. Trüeb RM, Pericin M, Winzeler B, et al. Eosinophilic myositis/perimyositis: frequency and spectrum of cutaneous manifestations. *J Am Acad Dermatol* 1997; 37: 385–391.
2. Roberts KE, Hanson P, Zaslow IM. Masticular myopathy in the dog. *Vet Med Small Anim Clinician* 1975; 70: 840–843.
3. Kaufman LD, Kephart GM, Seidman RJ, et al. The spectrum of eosinophilic myositis. *Arthritis Rheum* 1993; 36: 1014–1024.
4. Trüeb RM, Lübe J, Toriccelli R, et al. Eosinophilic myositis with eosinophilic cellulitis-like skin lesions. Association with increased serum levels of eosinophil cationic protein and interleukin-5. *Arch Dermatol* 1997; 133: 203–206.
5. Trüeb RM, Becker-Wegerich P, Hafner J, et al. Relapsing eosinophilic perimyositis. *Br J Dermatol* 1995; 133: 109–114.
6. Yonker RA, Panush RS. Idiopathic eosinophilic myositis with preexisting fibromyalgia. *J Rheumatol* 1985; 12: 165–167.
7. Fang MA, Verity MA, Paulus HE. Subacute perimyositis. *J Rheumatol* 1988; 15: 1291–1293.
8. Serratrice G, Pellissier JF, Cros D, et al. Relapsing eosinophilic perimyositis. *J Rheumatol* 1980; 7: 199–205.
9. Faugere MC, Mussini JM, Pellissier JF, et al. Myosites à eosinophiles et syndrome de Shulman. *Semin Hôpital Paris* 1981; 57: 158–162.
10. Serratrice G, Pellissier JF, Roux H, et al. Fasciitis, perimyositis, myositis, polymyositis, and eosinophilia. *Muscle Nerve* 1990; 13: 385–395.
11. Arase S, Kato S, Nakanishi H, et al. Eosinophilic polymyositis induced by tranilast. *J Dermatol* 1990; 17: 182–186.
12. Koch-Weser J, Sidel VW, Dexter M, et al. Adverse reactions to sulfisoxazole, sulfamethoxazole and nitrofurantoin. *Arch Intern Med* 1971; 128: 399–404.
13. Ellman L, Miller L, Rappeport J. Leucophoresis therapy of hypereosinophilic disorder. *JAMA* 1974; 230: 1004–1005.
14. Layzer RB, Shearn MA, Satya-Murti S. Eosinophilic polymyositis. *Ann Neurol* 1977; 1: 65–71.
15. Stark RJ. Eosinophilic polymyositis. *Arch Neurol* 1979; 36: 721–722.
16. Pena Segura JL, Adrados I, Jimenez Bustos JM, et al. Eosinophilic myositis in a 9-year-old boy. *Rev Neurol* 2001; 33(10): 960–963 [Spanish].

17. Sofat N, Pitcher M, Price A, et al. A case of weak muscles. *Ann Rheum Dis* 2002; 61: 10–12.
18. Zivkovic SA, Lacomis D, Clemens PR. Chronic eosinophilic perimyositis with persistent myalgias. *Muscle Nerve* 2002; 25(3): 461–465.
19. Dunand M, Lobrinus JA, Spertini O, et al. Eosinophilic perimyositis as the presenting feature of a monoclonal T-cell expansion. *Muscle Nerve* 2005; 31(5): 646–651.
20. Ishizawa K, Adachi D, Kuboi K, et al. Multiple organ involvement in eosinophilic polymyositis: an autopsy report. *Hum Pathol* 2006; 37(2): 231–235.

Eosinophilia–Myalgia Syndrome and Eosinophilic Fasciitis (Shulman Syndrome)

29

Severe myalgias, primarily of extremities with fasciitis, pulmonary, and cutaneous manifestations similar to those found in DM, occur in patients with eosinophilia–myalgia syndrome. The disease is associated with an ingestion of products containing L-tryptophan, an essential amino acid used over-the-counter for treatment of soft-tissue rheumatic syndromes, premenstrual syndrome, insomnia, depression, and avariety of neuropsychiatric disorders in some countries [1–3]. More than 1,000 cases with this syndrome have been reported in New Mexico, Oregon, and Minnesota, with symptoms of pain in the proximal muscles, stiffness, muscular weakness primarily of the extremities, occasional edema, prominent eosinophilia, and no evidence of parasitic disease [4–6]. Many features of eosinophilia–myalgia syndrome resemble the clinical manifestations occurring with the toxic oil syndrome observed in Spain during 1981, after the use of contaminated rape seed cooking oil [7–9]. A number of similarities exist between the acute phases of eosinophilia–myalgia syndrome and toxic oil syndrome. About one third of the cases with toxic oil syndrome progressed to a chronic form of the disease associated with scleroderma-like changes, joint contractures, sicca syndrome, Raynaud's phenomenon, peripheral neutropathy, pulmonary hypertension, and liver disease [10]. Toxic oil syndrome appeared in Spain, affecting more than 20,000 persons, predominantly female (61%), and causing over 2,500 deaths among people younger than 40 years of age [11]. When the Spanish toxic oil syndrome appeared, many authors asked why aniline or fatty acid anilides found in many samples of oil [7, 9] were permitted as an official adulterant for imported French rape seed oil, and why such adulterated oils were often illegally refined in Spain and marketed without difficulty [12]. Possible chemical links have been found between oil contaminants and those detected in L-tryptophan implicated in the eosinophilia–myalgia syndrome. On metabolic evidence, it is suggested that not one, but a group of toxic agents was responsible for toxic oil syndrome [12].

Cutaneous manifestations have been reported in 64–87% of patients with eosinophilia–myalgia syndrome [13, 14]. The most characteristic abnormality was the spectrum of sclerodermatous disease (50%), often after a subacute stage of peripheral or truncal edema. Eosinophilic fasciitis, consisting of induration and puckering of the skin was seen in 30% of cases, alopecia in 37%, and mucinous papules in 17% [14]. Histopathologic features in the skin included fibrosis in papillary dermis, dermal and fascial infiltrates consisting

29

of mononuclear cells, eosinophils in the perimysium, epineurium, and subcutaneous tissues and deposit of glycoaminoglycans in the dermis [14]. These findings suggested eosinophilic fasciitis in combination with sclerodermoid alterations [15, 16]. Muscle biopsy specimens showed type II muscle fiber atrophy and changes similar to the carcinoid myopathy [17]. Eosinophilia–myalgia syndrome does not appear to depend on daily dose, duration of administration, or total cumulative dose of L-tryptophan [2, 17]. The condition of all patients improves after L-tryptophan intake cessation, the initiation of corticosteroid therapy, or both [14, 17].

Recently, eosinophilia–myalgia syndrome-like symptoms have been associated with ingestion of or exposure to 5-hydroxy-L-tryptophan, a dietary supplement, an alternative to the previously banned L-tryptophan [18]. Using tandem mass spectrometric analysis, Klarskov et al. [19] were able to determine the chemical structure of a contaminant X1, previously found in eosinophilia–myalgia syndrome case-implicated 5-hydroxytryptophan. Peak X1 was identified as the putative neurotoxin 4,5-tryptophan-dione [19]. The presence of X1 varied from 0.5% to 10.3% of the amount of 4,5-tryptophan-dione present in case-implicated 5-hydroxytryptophan, and was found in samples of six over-the-counter commercially available products [19].

Recently, a case with non-L-tryptophan related eosinophilia–myalgia syndrome with hypoproteinemia and hypoalbuminemia has been reported [20].

It is suggested that L-tryptophan alone or its products can induce connective tissue matrix protein synthesis via a direct action on dermal fibroblasts or indirectly through the production of IL-1 and IL-4 cytokines, TNF-α, TGF-β, CTGF growth factors, or both [21]. Mast cells are prominent in the dermis of patients with eosinophilia–myalgia syndrome and the toxic oil syndrome [14, 22]. In vitro studies have suggested that the eosinophils are important factors in activation of DNA synthesis of fibroblasts [23].

29.1 Eosinophilic Fasciitis Syndrome (Shulman Syndrome)

In the same year when L-tryptophan was marketed in the USA as an over-the-counter food supplement, Shulman described the first case of "diffuse fasciitis with hypergammaglobulinemia and eosinophilia" [24]. Shulman Syndrome is a rare fibrosing disease characterized by the rapid onset of symmetric woody edema of extremities with a peau d'orange appearance and histologic presentation consistent with focal infiltration of muscle fascia by lymphocytes and eosinophils associated with L-tryptophan ingestion [15, 24–26]. In the study by Fujimoto et al. (1995), the skin thickening progressed to scleroderma-like changes of the shins and later of the face associated with myalgias and arthralgias, but without visceral involvement and Raynaud's phenomenon. Laboratory parameters included hypereosinophilia, hypergammaglobulinemia, and raised levels of serum aldolase [27].

Drug-induced eosinophilic fasciitis has been reported from phenytoin [28] and antituberculous therapy [29]. L-tryptophan is the first agent linked with eosinophilic fasciitis induction [25], despite the opinion that Shulman syndrome could be a drug- or toxin-induced condition [30].

References

1. Boman BL. L-tryptophan: a rational anti-depressant and a natural hypnotic? *Aust N Z J Psychiatry* 1988; 22: 83–97.
2. Hertzman PA, Blevins WL, Mayer J, et al. Association of the eosinophilia–myalgia syndrome with ingestion of tryptophan. *N Engl J Med* 1990; 322: 869–873.
3. Medsger TA. Tryptophan-induced eosinophilia–myalgia syndrome. *N Engl J Med* 1990; 322: 926–928.
4. Blevins WL, Hertzman P, Ting M, et al. Eosinophilia–myalgia syndrome — New Mexico. *MMWR* 1989; 38: 765–767.
5. Centers for Disease Control. Eosinophilia–myalgia syndrome and L-tryptophan–containing products — New Mexico, Minnesota, Oregon, and New York, 1989. *MMWR* 1989; 38: 785–788.
6. Eidson M, Philen RM, Sewell CM, et al. L-tryptophan and eosinophilia–myalgia syndrome in New Mexico. *Lancet* 1990; 335: 645–648.
7. Tabuenca JM. Toxic–allergic syndrome caused by ingestion of rapeseed oil denatured with aniline. *Lancet* 1981; 2: 567–568.
8. Toxic Epidemic Syndrome Study Group. Toxic epidemic syndrome, Spain, 1981. *Lancet* 1982; 2: 697–702.
9. Kilbourne EM, Rigau-Perez JG, Heath CW Jr, et al. Clinical epidemiology of toxic-oil syndrome. *N Engl J Med* 1983; 309: 1408–1414.
10. Phleps RG, Fleischmajer R. Clinical, pathologic, and immunopathologic manifestations of the toxic-oil syndrome. *J Am Acad Dermatol* 1988; 18: 313–324.
11. Sanchez-Porro Valades P, Posada de la Paz M, De Andres Copa P, et al. Toxic-oil syndrome: survival in the whole cohort between 1981 and 1995. *J Clin Epidemiol* 2003; 56: 701–708.
12. Diggle GE. The toxic-oil syndrome: 20 years on. *Int J Clin Pract* 2001; 55: 371–375.
13. Centers for Disease Control. Clinical spectrum of eosinophilia–myalgia syndrome — California. *MMWR* 1990; 39: 89–91.
14. Kaufman LD, Seidman RJ, Phillips ME, et al. Cutaneous manifestations of the l-tryptophan-associated eosinophilia–myalgia syndrome: a spectrum of sclerodermatous skin disease. *J Am Acad Dermatol* 1990; 23: 1063–1069.
15. Cotsarelis G, Werth V. Tryptophan-induced eosinophilic fasciitis. *J Am Acad Dermatol* 1990; 23: 938–940.
16. Senff H, Köllner A, Engelmann L, Woort-Menker M, et al. L-tryptophan-induziertes Eosinophilie–myalgie-Syndrome unter dem Bild einer diffusen Fasziitis mit Eosinophilie = Shulman-Syndrome. *Hautarzt* 1990; 41: 578–582.
17. Connolly SM, Quimby SR, Griffing WL, et al. A possible explanation of the eosinophilia–myalgia syndrome. *J Am Acad Dermatol* 1990; 23: 451–457.
18. Klarskov K, Johnson KL, Benson LM, et al. Eosinophilia–myalgia syndrome case-associated contaminants in commercially available 5-hydroxytryptophan. *Adv Exp Med Biol* 1999; 467: 461–468.
19. Klarskov K, Johnson KL, Benson LM, et al. Structural characterization of a case-implicated contaminant, "Peak X," in commercial preparations of 5-hydroxytryptophan. *J Rheumatol* 2003; 30: 89–95.
20. Margolin L. Non-L-tryptophan related eosinophilia–myalgia syndrome with hypoproteinemia and hypoalbuminemia. *J Rheumatol* 2003; 30: 628–629.
21. Varga J, Kahari VM. Eosinophilia–myalgia syndrome, eosinophilic fasciitis, and related fibrosing disorders. *Curr Opin Rheumatol* 1997; 8: 562–570.

22. Fonseca E, Solis J. Mast cells in the skin: progressive systemic sclerosis and the toxic-oil syndrome. *Ann Intern Med* 1985; 102: 864–865.
23. Pincus SH, Ramesh K, Wyler D. Eosinophils stimulate fibroblast DNA synthesis. *Blood* 1987; 70: 572–574.
24. Shulman LE. Diffuse fasciitis with hypergammaglobulinemia and eosinophilia: a new syndrome? *J Rheumatol* 1974; 1(Suppl): 46.
25. Martin R, Duffy J. Eosinophilic fasciitis associated with l-tryptophan (LT) use: a case control study. *Arthritis Rheum* 1990; 33(Suppl): R30.
26. Gordon ML, Lebwohl MG, Phelps RG, et al. Eosinophilic fasciitis associated with tryptophan ingestion: a manifestation of eosinophilia–myalgia syndrome. *Arch Dermatol* 1991; 127: 217–220.
27. Fujimoto M, Sato S, Ihn H, et al. Serum aldolase level is a useful indicator of disease activity in eosinophilic fasciitis. *J Rheumatol* 1995; 22(3): 563–565.
28. Buchanan RR, Gordon DA, Muckle TJ, et al. The eosinophilic fasciitis syndrome after phenytoin (dilantin) therapy. *J Rheumatol* 1980; 7: 733–736.
29. Seaman JM, Goble M, Madsen L, et al. Fasciitis and polyarthritis during antituberculous therapy. *Arthritis Rheum* 1985; 28: 1079–1084.
30. Lee P. Eosinophilic fasciitis – new association and current perspectives. *J Rheumatol* 1981; 8: 6–8.

Laboratory Manifestations of Dermatomyositis

Muscle Enzymes 30

Sarcoplasmic membrane muscle enzymes are released when damage of the muscle cell occurs or its membrane becomes defective. Serum muscle enzymes such as creatine kinase (CK), aspartate aminotransferase (AST), lactate dehydrogenase (LDH), alanine aminotransferase (ALT), and aldolase are often elevated in DM and PM. Changes in the levels of serum enzymes depend on the form and severity of inflammatory muscle disease, and the applied therapy.

Creatine kinase (CK) catalyze the formation of adenosine triphosphate and the donation of a phosphate group to creatine, the combination of which is used as a high-energy storage molecule responsible for the energy transport in muscle fiber according to the so-called "creatine phosphate shuttle" [1]. The enzyme is a dimer consisting of two subunits, M (muscle) and B (brain), either with sulfhydryl groups present at the active sites of the enzyme. CK isoenzymes MM, MB, and BB are characteristic for skeletal muscle, myocardium, and brain respectively. In addition to differences in the activity ratios of enzymes and isoenzymes, the extent of CK increase also provides important diagnostic clues. CK is found in numerous organs such as skeletal muscles, myocardium, and brain in the ratio 10:2.5:1 respectively, but also in thyroid gland, kidney, and liver. In inflammatory muscle disease such as PM or DM, CK levels in sera could be elevated more than 50-fold higher than the normal upper limit [2]. CK-MM subtype is the most sensitive and the most specific enzyme marker for skeletal muscle damage. The CK-MB isoenzyme, which is usually a hallmark of acute myocardial injury, may also increase in DM/PM [3–5]. Recently, Hamilton and Sharpe [5] reported two cases of inflammatory muscle disease presenting as either PM or DM with raised serum levels of CK-MB isoenzyme and troponin T in the absence of acute myocardial damage. B units of CK can be abnormally produced by regenerating skeletal muscle when these patients are treated with corticosteroids [4, 6]. Inflammatory muscle diseases are an important cause for the increasement of cardiac injury markers such as CK-MB and troponins, which are raised in up to 75% of PM/DM patients [7]. CK is not a specific marker for myositis; however, in inflammatory muscle diseases, as well as after physical exercise or traumatic muscle damage, it is the most often elevated enzyme [1] (Table 30.1).

The measurement of serum CK, which is widely used in the diagnosis and management of PM and DM, lacks both sensitivity [8] and specificity [3], leading to potential

30

Table 30.1 Causes of the elevated serum levels of creatine kinase (Adapted from Geigy Scientific Tables. Ed. C. Lentner, Ciba-Geigy, Basel 1984; 3: 173)

Conditions	References
I. Physical stress	
Sport and enlargement of skeletal muscle mass	Garcia W. *JAMA* 1974; 228: 1395
Acute psychosis and delirious states	Gosling et al. *Brit J Psychiat* 1972; 121: 351
Convulsions (e.g., in epilepsy or tetanus)	Mohr et al. *Med Klin* 1974; 69: 1112
Childbirth labor	Chemnitz et al. In: *Creatine Kinase Isoenzymes*, Springer, Berlin, 1984; 224
II. Traumatic muscle damage	
Direct injuries	Dubo et al. *Lancet* 1967; 2: 743
Extensive burns	Lafargue et al. *Biomedicine* 1977; 27: 244
Surgical interventions	Krafft et al. *Ann Clin Biochem* 1977; 14: 294
Intramuscular injections	Gloor et al. *Schweitz med Wschr* 1977; 107: 948
Diagnostic and therapeutic interventions	Reiffel et al. *JAMA* 1978; 239: 122
III. Hypoxic muscle damage	
Shock	Prellwitz and Neumier. *Internist* 1976; 17: 436
Myocardial infarction	Neumier et al. *Clin Chem Acta* 1977; 15: 131
Intoxications	Grabensee B. *Dtsch Med Wschr* 1976; 101: 976
IV. Toxic muscle damage	
Alcoholism	Song and Rubin. *Science* 1972; 175: 327
(Local) intoxications (intramuscular injections)	Gloor et al. *Schweitz Med Wschr* 1977; 107: 948
Drugs (anesthetics, bronchodilators, statins)	Schmidt et al. *Arzneimittel-Forsch* 1976; 26: 1455
V. Degenerative and inflammatory muscle diseases	
Myopathy	Hood et al. *Am J Clin Pathol* 1991; 95: 401
Myositis	Bohlmeyer. *Rheum Dis Clin North Am* 1994; 20: 845
Muscular dystrophy	Ohta et al. *Clin Chem* 1991; 36: 36
Myocarditis	Kinderman et al. *Dtsch Med Wschr* 1973; 98: 1609
Erysipelas	Nakafusa J et al. *Br J Dermatol* 2001; 145: 280
Trichinosis	Gentilini et al. *Bull Soc Path Exot* 1976; 69: 525
VI. Metabolic muscle damage	
Hyperthyroidism	Doran GR. *J Roy Soc Med* 1978; 71: 189

(continued)

Table 30.1 (continued)

Conditions	References
Hypothyroidism	Giampietro O et al. *Am J Med Sci* 1985; 289: 160
Myoglobinuria	Rose et al. *Neurology* 1996; 47: 119
Glycogenosis	Gerson et al. *Arch Path Lab Med* 1977; 101: 213
Hyperosmolar diabetes coma	Knight et al. *Diabetes* 1974; 23: 126
Malignant hyperpyrexia	Moulds and Denborough. *Br J Med* 1974; 2: 245

problems if the total serum CK concentration is interpreted as a direct measure of muscle disease activity. Furthermore, in such cases where the total CK is raised, an analysis of the CK isoforms is unreliable for determining the presence of myocardial involvement. This is because in chronic inflammatory muscle diseases, regenerating striated muscle contains up to 50% of the CK-MB isoform [9, 10]. This often results in an increase in the CK-MB to total CK ratio, with more than the 3% threshold commonly used to imply myocardial damage [10, 11].

CK levels in sera present sex and race variations, and are higher for healthy men than for women as well as being raised in African patients with inflammatory myopathies compared to Caucasian ones. Moreover, the elevation of the enzyme levels may at times precede the clinical symptoms of myositis. Fluctuations of serum level of CK usually correlate with changes in clinical manifestations of DM/PM. The MM subtype of creatine kinase is the most sensitive and the most specific enzyme marker for skeletal muscle damage. Determination of enzyme is used for confirmation of diagnosis, or for follow-up of the clinical course of disease and management of the treatment. According to Stonecipher et al. [12], CK levels in sera are elevated in 95% of patients with dermatomyositis at some point in their disease. These enzyme changes can give evidence themselves months before or after the changes in clinical course, as portending improvement or therapy failure [3, 13]. In a small number of cases, muscle enzyme measurements are not elevated even on repeated testing, and it is worth recalling that the serum level of CK tends to be low in some patients with CTD and high in some patients with hypothyroidism. Extreme elevations in CK are very rare in myositis, and should signal the need for a careful search for another diagnosis. Fudman and Schnitzer [14] reported that patients with DM who had a normal CK had a poor prognosis. Three of their seven patients had associated malignancy. Montagna et al. [15] also found that three of nine patients with normal CK had malignancy compared with five of 17 with elevated CK. CK levels can be normal in patients with concomitant CK activity inhibitors, early in the course of PM/DM, or after significant muscle atrophy [13, 16].

The levels of fructose-biphosphate aldolase (subtype A), an enzyme involved in glycolysis, lactate dehydrogenase (LDH isoenzymes 4 and 5), which converts lactate to pyruvate, and the aminotransferases — alanine aminotransferase (ALT) and aspartate aminotransferase (AST) — can be raised when the level of CK is normal in patients with inflammatory muscle disease [17, 18]. Aldolase (subtype A) in myositis patients is not a sensitive measure of muscle inflammation or response to therapy [18].

30

These enzymes are not sensitive measures for determination of muscle inflammation or response to therapy. Enzyme constellation of increased AST level > 50 U/L, CK/AST ratio > 40, and CK-MB fraction elevated more than 2% provide a specific and sensitive tool to separate PM [3]. Carbonic anhydrase isoenzyme III is found in slow-twitch skeletal muscles but not in the myocardium, and the enzyme is a more specific marker of inflammatory muscle disease than aminotransferases and LDH; however, the assay for this enzyme is not widely available [19].

In conclusion, muscle enzymes play an important role in diagnosing and monitoring of inflammatory muscle disease therapy. However, relying on any of these parameters alone yields either low sensitivity or low specificity for the evaluation of disease activity [20], particularly in those patients with amyopathic DM with normal enzyme levels and free from myositis.

References

1. Bohlmeyer TJ, Wu AH, Perryman MB. Evaluation of laboratory tests as a guide to diagnosis and therapy of myositis. *Rheum Dis Clin North Am* 1994; 20: 845–856.
2. Dalakas M. Polymyositis, dermatomyositis and inclusion body myositis. *N Engl J Med* 1991; 325(21): 1487–1498.
3. Hood D, Van Lente F, Estes M. Serum enzyme alterations in chronic muscle disease. *Am J Clin Pathol* 1991; 95: 401–407.
4. Kiely PD, Bruckner FE, Nisbet JA, et al. Serum skeletal troponin I in inflammatory muscle disease: relation to creatine kinase, CKMB and cardiac troponin I. *Ann Rheum Dis* 2000; 59: 750.
5. Hamilton JS, Sharpe PC. Two cases of inflammatory muscle disease presenting with raised serum concentrations of troponin T. *J Clin Pathol* 2005; 58: 1323–1324.
6. Bodor GS, Survant L, Voss EM, et al. Cardiac troponin T composition in normal and regenerating human skeletal muscle. *Clin Chem* 1997; 43: 476–484.
7. Prellwitz W, Hafner G, Rupprecht HJ, et al. Diagnostic and differential diagnostic value of troponins. *Med Klin* 1996; 91: 336–342.
8. Gunst JJ, Langlois MR, Delanghe JR, et al. Serum creatine kinase activity is not a reliable marker for muscle damage in conditions associated with low extracellular glutathione concentration. *Clin Chem* 1998; 44: 939–943.
9. Trask RV, Billadello JJ. Tissue specific distribution and developmental regulation of M and B creatine kinase mRNAs. *Biochem Biophys Acta* 1990; 1049: 182–188.
10. Panteghini M. Enzyme and muscle diseases. *Curr Opin Rheum* 1995; 7: 469–474.
11. Larca LJ, Coppola JT, Honig S. Creatine kinase MB isoenzyme in dermatomyositis: a non cardiac source. *Ann Intern Med* 1981; 94: 341–343.
12. Stonecipher MR, Callen JP, Jorizzo JL. The red face: dermatomyositis. *Clin Dermatol* 1993; 11: 261–273.
13. Kargen LJ, Aram S. Creatine kinase activity inhibitor in sera from patients with muscle disease. *Arthritis Rheum* 1987; 30: 213–217.
14. Fudman EJ, Schnitzer TJ. Dermatomyositis without creatine kinase elevation: a poor prognostic sign. *Am J Med* 1986; 80: 329–332.
15. Montagna GL, Manzo C, Califanc E, et al. Absence of elevated creatine kinase in dermatomyositis does not exclude malignancy. *Scand J Rheumatol* 1988; 17: 73–74.
16. Gran JT, Myklebast G. Adult idiopathic polymyositis without elevation of creatine kinase: case report and review of the literature. *Scand J Rheumatol* 1993: 22: 94.

17. Rosalki SB. Serum enzymes in disease of skeletal muscle. *Clin Lab Med* 1989; 9: 767–781.
18. Pachman LM. Juvenile dermatomyositis. *Pediatr Clin North Am* 1995; 42: 1071–1098.
19. Vuori J, Rasi S, Takala T, et al. Dual-label time-resolved fluoroimmunoassay for simultaneous detection of myoglobin and carbonic anhydrase III in serum. *Clin Chem* 1991; 37: 2087–2092.
20. Kroll M, Otis J, Kagen L. Serum enzymes, myoglobin and muscle strength relationship in polymyositis and dermatomyositis. *J Rheumatol* 1986; 13: 349–355.

Autoantibodies 31

DM and PM belong to a heterogeneous group of idiopathic inflammatory myopathies with autoimmune origin. Various characteristic autoantibodies against defined nuclear ribonucleic acids, and certain cytoplasmatic antigens involved in the process of protein synthesis, are found in up to 55% of patients with PM and DM [1]. The heterogeneity of the idiopathic inflammatory myopathies is also reflected over the autoantibody spectrum in the patient's sera. Anti-Jo-1 antibodies are the first characterized antibodies in patients with PM/DM [2]. Since the initial observation that interstitial lung disease is particularly frequent in patients with anti-Jo-1 autoantibodies [3–5], it has been recognized that several autoantibodies are strongly associated with certain clinical features [1].

Antibodies in DM are categorized in two groups: myositis-specific autoantibodies (MSAs) and myositis-associated autoantibodies (MAAs) [6]. The autoantibodies that are found only in patients with myositis and are specific for IIM are known as **myositis-specific autoantibodies (MSAs)** [1, 7, 8]. Others autoantibodies are commonly encountered in other CTDs without clinical signs of myositis. They are not specific for IIM, and are referred to as **myositis-associated autoantibodies (MAAs)**. The prevalence of these various autoantibody specificities have been studied in a large group of 181 European patients with dermatomyositis [9] and compared with similar studies of American and Japanese patients [1, 10, 11].

31.1 Myositis-Specific Autoantibodies

The myositis-specific autoantibodies are antigen-driven, arise months before the onset of myositis, remain of the same type over many years, correlate in titer with disease activity, disappear after prolonged remission, and bind to and inhibit the function of targeted human autoantigenic enzymes in in vitro assays [8]. There is no direct evidence that the MSAs play a pathological role, but the correlation of their titers with disease activity suggests that they are regulated by immune responses linked to those responsible for IIM. Most of these MSAs were arbitrarily named, before their target antigens were identified, by the letters of the name of the first patient in whom they were detected, followed by the number of the antibody seen in that patient (i.e., Jo-1, Mi-2), or by the number of the antibody immunodiffusion precipitin line found to be associated with a disease (i.e., Pl-7, PL-12) [8]. For example, "Mi" denotes the first two initials of the surname Mitchell of a 60-year-old patient with classic DM in whom the antibody was initially detected [12]. Myositis-specific autoantibodies are identified in approximately one third of the patients with PM/DM [7]. They are not associated with malignancy, and are less commonly associated with other myositis syndromes [1, 8]. These antibodies are directed against certain cytoplasmatic proteins, and transport RNA involved in the process of protein synthesis. It is noteworthy that juvenile MSA-positive patients exhibit similar clinical characteristics to adult patients with identical autoantibody profiles [13]. MSA have a strong genetic background. For example, Jo-1 antibodies are highly HLA DR3 associated [1, 14], whereas the HLA DR3 genotype is completely absent in all Mi-2 positive patients with dermatomyositis published so far in literature [1, 15, 16].

MSAs described in patients with idiopathic inflammatory myopathies are divided into four groups [8]. Their targets are: (i) the nuclear helicase/ATPase Mi-2, an anti-nuclear helicase complex composed of eight proteins [12, 17–19], (ii) aminoacyl-tRNA synthetases, transfer RNAs [3–5, 20, 21], (iii) components of the signal recognition particle (SRP) [22–24], and (iv) other rare, less-studied, and not well-determined MSAs such as anti-56 kDa, "MJ" antibody etc. [6, 25–27]. In fact, none of the MSAs occur with greater prevalence than one in five DM patients, which makes routine clinical testing for these autoantibodies relatively seldom used [28]. Nevertheless, positive MSAs have a highly predictive value for myositis [1, 6].

A first group includes autoantibodies to a 240 kD nuclear helicase protein complex of known as **anti-Mi-2** [8, 12]. Two autoantigenic forms of the Mi-2 antigen (Mi-2α and Mi-2β) have been reported [29]. The precipitating autoantibodies against a nuclear helicase or protein complex Mi-2 antigen detected by ELISA or Ouchterlony's immunodiffusion analysis are highly [30, 31], but not absolutely specific for DM [12, 32]. Autoantibodies against Mi-2 antigen are detected in approximately 20% of the sera of idiopathic inflammatory myopaties, and occur primarily in patients with treatment-responsive form of DM [30, 32], with prominent shawl sign and cuticular changes [33], and seldom in PM and IBM patients [6]. Anti-Mi-2 strongly associated with HLA-DR7 (88%), HLA-DQA1*0201 (86%) and a tryptophan on residue 9 of DRB1 was found in all patients with Mi-2 antibodies in sera [34]. HLA-DRB1*07, DQA1*02, and DQB1*02 were strong risk factors for the presence of anti-Mi-2 antibodies in sera versus controls [35].

The prevalence of anti-Mi-2 autoantibodies in European patients with classic DM in adults found in Brouwer et al.'s 2001 study was 21% [9], and its sensitivity is rather low. Anti-Mi-2 antibodies are found in between 5% and 10% of patients; however, over 95% of patients with positive anti-Mi-2 sera have had characteristic cutaneous features of classic DM in adults [7]. Approximately 10% of juvenile DM patients also possess this antibody. Anti-Mi-2 antibody is seldom present in DM associated with malignancy. Thus, this is the only autoantibody which is highly, but not absolutely specific for DM. Brouwer et al. [9] succeeded in finding anti-Mi-2 antibodies in 9% of patients with PM. Since anti-Mi-2 antibody is found in less than a quarter of DM patients it was not found useful in routine clinical testing [36].

The second group of autoantibodies is directed against one of six aminoacyl-transfer RNAs synthetases [2–5, 21], whose enzymes are critical components of the binding and

Table 31.1 Subsets of autoantibodies in DM

I. MSAs	1. Antisynthetase	Anti-Jo-1	Antisynthetase syndrome
		Anti-PL-7	Adult PM, DM
		Anti-PL-12	Adult PM, DM
		Anti-OJ	Adult PM, DM
		Anti-EJ	Adult PM, DM
		Anti-KS	Interstitial pneumonitis
	2. Anti-SRP		Anti-SRP syndrome
	3. Anti-Mi-2	Mi-2α, Mi-2β	Classic DM
	4. Other	Anti-56 kDa	Juvenile DM
		"MJ", anti-140 kD	Amyopathic DM
		Anti-CADM-140	Amyopathic DM
		Anti-Se antigen	Amyopathic DM
II. MAAs	1. PM/Scl		PM/SS, scleromyositis
	2. Mas		PM/SS overlap
	3. Ro/SS-A	Ro52	Adult PM, DM
		Ro60	Adult PM, DM
	4. La/SS-B		
	5. U1RNP		
	6. U2RNP		
	7. U3RNP	Anti-Myo 22/25	
	8. Anti-Ku		Scleromyositis

of the translation machinery, and each enzyme catalyzes the esterification of one amino-acid to its cognate tRNA (Table 31.1). These antibody systems predominantly occur in PM, but have also been detected in a small percentage of patients with DM. Furthermore, an individual PM/DM patient generally makes autoantibodies against only one of these synthetases.

The most commonly detected and best characterized MSA is the **anti-Jo-1 antibody** (anti-histidyl-tRNA synthetase), which is found in up to 25% of the myositis and 16% of the DM sera [1, 9, 20, 21, 37]. The Jo-1 antigen, histidyl-tRNA synthetase, is a cytoplasmatic protein that is usually visualized with speckled cytoplasm pattern fluorescence on ANA testing using HEp-2 cells [3, 20, 21, 38]. Identification of histidyl-tRNA synthetase was demonstrated by the evidence that anti-Jo-1 antibodies precipitated tRNA containing anticodon for histidine along a 50 kD immunoreactive protein dimer [39], and that IgG from anti-Jo-1 containing sera specifically inhibited the binding of histidine to the corresponding tRNA [21]. Anti-Jo-1 antibodies are detectable with different immunological methods, such as Ouchterlony's double immunodiffusion method [3, 20], immunoelectrophoresis [11, 40], ELISA [12, 41], and Western blot [42]. Anti-Jo-1 is 2–10 times more common in PM than in DM [7]. This antibody almost never occurs in patients with the myositis associated with malignancy, and has never been found in juvenile DM [43]. It has been suggested that anti-Jo-1 antibody is a marker for myositis with ILD [5].

Autoantibodies directed toward five other synthetases specific for alanine (**anti-PL12**), glycine (**anti-EJ**), isoleucine (**anti-OJ**), threonine (**anti-PL7**), and aspargine (**anti-KS**) have been reported to occur much less commonly [1, 9, 44–46]. These tRNA synthetase antibodies compose approximately 10% of patients with PM/DM in USA [43]. A new class of autoantibodies to aminoacyl-tRNA synthetase termed anti-KS, that recognized asparaginyl-tRNA synthetase, was recently described [44]. Unlike other antisynthetases, anti-KS antibodies were detected almost exclusively in patients with idiopathic interstitial pneumonitis without myositis [44, 47].

The third group of autoantibodies is directed against proteins of the signal recognition particle (**anti-signal recognition particle, anti-SRP**), and are a complex of RNA molecules and six proteins that escort newly synthesized proteins to the membrane of the endoplasmatic reticulum [22, 23, 48]. Anti-SRP autoantibodies have been detected in approximately 4% of patients with IIM, who show a distinct seasonal onset of disease, no association with other MSAs, and significant clinical prevalence of PM rather than DM and IBM [1, 22, 24]. The prevalence of SRP in European classic DM was 3% [9].

Novel autoantibodies against **7SL RNA of SRP** are identified in patients with PM/DM, and the presence of these antibodies was correlated to ethnic background, clinical features, and season of disease onset [48]. The immunoprecipitation analysis indicated that 50% of Japanese and 5% of North American patients with anti-SRP antibodies had these autoantibodies [48].

A fourth group of MSAs consists of rarer, unconnected autoantibodies such as an antibody against a nuclear 56-kDa protein, annexin XI [25–27], the "MJ" antibody, which reacts with a 140-kD protein [6], and PMS1, which reacts with a DNA repair enzyme [49].

MSAs to a **56-kD nuclear antigen**, annexin XI, are the most sensitive immunology marker for juvenile DM [27, 50]. Approximately 60% of patients with the classic form of juvenile DM have antibody against a 56-kD autoantigen, whose specificity correlates with the presence of the HLA-DQA*0501 allele [27]. This allele has been associated with the presence of maternal fetal microchimerism [51]. Autoantibodies to annexin XI have been associated with thrombosis in a broad spectrum of systemic autoimmune diseases [52].

Antibodies to 140 kD cytoplasm proteins have been reported in Japanese patients with amyopathic DM having interstitial lung disease [53, 54]. Since all eight patients with anti 140 kD antibodies in sera had clinically amyopathic DM (CADM), Sato et al. [54] have proposed the term **anti-CADM-140**. Anti-CADM-140 antibodies were detected in eight of 42 patients with DM, but not in patients with other connective tissue diseases [54].

Preliminary studies have indicated that a unique pair of new antibody specificities (155 kD and Se antigen) might also serve as serologic markers of patients with amyopathic DM [6, 55]. Recently, however, the autoantibodies 155-kD protein (**anti-p155**) have been found strongly associated with increased risk of malignancy in Caucasians with DM and

HLA – DQA1*0301 genotype [56]. Adult and juvenile DM patients with anti-p155 demonstrated a high incidence of cutaneous ulcers and other vasculitic skin lesions, as well as erythroderma and lipodystrophy [57].

A classification system based on the MSA profiles has been proposed as a useful alternative for classification into clinical groups [1]. Recent advances in serology suggest that a disease entity should be established by its serological characteristics as well as by its clinical and pathological features. Epidemiologic and clinical studies of more than 200 patients suggest that each group of these autoantibodies defines an IIM syndrome that is sufficiently distinguishable from the others in terms of immunogenetics, clinical manifestations, severity of disease, prognosis, and influence of therapy as to be considered a distinct disorder [1, 8, 24].

The most important clinical association is referred to as the "**antisynthetase syndrome**", which is characterized by the presence of autoantibodies toward a subset of aminoacyl-tRNA synthetases and clinically presents with myositis, symmetric nonerosive arthritis, interstitial lung disease, Raynaud's phenomenon, mechanic's hands, unexplained low-grade fever, and other clinical features [1, 7].

The prevalence of other antisynthetases, different from aminoacyl-tRNA in European classic DM, was less than 3% [9]. All the antisynthetase antibody-positive patients have a clinical picture similar to patients with anti-Jo-1. Myositis can be mild, and the cutaneous manifestations of DM are more common in these antisynthetase patients than observed in anti-Jo-1 antibody-positive patients. The pulmonary interstitial disease, however, is very common and may be rapidly progressive [58]. These antisynthetase DM/PM patients generally have recalcitrant disease with frequent relapses. Patients with the antisynthetase syndrome can be refractory to treatment [1, 8]. However, the prognosis of this syndrome is similar to those of seronegative classic DM if early and aggressive treatment with corticosteroids or immunosuppressive drugs is prescribed [59].

Recently, in a study of seven Japanese patients with anti-PL-7 autoantibodies, it was reported that these autoantibodies are closely associated with PM-SSc overlap as well as with ILD, arthritis, and sclerodactyly [45].

Another remarkable clinical association is the high incidence of anti-Mi-2 auto antibodies in sera of patients with classic DM, termed **anti-Mi-2 antibody syndrome**. Anti-Mi-2 antibodies are not completely specific for DM as has been suggested above, and also occur in 9% of patients with PM [9] (Table 31.2).

Patients with **anti-signal recognition particle syndrome** have an acute severe PM with myalgias and cardiac involvement with palpitations. Antibodies to the signal recognition particle are found almost exclusively in adult PM. Whereas the overwhelming majority of patients with anti-SRP up to now were reported to have PM [1, 22], and anti-Mi-2 was almost completely specific for DM [1, 12, 34], Brouwer et al. [9] mentioned several anti-SRP-positive DM and anti-Mi-2-positive PM cases, and even some patients with these autoantibodies and IBM. Moreover, a seasonal onset of the disease was observed for Japanese PM/DM patients with anti-7SL RNA antibodies, who developed the illness between October and January, in contrast to patients without these antibodies in sera, who had increased disease activity between June and August [48].

Table 31.2 Antisynthetase autoantibodies in DM/PM

Antibody	Target	Frequency (%)	Clinical features
Anti-Jo-1	Histidyl-tRNA synthetase	~20	Adult PM, DM, HLA-DR3, DRw52, DQA 1050, antisynthetase syndrome
Anti-PL-7	Threonyl-tRNA synthetase	~3	Adult DM, PM, antisynthetase syndrome
Anti-PL-12	Alanyl-tRNA synthetase	~3	Adult DM, PM, interstitial lung disease, antisynthetase syndrome
Anti-OJ	Isoleucyl-tRNA synthetase	~1	Adult DM, PM, interstitial lung disease, antisynthetase syndrome
Anti-EJ	Glycyl-tRNA synthetase	~1	Adult DM, PM, antisynthetase syndrome
Anti-KS	Asparginyl-tRNA synthetase	<1	Idiopathic interstitial pneumonitis without myositis

31.2 Myositis-Associated Autoantibodies

Antigens recognized by myositis-associated autoantibodies (MAAs) include the PM/Scl autoantigens, the Mas autoantigens, and components of the U1 small nuclear RNP (snRNP) with target spliceosome U1RNP particle or the cytoplasmatic Ro RNPs such as Ro60/SS-A, La/SS-B, and Ro52 [7, 9]. There are also myositis syndromes associated with autoantibodies that are not specific for myositis, such as anti-RNP [60].

Anti-PM/Scl autoantibodies recognize two components, PM/Scl-100 and PM/Scl-75, consisting of an RNA processing nuclear protein complex (11–16 proteins) named the exosome [61]. The Mas autoantigen is a $tRNA^{Sel}$-binding protein of about 48 kDa molecular weight, which plays a part in the pathway of seleno-cysteine incorporation [62, 63]. The U1 snRNP is involved in pre-messenger RNA splicing (mRNA splicing factor) [64] and is widely detected in patients with connective tissue diseases [40]. The function of the Ro RNPs has not been identified yet [65]. A very strong relationship has been identified between anti-Jo-1 antibody and Ro52 in DM patients [6, 37, 66, 67].

On rare occasions, anti-KJ antibodies against unidentified cytoplasmic protein have been detected in patients with PM and ILD, who developed clinical manifestations similar to the antisynthetase syndrome [43, 67].

A group of antibodies with distinct specificity have been detected in patients with a myositis–scleroderma overlap syndrome. These antibodies are anti-PM-Scl (PM-Scl), anti-Ku, anti-U1RNP, and anti-U2RNP [40].

Anti-PM-Scl antibodies are strongly associated with the HLA-DR3 haplotype, which is found in 75–100% of patients with anti-PM-Scl but in 30% of the normal Caucasian population [40]. Scleromyositis is a syndrome combining clinical features of DM and SSc, but differing from both by a chronic and relatively benign course and association with highly characteristic PM-Scl antibody [68]. Almost all patients with scleromyositis associated with PM-Scl antibodies had HLA- DQA1*0501 and 94% HLA-DRB1*0301 suballeles [69]. It has been reported that almost 50% of patients with anti-PM-Scl have myositis–scleroderma overlap and about 85% of them are HLA- DQw2 allele carriers [70]. Since HLA-DR3 is found in less than 1% of the Japanese population, anti-PM-Scl antibodies are not detected in Japanese patients with myositis overlap syndrome. One of the reasons for this ethnic discrepancy of anti-PM-Scl appears to be attributed to the genetic background [40].

Anti-Ku antibodies were first described in patients with PM/DM-Scl overlap syndrome in the Japanese population [71]. Later, the same autoantibodues were described in the Caucasian population [72] and in patients with scleromyositis (DM-SSc overlap syndrome), who had a good prognosis [73]. The target antigen of anti-Ku antibodies is a regulatory subunit of DNA-dependent protein kinase (DNA-PK) [74, 75] (Table 31.3).

In addition, rare antibodies including anti-KJ, anti-Fer, anti-Mas, and anti-U2 small nuclear ribonucleoprotein (snRNP) antibodies have also been reported in patients with PM-Scl overlap syndrome [7]. Anti-KJ antibody has been reported also in patients with PM and ILD [67].

Anti-Myo 22/25 antibodies against a U3 snRNP were detected in four (8%) of 53 serum samples from patients with PM/DM by RNA immunoprecipitation [76]. Three of the four PM/DM patients had other identified autoantibodies including anti-PL-12 antibodies, antihistone antibodies (AHA), anti-SS-A antibodies and anti-SS-B antibodies defined by double immunodiffusion, ELISA, or RNA immunoprecipitation. There were no significant correlations between the presence of anti-Myo 22/25 antibodies and distinct clinical or laboratory findings [76].

An overlap syndrome of myositis with Sjögren's syndrome or systemic lupus erythematosus (SLE) has been found to be associated with anti-Ro (SS-A) antibodies [43] (Table 31.4).

The determination of ANA on HEp-2 cells substrate is widely used as a screening test for different autoimmune diseases, particularly the idiopathic inflammatory myopathies. Approximately 80–90% of DM/PM patients demonstrate significant ANA titers [37, 77]. ANA, however, are not useful in distinguishing from other connective tissue diseases such as systemic LE and systemic sclerosis [77]. Solomon et al. [78] analyzed all studies concerning ANA in association with PM/DM and concluded that the sensitivity was 61% and specificity 63%, and the positive and negative likelihood ratios were 1.7 and 0.6 respectively. Moreover, ANA with low titers may appear in sera of healthy individuals [79] in some physiological conditions such as pregnancy, could be identified in the course of chronic infections or malignancies, or may be induced by certain drugs, such as procainamide and hydralazine [80]. In juvenile DM, ANA titers greater than 1:160, occurring in a minority of patients, do not correlate with disease activity, usually return to normal after successful treatment, and are associated with the presence of immune complexes [81]. These antibodies are found positive also in most of published patients with amyopathic DM [28]. ANA testing is, therefore, not a valid parameter for establishing a diagnosis of PM/DM. The results of tests for ANA frequently are positive in juvenile DM, but MSA are much less frequently found in juvenile DM than in adult patients [13].

Other autoantibodies have been reported in serum of adults and children with DM. Cases of circulatory antibodies to human myoglobin [2] and skeletal muscle myosin [82] in PM patients have been published. Antibodies directed against endothelial cells have also been reported, and these patients have a statistically significant increased risk for ILD [83].

Table 31.3 Prevalence of autoantibodies in European patients with myositis

Autoanti-bodies	DM			PM			IBM	OS	Total		
	Brouwer R. et al. (2001)[a]	Ghirardello A. et al. (2005)[b]	Dourmishev L. et al. (2006)[c]	Dourmishev L. et al. (2006)[c]	Ghirardello A. et al. (2005)	Dourmishev L. et al. (2006)[c]	Brouwer R. et al. (2001)	Ghirardello A. et al. (2005)	Brouwer R. et al. (2001)	Ghirardello A. et al. (2005)	Dourimishev L. et al. (2006)[c]
Total	181 (100%)	22 (100%)	18 (100%)	198 (100%)	21 (100%)	6 (100%)	38 (100%)	3 (100%)	417 (100%)	46 (100%)	24 (100%)
MSAs											
Antisynthetase											
Anti-Jo-1	28 (16%)	3 (14%)	2 (11%)	43 (22%)	12 (57%)	1 (17%)	2 (5%)	0	73 (18%)	15 (33%)	3 (13%)
Other	5 (3%)	1 (4%)	n.d.	6 (3%)	2 (9%)	n.d.	1 (3%)	0	12 (3%)	3 (6%)	n.d.
Anti-SRP	5 (3%)	n.d.	n.d.	14 (7%)	n.d.	n.d.	1 (3%)	n.d	20 (5%)	n.d	n.d.
Anti-Mi-2	38 (21%)	6 (27%)	n.d.	17 (9%)	0	n.d.	3 (8%)	0	58 (14%)	6 (13%)	n.d.
MAAs											
PM/Scl	16 (9%)	0	0	18 (10%)	0	0	0	1 (33%)	34 (8,2%)	1 (2%)	0
Mas	2 (1%)	n.d	n.d	6 (3%)	n.d	n.d	0	n.d	8 (2%)	n.d	n.d
Ro/SS-A		5 (23%)	2 (11%)		8 (38%)	2 (33%)		0		13 (28%)	4 (17%)
Ro52	44 (24%)	n.d	2 (11%)	54 (27%)	n.d	1 (17%)	8 (21%)	n.d	106 (25%)	n.d	3 (13%)
Ro60	8 (4%)	n.d	0	5 (3%)	n.d	0	4 (11%)	n.d	17 (4%)	n.d	0
La/SS-B	6 (3%)	n.d	0	12 (6%)	n.d	1 (16,7%)	3 (8%)	n.d	21 (5%)	n.d	1 (4%)
U1RNP	7 (4%)	1 (4%)	1 (6%)	17 (9%)	1 (5%)	0	1 (3%)	2 (67%)	25 (6%)	4 (9%)	1 (4%)
Anti-Ku	n.d	0	0	n.d	0	1 (17%)	n.d.	1 (33%)	n.d	1 (2%)	1 (4%)

[a] Brouwer R et al. Autoantibody profiles in the sera of European patients with myositis. *Ann Rheum Dis* 2001; 60: 116.
[b] Ghirardello A et al. Myositis-specific and myositis-associated autoantibodies in idiopathic inflammatory myopathies: a serologic study of 46 patients. *Reumatismo* 2005; 57(1): 22–28.
[c] Dourmishev L, Wollina U, Hipler UC, et al. Myositis-specific and myositis-associated autoantibodies in dermatomyositis and polymyositis. *Clin Appl Immunol* 2006; 5(1): 533–537.

Table 31.4 Autoantibodies associated with scleroderma–myositis overlap syndrome

Antibody	Target	Frequency (%)	Clinical features
Anti-PM-Scl	Nucleolar protein complex	10	Scleromyositis, PM, SSc, increased frequency HLA-DR2
Anti-U1RNP	Splicesome U1RNP	10	MCTD; particle features of myositis, SSc, and SLE
Anti-Ku	DNA-dependent protein kinase	10	Scleromyositis, SLE, SSc, more common in Japanese

PM = polymyositis; SSc = systemic scleroderma; SLE = systemic lupus erythematosus; MCTD = mixed connective tissue disease

Antibodies (anti-ADAM 10) against 62 KD antigen in bronchial epithelial cells have been determined in serum of a patient with pulmonary fibrosis associated with DM [84].

Anticardiolipin (aCl) antibodies were found in juvenile and adult DM patients [85, 86]. In a study of 14 patients with juvenile DM, three patients were anticardiolipin antibodies positive, and in two of them severe vascular complications were observed [85]. The prevalence of either IgG or IgM aCL in PM or DM has been reported to be 8.3% [86]. In three of 18 cases with adult DM, both anti-cardiolipin IgM and IgG antibodies were found in 16.7% of cases respectively, but in none of six patients with PM [37]. The other study reported three patients with PM and DM associated with antiphospholipid syndrome (APS), suggesting the novel DM/PM + antiphospholipid overlap syndrome [87].

Widespread use of autoantibody testings however are not widely recommended, because it neither confirms nor excludes diagnosis. Autoantibodies are uncertain predictors of the prognosis, and in general are not helpful in monitoring therapy [88].

References

1. Love LA, Feff RL, Fraser DD, et al. A new approach to the classification of idiopathic inflammatory myopathy: myositis-specific autoantibodies define useful homogeneous patient group. *Medicine (Baltimore)* 1991; 70: 360–374.
2. Nishikai M, Homma M. Circulatory autoantibody against human myoglobin in polymyositis. *JAMA* 1977; 237: 1842–1844.
3. Yoshida S, Akizuki M, Mimori T, et al. The precipitating antibody to an acidic nuclear antigen protein, the Jo-1, in connective tissue diseases: a marker for a subset of polymyositis with interstitial pulmonary fibrosis. *Arthritis Rheum* 1983; 26: 604–611.
4. Hochberg MC, Feldman D, Stevens MB, et al. Antibody to Jo-1 in polymyositis/dermatomyositis: association with interstitial pulmonary disease. *J Rheumatol* 1984; 11: 663–665.
5. Bernstein RM, Morgan SH, Chapman J, et al. Anti-Jo-1 antibody: a marker for myositis with interstitial lung disease. *Br J Med* 1984; 289: 151–152.
6. Targoff IN. Update on myositis-specific and myositis-associated autoantibodies. *Curr Opin Rheumatol* 2000; 12: 475–481.

31

7. Targoff IN. Humoral immunity in polymyositis/dermatomyositis. *J Invest Dermatol* 1993; 100: 116s–123s.
8. Miller FW. Myositis-specific autoantibodies: touchstones for understanding the inflammatory myopathies. *JAMA* 1993; 270: 1846–1849.
9. Brouwer R, Hengstman GJD, Vree Egberts W, et al. Autoantibody profiles in the sera of European patients with myositis. *Ann Rheum Dis* 2001; 60: 116–123.
10. Hirakata M, Mimori T, Akizuki M, et al. Autoantibodies to small nuclear and cytoplasmatic ribonucleoproteins in Japanese patients with inflammatory muscle disease. *Arthritis Rheum* 1992; 35: 449–456.
11. Arnett FC, Targoff IN, Mimori T, et al. Interrelationship of major histocompatibility complex class II alleles and autoantibodies in four ethnic groups with various forms of myositis. *Arthritis Rheum* 1996; 39: 1507–1518.
12. Targoff IN, Reichlin M. The association between Mi-2 antibodies and dermatomyositis. *Arthritis Rheum* 1985; 28: 796–803.
13. Rider LG, Miller FW, Targoff IN, et al. A broadened spectrum of juvenile myositis. Myositis-specific autoantibodies in children. *Arthritis Rheum* 1994; 37: 1534–1538.
14. Goldstein R, Duvic M, Targoff IN, et al. HLA-D region genes associated with autoantibody responses to histidyl-transfer RNA synthetase (Jo-1) and other translation-related factors in myositis. *Arthritis Rheum* 1990; 33: 1240–1248.
15. Mierau R, Dick T, Genth E, et al. An update on HLA association of Mi-2 autoantibodies: the association with a tryptophan at position 9 of the HLA-DR beta chain is strong but not absolute. *Arthritis Rheum* 1999; 42: 1552–1553.
16. Mierau R, Dick T, Genth E. Less specific myositis autoantibodies? *Ann Rheum Dis* 2001; 60: 810.
17. Targoff IN. Immune manifestations of inflammatory muscle disease. *Rheum Dis Clin North Am* 1994; 20: 857–880.
18. Nilasena DS, Trieu EP, Targoff IN. Analysis of the Mi-2 autoantigen of dermatomyositis. *Arthritis Rheum* 1995; 38: 123–128.
19. Komura K, Fujimoto M, Matsushita T, et al. Prevalence and clinical characteristics of anti-Mi-2 antibodies in Japanese patients with dermatomyositis. *J Dermatol Sci* 2005; 40(3): 215–217.
20. Nishikai M, Reichlin M. Heterogeneity of presenting antibodies in polymyositis and dermatomyositis. Characterization of the Jo-1 antibody system. *Arthritis Rheum* 1980; 23: 881–888.
21. Mathews MB, Bernstein RM. Myositis autoantibody inhibits histidyl-tRNA synthetase: a model for autoimmunity. *Nature* 1983; 304: 177–179.
22. Targoff IN, Johnson AE, Miller FW. Antibody to signal recognition particle in polymyositis. *Arthritis Rheum* 1990; 33: 1361–1370.
23. Lütcke H, Dobberstein B. Structure and function of signal recognition particle (SRP). *Mol Biol Rep* 1993; 18(2): 143–147.
24. Leff RL, Burgess SH, Miller FW, et al. Distinct seasonal patterns in the onset of adult idiopathic inflammatory myopathy in patients with anti-Jo-1 and anti-signal recognition particle autoantibodies. *Arthritis Rheum* 1991; 34: 1391–1396.
25. Arad-Dann H, Isenberg D, Ovadia E. Autoantibodies against a nuclear 56-kDa protein: a marker for inflammatory muscle disease. *J Autoimmun* 1989; 2: 877–878.
26. Miller FW. Humoral immunity and immunogenetics in the idiopathic inflammatory myopathies. *Curr Opin Rheum* 1991; 3: 902–910.
27. Lutz JL, Fedczyna TO, Isenberg D, et al. The association of the DQA * 0501 allele and antibody to a 56 kD nuclear proteins in sera from patients with juvenile dermatomyositis. *Arthritis Rheum* 2001; 44: S293.
28. Sontheimer RD. Dermatomyositis: an overview of recent progress with emphasis on dermatologic aspects. *Dermatol Clin* 2002; 20(3): 387–408.

29. Seeling HP, Renz M, Targoff IN, et al. Two forms of the major antigenic protein of the dermatomyositis-specific Mi-2 autoantigen. *Arch Rheum* 1996; 39: 1769–1771.
30. Seeling HP, Moosbruger I, Ehrfeld H, et al. The major dermatomyositis-specific Mi-2 autoantigen is a presumed helicase involved in transcriptional activation. *Arthritis Rheum* 1995; 38: 1389–1399.
31. Zhang Y, LeRoy G, Seelig HP, et al. The dermatomyositis-specific autoantigen Mi2 is a component of a complex containing histone deacetylase and nucleosome remodeling activities. *Cell* 1998; 95(2): 279–289.
32. Roux S, Seelig HP, Meyer O. Significance of Mi-2 autoantibodies in polymyositis and dermatomyositis. *J Rheumatol* 1998; 25(2): 395–396.
33. Koler RA, Montemarano A. Dermatomyositis. *Am Fam Physician* 2001; 64(9): 1565–1572.
34. Mierau R, Dick T, Bartz-Bazzanella P, et al. Strong association of dermatomyositis-specific Mi-2 autoantibodies with a tryptophan at position 9 of the HLA-DRβ chain. *Arthritis Rheum* 1996; 39: 868–876.
35. Chinoy H, Salway F, Fertig N, et al.(AOMIC). In adult onset myositis, the presence of interstitial lung disease and myositis specific/associated antibodies are governed by HLA class II haplotype, rather than by myositis subtype. *Arthritis Res Ther* 2006; 8(1): R13.
36. Feldman BM, Reichlin M, Laxer RM, et al. Clinical significance of specific autoantibodies in juvenile dermatomyositis. *J Rheumatol* 1996; 23: 1794–1797.
37. Dourmishev L, Wollina U, Hipler UC, et al. Myositis-specific and myositis-associated autoantibodies in dermatomyositis and polymyositis. *Clin Appl Immunol* 2006; 5(1): 533–537.
38. Shi MH, Tsui FW, Rubin LA. Cellular localization of the target structures recognized by the anti-Jo-1 antibody: immunofluorescence studies on cultured human myoblasts. *J Rheumatol* 1991; 18: 252–258.
39. Rosa MD, Hendrick JP, Lerner MR, et al. A mammalian tRNAhis-containing antigen is recognized by polymyositis-specific antibody anti-Jo-1. *Nucleic Acid Res* 1983; 11: 853–870.
40. Mimori T. Autoantibodies in connective tissue diseases: clinical significance and analysis of target autoantigens. *Internal Med* 1999; 38: 523–532.
41. Nishikai M, Ohya K, Kosaka M, et al. Anti-Jo-1 antibodies in polymyositis or dermatomyositis: evaluation by ELISA using recombinant fusion protein Jo-1 antigen. *Br J Rheum* 1998; 37: 157–161.
42. Elkon K, Jankowski P. Fine specificities of autoantibodies directed against the Ro, La, Sm, RNP, and Jo-1 proteins defined by two-dimensional gel electrophoresis and immunoblotting. *J Immunol* 1985; 134: 3819–3824.
43. Provost TT, Flyn JA. Dermatomyositis. In: *Cutaneous Medicine, Cutaneous Manifestations of Systemic Diseases*, BC Decker, Hamilton/London, 2001; 82–103.
44. Hirakata M, Suwa A, Nagai S, et al. Anti KS. Identification of autoantibodies to asparginyl-transfer RNA synthetase associated with interstitial lung disease. *J Immunol* 1999; 162: 2315–2320.
45. Sato S, Hirakata M, Kuwana M, et al. Clinical characteristics of Japanese patients with anti-PL-7 (anti-threonyl-tRNA synthetase) autoantibodies. *Clin Exp Rheumatol* 2005; 23: 609–615.
46. Sato S, Kuwana M, Hirakata M. Clinical characteristics of Japanese patients with anti-OJ (anti-isoleucyl-tRNA synthetase) autoantibodies. *Rheumatology (Oxford)* 2007; 46(5): 842–845.
47. Hirakata M, Suwa A, Takada T, et al. Clinical and immunogenetic features of patients with autoantibodies to asparaginyl-transfer RNA synthetase. *Arthritis Rheum* 2007; 56(4): 1295–1303.
48. Satoh T, Okano T, Matsui T, et al. Novel autoantibodies against 7SL RNA in patients with polymyositis/dermatomyositis. *J Rheumatol* 2005; 32: 1727–1733.
49. Rosen A, Casciola-Rosen L. Clearing the way to mechanism of autoimmunity. *Nat Med* 2001; 7: 664–665.

50. Rider LG, Miller FW. Classification and treatment of juvenile idiopathic inflammatory myopathies. *Rheum Dis Clin North Am* 1997; 23: 619–655.
51. Artlett CM, Miller FW, Rider LG. Persistent maternally derived peripheral microchimerism is associated with the juvenile idiopathic inflammatory myopathies. *Rheumatology* 2001; 20: 1279–1284.
52. Jorgensen CS, Levantino G, Houen G, et al. Determination of autoantibodies to annexin XI in systemic autoimmune diseases. *Lupus* 2000; 9: 515–520.
53. Sathoh S, Hirakata M, Suwa A, et al. Antibodies to 140 kD proteins in Japanese patients with amyopathic dermatomyositis [abstract]. *Arthritis Rheum* 2001; 44: S205.
54. Sato S, Hirakata M, Kuwana M, et al. Autoantibodies to a 140-kd polypeptide, CADM-140, in Japanese patients with clinically amyopathic dermatomyositis. *Arthritis Rheum* 2005; 52(5): 1571–1576.
55. Sontheimer RD, Targoff IN, Trieu EP, et al. Antibodies to 155 kD and Se antigens in patients with clinically amyopathic dermatomyositis [abstract]. *J Invest Dermatol* 2001; 117: 466.
56. Targoff IN, Mamyrova G, Trieu EP, et al. A novel autoantibody to a 155-kd protein is associated with dermatomyositis. *Arthritis Rheum* 2006; 54(11): 3682–3689.
57. Santmyire-Rosenberger B, Dugan EM. Skin involvement in dermatomyositis. *Curr Opin Rheumatol* 2003; 15(6): 714–722.
58. Lamedica G, Parodi A, Peris G, et al. Polymyositis and pulmonary fibrosis associated with anti-PL-7 antibody. *J Am Acad Dermatol* 1988; 19: 567–568.
59. Herrero C, Grau JM, Lecha M. Anti-synthetase syndrome. *J Eur Acad Dermatol Venereol* 2000; 14(Suppl 1): 17.
60. Targoff IN. Idiopathic inflammatory myopathy: autoantibody update. *Curr Rheumatol Rep* 2002; 4: 434–441.
61. Allmang C, Petfalski E, Podtelejnikov A, et al. The yeast exosome and human PM-Scl are related complexes of 3 →5 exonucleases. *Genes Dev* 1999; 13: 2148–2158.
62. Gelpi C, Sontheimer EJ, Rodrigez Sanchez JI. Autoantibodies against a serine tRNA-protein complex implicated in contranslational seleno cysteine insertion. *Proc Natl Acad Sci USA* 1992; 89: 9739–9743.
63. Low SC, Berry MJ. Knowing when not to stop: selenocysteine incorporation in eukaryotes. *Trends Biochem Sci* 1996; 21: 203–208.
64. Klein Gunnenwiek J, van de Putte LB, van Verooij WJ. The U1 snRNP complex: an autoantigen in connective tissue diseases. An update. *Clin Exp Rheumatol* 1997; 74: 123–132.
65. Pruijn GJ, Simons FH, van Venroij WJ. Intracelullar localisation and nucleocytoplasmatic transport of Ro RNP components. *Eur J Cell Biol* 1997; 74: 123–132.
66. Frank MB, McCubbin V, Trieu E, et al. The association of antiRo52 autoantibodies with myositis and scleroderma autoantibodies. *J Autoimmun* 1999; 12: 137–142.
67. Targoff IN, Arnett FC, Berman L, et al. Anti-KJ: a new antibody associated with syndrome and polymyositis and interstitial lung disease. *J Clin Invest* 1989; 84: 162–172.
68. Jablonska S, Chorzelski TP, Blaszcyk M, et al. Scleroderma/polymyositis overlap syndrome and their immunologic markers. *Clin Dermatol* 1993; 10: 457–472.
69. Hausmanowa-Petrusewicz I, Kowalska-Oledzka E, Miller FW, et al. Clinical, serological and immunogenetic features in Polish patients with idiopathic inflammatory myopathies. *Arthritis Rheum* 1997; 40: 1257–1266.
70. Oddis CV, Okano Y, Rudert WA, et al. Serum autoantibody to the nuclear antigen PM-Scl. Clinical and immunogenetic associations. *Arthritis Rheum* 1992; 35: 1211–1217.
71. Mimori T, Akizuki M, Yamagata H, et al. Characterization of a high molecular weight acidic nuclear protein recognized by autoantibodies in sera from patients with polymyositis–scleroderma overlap. *J Clin Invest* 1981; 68: 611–620.

72. Reichlin M, Maddison PJ, Targoff I, et al. Antibodies to a nuclear/nucleolar antigen in patients with polymyositis-overlap syndrome. *J Clin Immunol* 1984; 4: 40–44.
73. Parodi A, Rebora A. Anti-Ku antibodies in connective tissue diseases. Report of three cases. *J Am Acad Dermatol* 1989; 21: 433–435.
74. Gottlieb TM, Jackson SP. The DNA-dependent protein kinase. Requirement for DNA ends and association with KU antigen. *Cell* 1993; 72: 131–142.
75. Suwa A, Hirakata M, Takeda Y, et al. Autoantibodies to DNA-dependent protein kinase. Probes for the catalytic subunit. *J Clin Invest* 1996; 97 (6): 1417–1421.
76. Kubo M, Ihn H, Kuwana M, et al. Prevalence in myositis of antibodies recognizing anti-U3 RNA probably in a novel complex with 22/25 kD protein and not fibrillarin. *Clin Exp Immunol* 2001; 126: 339–344.
77. Drake LA, Dinehart SM, Farmer ER, et al. Guidelines of care for dermatomyositis. *J Am Acad Dermatol* 1996; 34: 824–829.
78. Solomon DH, Kavanaugh HJ, Schur PH. Evidence-based guidelines for the use of immunologic tests: antinuclear antibody testing. *Arthritis Rheum* 2002; 47: 434–444.
79. Tan EM, Feltkamp TE, Smolen JS, et al. Range of antinuclear antibodies in "healthy individuals." *Arthritis Rheum* 1997; 40: 1601–1611.
80. van Paassen P, Damoiseaux J, Tervaert JWC. Laboratory assessment in musculoskeletal disorders. *Best Pract Res Clin Rheumatol* 2003; 17: 475–494.
81. Kovacs SO, Kovacs SC. Dermatomyositis. *J Am Acad Dermatol* 1998; 39(6): 899–920.
82. Wada K, Ueno S, Hazama T, et al. Radioimmuno-assay for antibodies to human skeletal muscle myosin in serum from patients with polymyositis. *Clin Exp Immunol* 1983; 52: 297–304.
83. Cervera R, Ramirez G, Fernandez-Sola J, et al. Antibodies to endothelial cells in dermatomyositis: association with interstitial lung disease. *BMJ* 1991; 302: 880–881.
84. Fujita J, Takeuchi T, Dobashi N, et al. Detection of anti-ADAM 10 antibody in serum of a patient with pulmonary fibrosis associated with dermatomyositis. *Ann Rheum Dis* 1999; 58: 770–772.
85. Montecucco C, Ravelli A, Caporali R, et al. Autoantibodies in juvenile dermatomyositis. *Clin Exp Dermatol* 1990; 8: 193–196.
86. Merkel PA, Chang Y, Pierangeli SS, et al. The prevalence and clinical associations of anticardiolipin antibodies in a large inception cohort of patients with connective tissue diseases. *Am J Med* 1996; 101: 576–583.
87. Sherer Y, Livenh A, Levy Y, et al. Dermatomyositis and polymyositis associated with the antiphospholipid syndrome — a novel overlap syndrome. *Lupus* 2000; 9: 42–45.
88. Trüeb RM. Dermatomyositis. *Dermatol Ther* 2001; 14: 70–80.

Laboratory Assessments of Disease Activity in DM

32

Various laboratory methods have been used in DM patients for determination of disease activity: (i) in the onset of disease — for confirmation of diagnosis, (ii) in course of disease — to find the complications of disease (ILD, acute renal failure, or malignancy), and (iii) in all phases of the therapeutic management. Since serum enzymes as an indicator of muscle inflammation can normalize rather quickly after the onset of systemic therapy, other substitute markers of DM disease activity are used by some to guide therapy [1]. Such markers include ESR, rheumatoid factor, C-reactive protein, sCD30 levels, neopterin, von Willebrand factor, hyaluronate, bFGF (basic fibroblast growth factor), procollagen type I polypeptide, vascular endothelial growth factor (VEGF), soluble vascular cell adhesion molecules (VCAM-1 and E selectin), KL-6, troponin T, myoglobin, and creatine in blood serum and urine.

Erythrocyte sedimentation rate (ESR) is elevated in 50% of DM patients in the active phase [2]. Patients with DM had significantly higher ESR than PM patients and it could represent, as previously mentioned, a more intense systemic repercussion in DM [3]. ESR does not correlate well with disease activity, but was suggested as a potential marker of malignancy in association with cutaneous necrosis [2]. The high levels are seen in patients with a severe ulcerative/vasculopathic juvenile DM, or in DM associated with infection [4].

Rheumatoid factor (RF) is elevated in 10–20% of DM patients and often in those with overlap syndrome [5]. RF are antibodies that react with the Fc-portion of IgG molecules. Although RF assays are primarily used in evaluating patients with rheumatoid arthritis, RF are not specific for RA, and can be observed in other musculoskeletal disorders.

Elevated serum levels of **C-reactive protein** are suggested as a predictive sign of malignancy in adult DM [6]. They are often modestly elevated in juvenile DM [4].

A significant elevation of circulating serum **soluble CD30** concentrations has been found in 64% of 33 patients with DM as compared with healthy controls [7]. Soluble CD30 levels were significantly elevated in DM associated with neoplasia and in juvenile DM. The presence of pruritus was significantly correlated with elevated sCD30 [7].

Neopterin and **factor VIII-related antigen** (von Willebrand factor) are suggested as serological indicators of disease activity [8]. They are elevated in more than 60% of patients with juvenile DM and correlated with disease activity [9]. Factor VIII-related antigen (von Willebrand factor) levels are elevated in many patients, probably due to small

32

blood vessel endothelial cell damage; however, they are not specific to juvenile DM. They may indicate ongoing inflammation when muscle enzymes may returned to normal [10], and thus are useful for monitoring disease activity in some patients.

Serum hyaluronate level is elevated in patients with DM and correlated with disease activity [11, 12]. Hyaluronate is an extracellular matrix component, consisting of repeating disaccharide units of *N*-acetyl-D-glucosamine linked by glycosidic linkages. Hyaluronate is produced mainly in fibroblasts, enters the circulation through lymph, and is degraded in hepatic sinusoidal endothelial cells. Raised serum concentrations of hyaluronate have been reported in patients with internal malignancy. The hyaluronate level is decreased by systemic corticosteroid therapy in classic DM or after surgical resection of neoplasma and subsequent chemotherapy in paraneoplastic DM [12].

Serum factors related to fibrosis, including basic **fibroblast growth factor** (bFGF) [13] and procollagen type I polypeptide [14], were detected recently in patients with DM without lung fibrosis. The patients with DM had significantly elevated serum bFGF compared with normal healthy controls [13], which correlated with serum CK levels and the frequency of lung fibrosis in PM/DM patients.

Vascular endothelial growth factor (VEGF) is another angiogenic mitogen, which specially targets vascular endothelial cells and plays an important part in wound healing. The levels of VEGF in Japanese patients with PM/DM were significantly higher than in normal controls, and the serum concentration of the marker was elevated in 45% (21/49) of these patients [15]. The elevation of bFGF level in PM/DM patients correlates significantly with the increased VEGF levels. In DM, bFGF is more important in the angiogenic process than VEGF; nevertheless, both markers are synergically involved in tissue processes such as the vascular abnormalities and the variable degrees of hypoxia.

Elevated levels of other markers of vascular activation including soluble **vascular cell adhesion molecules** (VCAM-1) and E selectin in the circulation of patients with classic DM [16], amyopathic DM [17] and other inflammatory myopathy [18] have also been reported. Serum VCAM-1 levels may reflect an acute phase of inflammatory reaction similar to ESR or C-reactive protein in inflammatory diseases [16]. The elevated serum VCAM-1 levels in PM/DM correlated with elevated ESR and increased concentration of hyaluronate in sera [16]. The elevated serum E-selectin levels also correlate with CK activities. However, no correlation was found between the elevated serum levels of these soluble adhesion molecules and the presence of clinical features, including cutaneous eruptions, muscle weakness, lung fibrosis, or internal malignancy [16]. The upregulation of adhesion molecules has been reported in muscle biopsy specimens in inflammatory myogenic diseases [19, 20] and in cutaneous biopsy specimens in DM [21, 22].

Serum levels of **KL-6** (a human MUV-1 class mucin that is preferentially expressed on pneumocytes type II) is a sensitive marker of classic DM in adults associated with ILD [23–25] and juvenile DM [26], but also as a tumor marker in hematologic malignancy [27].

Skeletal troponin I has been found to correlate with total CK in exercising athletes [28, 29] and was increased in a small series of patients with PM [28]. A highly significant correlation was found between the concentrations of skeletal troponin I and both total CK and CK-MB in patients with PM and DM [30]. Elevated serum levels of troponin I (>0.1 mg/l) and CK-MB, highly sensitive markers of myocardial injury, have been reported in patients with DM/PM in the absence of acute myocardial damage [30–34]. A raised serum concentration of skeletal troponin I has been determined in up to 75% of patients with inflammatory muscle disease including Duchenne dystrophy [35]. The cardiac troponin I is of particular use in distinguishing between a striated muscle and myocardial origin of a raised CK-MB/total CK ratio, as it is expressed only in cardiac muscle [36].

Levels of **myoglobin** [37] and **creatine** [38] in blood serum may also be elevated in DM patients. Sometimes myoglobinuria (>1 mg/ml) results from extensive muscle fiber necrosis (rhabdomyolysis) and associates with elevated CK (>500 U/l) [6, 38]. In these patients, the determination of myoglobin clearance as correlation from the urinary myoglobin concentration to urine volume and the serum is useful as a better predictor for the development of acute renal failure [39]. The estimation of 24-h urinary creatine excretion as marker of muscle damage is elevated in patients with myositis, providing even better information of disease activity than serum CK levels [40, 41]. Excretion of gamma carboxyglutamate in urine is a sensitive indicator of disease activity in calcinosis secondary to juvenile DM [42].

Peripheral blood B cells increase and CD8 + T cells decrease during the acute phase of juvenile DM [43–46], suggesting that some autoimmune mechanism is involved in the pathogenesis of this childhood illness. In DM in adults, a general lymphopenia has been observed which led to a decreased absolute number of all T-lymphocyte subsets [47].

Leukocyte activation markers have been found to correlate with disease activity in DM [48]. Serum levels of cytokines and soluble cytokine receptors may also serve as indicators of macrophage (e.g., IL-6, TNF-α) and T-lymphocyte (e.g., IFN-γ, IL-2, and IL-2R receptor) activation [49]. Serum level of soluble IL-2 receptor (sIL-2R) is a sensitive indicator of disease activity in DM [49] and PM [50]. In patients with DM, a decrease in IL-2R levels corresponds with the therapeutical response to IVIG [49].

32.1 Instrumental Assessments of Disease Activity in Myositis

32.1.1 Electromyography

Electromyography (EMG) shows myopathic potentials in most DM patients. The myopathic pattern in needle electromyography is characterized by short-duration, low-amplitude polyphasic units on voluntary action and increased spontaneous activity with fibrillations, complex repetitive discharges, and positive sharp waves. The voluntary motor units consist of low-amplitude polyphasic units of short duration [51, 52]. An abnormal electromyography was recorded in 90% of patients with DM/PM [53]. Although not disease-specific, these findings are useful to confirm active myopathy. Normal electromyography is found among some patients with mild–early DM that correlated with the beginning of the disease. There were also some patients who presented EMG showing mixed myopathic and neurogenic potentials. High-amplitude, long-duration polyphasic motor unit action potentials (MUAP) were present in 14% of the 102 patients with mild–early DM [3]. The neurogenic potentials usually represent a consequence of the regeneration of muscle fibers during the chronic course of disease [51, 54]. The relatively high incidence of neurogenic potentials among the patients with mild–early DM can be due to the different phases of the disease in which EMG had been carried out, including cases with initiated treatment when the regeneration of muscle fibers can occur. Abnormal EMG with short-duration, polyphasic motor unit potentials with spontaneous fibrillation potentials is helpful in distinguishing myopathy from neuropathy [55]. The presence of spontaneous activity can help to discriminate active disease from steroid-induced myopathy [38].

32.1.2 Magnetic Resonance Imaging

Magnetic resonance imaging (MRI) is an excellent noninvasive method for characterization of severity, distribution, and extent of inflammatory processes in muscle [56–58], as well as providing an assessment of disease activity and damage [59]. It was introduced in examination of muscle disease in patients with DM by Kaufman et al. [60]. Inflamed muscle is edematous, leading to increased (hyperintense) signal intensity on T2-weighted images or short tau inversion recovery [61]. T2-weighted images of the thigh muscles showed increased signal intensity, with focal and inhomogeneous involvement predominantly in the vastus lateralis. T1-weighted images are useful to show fibrosis atrophy and fatty infiltration. Muscle edema may be focal, with ill-defined and poorly circumscribed margins or diffusely involving a muscle [58]. A finding of muscle edema on MR images is almost always due to increased intracellular or extracellular free water [58]. The accumulation of abnormal metabolites that may occur in some pathologic conditions might also contribute to T2 prolongation, and thus contribute to increased signal intensity on T2-weighted images [62]. T2-weighted images of the thigh muscles showed increased signal intensity, with focal and inhomogeneous involvement predominantly in the vastus lateralis; T1 and T2 values of the vastus lateralis were significantly higher than those of the control subjects [62].

Muscle edema is observed in PM and DM [56, 63, 64], amyopathic DM [65, 66], IBM [67, 68], infectious myositis without phlegmon or abscess formation [64], rhabdomyolysis [69] and as a transient, physiologic finding during and briefly following muscle exercise [70].

MRI of muscle can be very useful to demonstrate the severity, distribution, and extent of the muscle inflammation, but can also demonstrate the presence of disease in other tissues, including fat and fascia [57]. T1-weighted images are useful to show fibrosis atrophy and fatty infiltration. MRI may be very useful to guide biopsies demonstrating active myositis, in patients with suspected myositis without muscle enzyme elevation, and to monitor myositis patients with complex response to treatment [56, 59, 62].

Typical MR imaging findings early in the course of DM/PM are bilateral and symmetric edema in pelvic and thigh musculature, especially in the vastus lateralis and vastus intermedius muscles [56, 61, 63, 64]. Progression to fatty infiltration, often with atrophy, occurs over months to years. Fat-suppressed images are needed to distinguish fat from edema, since the fat gives rise to hyperintense signals in both T1- and T2-weighted images. The severity of muscle edema on MR images has been shown to correlate with the severity of the disease [56, 62]. Relative sparing of the rectus femoris and biceps femoris muscles has been noted in DM patients [56]. It has been shown that inflammation, characteristic of active juvenile DM, is visible as a high signal intensity on fat-suppressed T2-weighted and short T1 inversion recovery MRI images [56]. These signals enable the use of MRI as a tool in establishing the diagnosis of juvenile DM, and monitoring the progression of the disease. On T2 MRI images, an increase in water content, repressing inflammation, appears as white within muscles that should have dark image areas [71]. These areas can be quantified by computer generation of the MRI T2 relaxation times [62, 72]. Sheetlike calcifications may develop, especially in DM, which are best appreciated on radiographs [58]. One third of patients with amyopathic DM demonstrated abnormal signal intensity in muscle on both T2 and fat-suppression sequences [66]. Patients with DM and clinically normal muscles may have detectable muscle inflammation on MR images, indicating that MRI is a potential tool for locating the relevant biopsy site and for longitudinal follow-up [66].

32.1.3 Magnetic Resonance Spectroscopy (MRS)

Phosphorus-31-MR spectroscopy show that the concentration of adenosine triphosphate (ATP) and phosphocreatine (PCr) in the diseased muscles were 30% below normal values, and the inorganic phosphate to PCr ratio was increased in the patient's muscles at rest and through exercise [62]. Based on the observations detected by MRS, it is concluded that factors other than the inflammatory process are involved in the mechanisms of muscle weakness, and it is hypothesized that metabolic abnormalities such as reduced levels of phosphocreatine (PCr) and adenosine triphosphate (ATP) are responsible for inducing a defective energy metabolism in DM and PM [73–75]. In a study by Park et al., in amyopathic DM, resting ATP and PCr levels and Pi/PCr ratio were similar to controls, but during the exercise the Pi/PCr ratio was elevated with no significant ATP loss [76]. With the developments of MRI techniques and MR spectroscopy, the understanding of the biochemical basis of the muscle dysfunction in juvenile DM is gained. Biochemical defects in energy metabolism and magnesium levels correlate closely with weakness and fatigue [73, 77]. Spectroscopy is a potentially noninvasive tool which may prove useful for monitoring response to therapy as well as provide valuable insights into mechanisms of pathogenesis.

32.1.4 Proton Magnetic Resonance Spectroscopy

In one case report of juvenile DM, proton MRS determined an abnormally low lipid-to-water ratio at the onset of the disease, and the latter ratio became abnormally high compared to controls at 3 months of treatment [78]. The metabolite ratios, such as cholin/lipid and creatine/lipid were significantly different in chronic PM and DM patients compared to controls [74].

Abnormal metabolic profiles were recorded in the urinary proton MR spectra of IIM patients [79]. Levels of muscle metabolites, such as creatine, cholin-containing compounds, glycine, taurine, and betaine, were significantly higher then in controls [79, 80]. High levels of urinary creatinine were recognized early in inflammatory myopathies, using standard methods for many decades [81]. Creatine, cholin-containing compounds, glycine, and taurine levels were reduced with treatment of PM and DM patients, and their levels seem to be related to clinical outcome [80]. It is suggested that urinary proton MRS metabolic profile may be a potential objective method for assessment of disease activity in PM/DM patients and for monitoring the efficacy of treatment [75].

32.1.5 Ultrasound

High-frequency muscle ultrasound (20 MHz) is also being used to show active muscle inflammation and fascial involvement, and Doppler studies may give indications of increased blood flow in inflamed tissues [65, 82, 83]. Ultrasound may also show the hyperechogenicity of the affected muscle group and the earliest indications of calcinosis before obvious X-ray changes, with characteristic signal dropout.

Power Doppler and contrast-enhanced ultrasound are useful tools for measuring increased skeletal muscle perfusion, with specificity of 91% [84], and for monitoring of muscle activity [85].

Non-invasive examinations such as MRI and ultrasound are beneficial as an objective means of examination in the evolution of patients with amyopathic and classic DM [65]. Ultrasound appears to be more a cost-effective and simple test, whereas MRI may be more expensive, but may be more sensitive and specific [65].

32.1.6 Anti-Myosin Scintigraphy

Scintigraphy with antimyosin antibody is a useful and safe method of detecting inflammatory lesions in muscles of PM and DM patients, as well as evaluating the efficacy of drug therapy [86] in dermatomyositis. The mechanism of action involves the revealing of insoluble myosin to anti-myosin antibodies, which increases their uptake and indicates the integrity of muscle cell membranes as a marker of the inflammatory processes in muscles. A high correlation has been found between the uptake of antimyosin antibody and serum CK activity, which favors scintigraphy as the method of choice for the assessment of the severity of inflammation [86]. An advantage of MRI compared with scintigraphy was the possibility of distinguishing between lesions in extensor and flexor muscles, and the observation that intramuscular fatty degeneration causing increased signal intensity on T_1-weighted MRI is not reflected in antimyosin scintigraphy [86].

32.1.7 Functional Assessment

Muscle weakness is a complex result of decreased strength and endurance. A test which measures muscle endurance is more sensitive and is more likely to detect impaired muscle function than a strength test [75]. The most commonly used technique for assessing

Table 32.1 The Rose–Walton scale of muscle strength [95]

Score	Clinical findings
0	No abnormality
1	No abnormality on examination, but easy fatigability
2	Minimal degree of muscle atrophy without functional impairment
3	Waddling gait, unable to run but able to climb stairs without support
4	Marked waddling gait, lordosis, unable to climb stairs or rise from chair without arm support
5	Marked waddling gait, unable to climb stairs or rise from the chair without arm support
6	Unable to walk without assistance

muscle function is the manual muscle test (MMT) with the Medical Research Council (MRC) scale [87, 88]. A more sensitive technique to measure muscle strength is the modified sphygmomanometer [89]. Another tool to measure muscle strength is the handheld pullgauge [90]. The isokinetic dynamometer is also a sensitive tool for measuring muscle strength and endurance [75]. The most useful and reliable functional test for clinical practice is the Functional Index of Myositis [91], which measures muscle strength and endurance and is feasible to use in a follow-up study of exercise [92]. Functional tests based on questionnaires have also been used [93].

Muscle strength was evaluated using a combination of two methods, the manual muscle test (MMT) [88] and handheld myometer [94] (Table 32.1).

32.2 Instrumental Assessments of Cutaneous Disease Activity of DM

32.2.1 Nailfold Capillary Microscopy

Nailfold capillary changes are better seen with magnification (capillary microscopy), and may share some similarities to those seen in other connective tissue diseases [96–99].

Nailfold capillaroscopy (NFC) is a simple and noninvasive screening test for the differential diagnosis of Raynaud's phenomenon. It has been established for investigation in adults and children with a variety of connective tissue diseases such as systemic sclerosis, lupus erythematosus, and DM. During the past 2 decades, several methods of nailfold capillaroscopy including direct in vivo capillaroscopy, wide field (panoramic) photomicrography [100–102], or videocapillaroscopy and computer-based image analysis [103] have been reported.

It is believed that morphological changes of the nailfold capillaries correspond with the microvascular abnormalities present in DM. Significant changes in capillary morphology (mainly capillary density, avascularity, and abnormal capillaries) are present in more than 80% of adult patients with systemic sclerosis and related disorders such as DM [96, 97]. In DM the capillary microscopy identifies bushy capillaries, sausage-shaped loops of dilated capillaries, or giant capillary loops interspersed with capillary loss, avascular areas, thromboses, and hemorrhage [104]. These changes may be seen in juvenile and adult DM, but also in some cases with PM [105]. Enlarged capillary loops are more frequently seen in patients with DM (56%) than in those with PM (21%) [105]. The distinctive microvascular pattern (dilated and distorted capillary loops alternating with avascular areas) is present in between 20% and 60% of patients with DM/PM [96, 106, 107]. In a study by Ohtsuka, all DM/PM patients showed abnormal values of capillary width [108]. The frequency of nailfold bleeding in DM/PM (58%) was found to be significantly higher [108] than that in normal controls and other connective tissue diseases such as systemic lupus erythematosus, Sjögren's syndrome, secondary Raynaud's phenomenon, diabetes mellitus, and psoriasis. Regarding to the avascular areas, an extensive loss of capillaries in the nailfold was found in 15.4% of cases with DM/PM [107]. The extent of microangiopathy detected by nailfold capillaroscopy has been shown to correlate with disease severity and prognosis [96]. Furthermore, microangiopathy in nailfold is a potential marker for more persistent disease in children with DM [100], and correlates with the degree of vasculopathy [102]. The clinical appearance of the periungual telangiectases varies from extremely prominent in DM to detectable only by capillary microscopy [98]. Nailfold capillary microscopy, with or without more advanced image analysis, is useful tool for monitoring of the overall disease activity and predicting severity and clinical course in classical adult and juvenile DM [109].

32.2.2 Photosensitivity in Dermatomyositis

The cutaneous features of DM strongly suggest that ultraviolet (UV) radiation in the sunlight spectrum plays an important role in the pathogenesis of the disease [110, 111]. The characteristic skin changes, particularly a persistent erythema, are prominent on the sunlight-exposed parts of face (heliotrope pattern) [112], as well on as the neck and shoulders (Gottron's sign), and disease photoaggravation in DM patients is common [113–115]. The relative prevalence of DM increases significantly with decreasing geographical latitude from northern Europe (Reykjavik) to southern Europe (Athens) [116]. Terrestrial surface UV irradiance was found in one study to contribute to the relative prevalence of DM, and was strongly related to the proportion of anti-Mi-2 autoantibodies [117]. The incidence of increased cutaneous photosensitivity in DM patients has been relatively poorly documented, and the photosensitivity has only been tested in a few cases [113, 115, 118]. Everett and Curtis (1957) [113] reported that seven of their 19 DM patients had sunlight-induced aggravation of the cutaneous lesions. Later, Harber and Bickers (1989) [119] marked a lack of correlation between light exposure and the occurrence of cutaneous lesions, but pointed out that the initial complaints in four of their patients began after sun exposure. Woo et al. [120] observed a case of recurrent photosensitive dermatitis preceding juvenile DM, and Badawy Abdel-Nasser et al. [121] reported induction of amyopathic DM in a patient treated for atopic dermatitis with UV light therapy. Photoinduction of PM has been reported in an adult black man with vitiligo who was treated with PUVA (psoralen and ultraviolet A) therapy [122]. Cheong et al. [115] showed that five of ten confirmed DM patients appeared photosensitive, with disease photoaggravation in three and sunlight-provoked skin lesions in two of them. Monochromatic irradiation testing demonstrated reduced MEDs in two patients, at 307.5 nm, and at 340 and 360 nm respectively [115]. In one study of 75 Caucasians with skin types II and III according to the Fitzpatrick classification divided into three different subject groups (19 patients with DM, 30 patients with lupus erythematosus, and 26 healthy control volunteers) were tested for photomanifestation on non-irradiated suprascapular back skin with an ETG-1 Erythemtester [118]. The MEDs were determined 24 h after irradiation, adjusted according to skin type. Nine of DM patients (47.4%) demonstrated reduced MEDs to UVB radiation; seven of them (36.8%) had a history of increased cutaneous photosensitivity, and in four DM patients an aggravation after sun exposure was reported. Both the DM and LE patient groups showed reduced MED to UVB radiation ($p < 0.05$) compared with the control group (Table 32.2, Fig. 32.1). According to various other clinical studies, photosensitivity in DM patients was present in 29% [123], 50% [113, 115], and 100% [114].

Table 32.2 Clinical photosensitivity and phototest results in 19 DM patients [118]

Patient No.	Sex	Age	Clinical photosensitivity	MED (J/m^2)	Medications
1	F	57	III type, increased, aggravation	163	Methylprednisolone 40 mg/day
2	F	41	II type	175	Methylprednisolone 12 mg/day
3	F	68	II type	163	No
4	M	14	II type	175	No
5	F	57	III type, increased, aggravation	200	Chloroquine 250 mg/day
6	F	15	III type	250	Methylprednisolone 8 mg/day
7	F	76	III type, increased	200	No
8	F	58	III type	250	Methylprednisolone 8 mg/day; Azathioprine 100 mg/day
9	M	67	III type, increased	200	No
10	F	54	III type	225	No
11	M	65	III type	250	No
12	M	75	III type, increased, aggravation	138	No
13	F	59	III type	225	No
14	M	21	III type	225	Dapsone 200 mg/day

(continued)

Table 32.2 (continued)

Patient No.	Sex	Age	Clinical photosensitivity	MED (J/m²)	Medications
15	M	21	III type, increased, aggravation	200	Methylprednisolone 8 mg/day; Chloroquine 250 mg/day
16	F	52	III type	300	Methylprednisolone 60 mg/day
17	M	65	III type	300	Methylprednisolone 20 mg/day
18	F	74	III type	250	No
19	M	43	III type, increased	225	No

DM — dermatomyositis; MED — minimal erythema dose

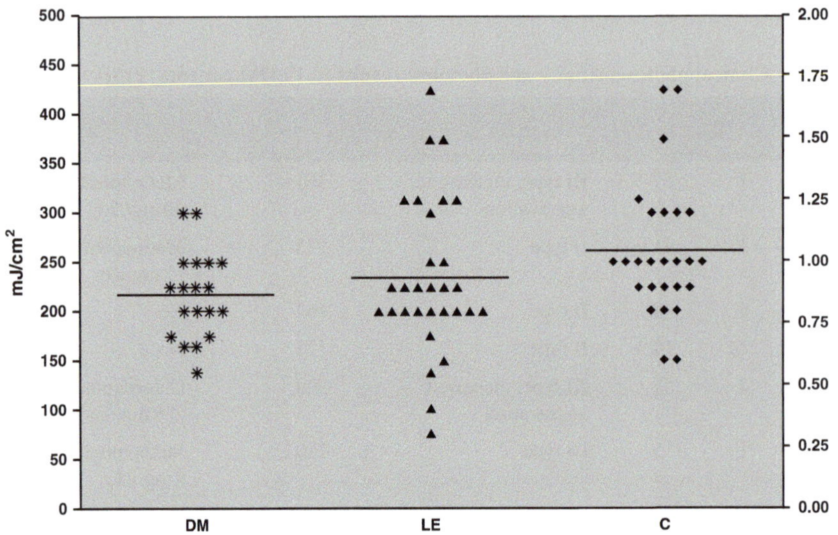

Fig. 32.1 Distribution of data from phototest in patients with DM, LE, and healthy persons (Adapted from [118])

The majority of MED determination techniques are based on stepwise increasing UV dosages over separate skin fields, which cause a systematic error at least of the magnitude of this step. Phototests are normally performed on the skin of the back, which allows a large number (often more than 30) of test exposures [124]. Because of variances in radiation sources, different tested cutaneous areas, and diverse protocols for MED determination, conflicting results may increase [124, 125].

The pathophysiology of photosensitive autoimmune skin reactions in DM patients could be explained by UV-induced production of TNF-α, which leads to keratinocyte apoptosis and translocation of previously sequestered cellular antigens, which then activate the immune system [110, 126]. An association of the overproducing of TNF-α-308A variant is found in adult DM and in LE patients [126]. The number of apoptotic keratinocytes in the disrupted basal zone of skin in DM and discoid lupus erythematosus was significantly increased compared with normal skin demonstrated by immunohistochemistry [127, 128]. The DM is more severe and therapeutically resistant, and disease course is prolonged in TNF-α-308A homozygous patients [8, 126].

32.2.3 Skin Assessment Instruments

Based on the need for independent evaluation of skin manifestations in DM, research instruments have been developed aimed at teaching clinicians to recognize and assess cutaneous involvement with regard to activity and damage [129, 130]. Since this myositis cutaneous assessment tool (MCAT) was reported, several studies have emphasized the importance of independent skin evaluation by demonstrating direct correlation between cutaneous and overall disease activity as reflected by nailfold capillary changes and other laboratory parameters [131, 132].

The International Myositis Assessment and Clinical Studies Group has developed a quantitative assessment tool that incorporates evaluation of cutaneous findings [133, 134]. This instrument includes evaluation of both disease activity (Myositis Disease Activity Assessment Tool, MITAX) and damage (Myositis Damage Index, MDI). Finally, the juvenile DM Disease Activity Score (DAS) includes a skin involvement distribution and severity assessment [135] (Table 32.3).

Table 32.3 Photosensitivity in DM and LE patients compared with healthy volunteers

	N	Positive phototest	Aver-ageMED	Average MED (J/m²)	STD (J/m²)
Dermatomyositis	19	9 (47.4%)	0.87	216.4	44.3
Amyopathic DM	2	1	0.85	212.5	17.7
Classic DM in adult	11	5 (45.5%)	0.90	226.1	45.6
Paraneoplastic DM	2	1	0.78	193.8	92.5
Juvenile DM	3	1	0.87	216.7	38.2
Overlap syndrome	1	1	0.7	163	–
Lupus erythematosus	30	14 (46.7%)	0.94	233.8	78.8
Systemic LE	13	6 (46.2%)	0.95	237	61.5
Chronic DLE	11	6 (54.5%)	0.87	218	101.5
Subacute CLE	6	2 (33.3%)	1	256	71.5
Control group	26	5 (19.2%)	1.04	260	68.9
P		<0.05			

SLE — systemic lupus erythematosus; CDLE — chronic cutaneous discoid lupus erythematosus; SCLE — subacute lupus erythematosus

32

References

1. Sontheimer RD. Dermatomyositis: an overview of recent progress with emphasis on dermatologic aspects. *Dermatol Clin* 2002; 20: 387–408.
2. Basset-Seguin N, Roujeau J, Gherardi R, et al. Prognostic factors and predicative signs of malignancy in adult dermatomyositis. *Arch Dermatol* 1990; 126: 633–637.
3. Scola RH, Werneck LC, Prevedello DM, et al. Diagnosis of dermatomyositis and polymyositis. A study of 102 cases. *Arq Neuropsiquiatr* 2000; 58(3-B): 789–799.
4. Murray KJ. Juvenile dermatomyositis: advances in understanding and management. *APLAR J Rheumatol* 2003; 6: 50–63.
5. Van Paassen P, Damoiseaux J, Tervaert JW. Laboratory assessment in musculoskeletal disorders. *Best Practice Res Clin Rheumatol* 2003; 17: 475–494.
6. Rose MR, Kissel JT, Bickley LS. Sustained myoglobinuria: the presenting manifestation of dermatomyositis. *Neurology* 1996; 47: 119–123.
7. Yazawa N, Ihn H, Yamane K, et al. Elevated circulating soluble CD30 levels in patients with polymyositis/dermatomyositis. *Br J Dermatol* 2001; 145: 676–678.
8. Pachman LM, Liotta-Davis MR, Hong DK, et al. TNFalpha-308A allele in juvenile dermatomyositis: association with increased production of tumor necrosis factor alpha, disease duration, and pathologic calcifications. *Arthritis Rheum* 2000; 43: 2368–2377.
9. Pachman LM. Juvenile dermatomyositis (JDMS): new clues to diagnosis and pathogenesis. *Clin Exp Rheumatol* 1994; 12(Suppl 10): S69–S73.
10. Bloom BJ, Tucker LB, Miller LC, et al. von Willebrand factor in juvenile dermatomyositis. *J Rheumatol* 1995; 22: 320–325.
11. Kubo M, Kikuchi K, Yazawa N, et al. Increased serum concentration of hyaluronate in dermatomyositis patients. *Arch Dermatol Res* 1998; 290: 579–581.
12. Kubo M, Ihn H, Matsukawa A, et al. Dermatomyositis with elevated serum hyaluronate. *Clin Exp Dermatol* 1999; 24: 275–278.
13. Kadono T, Kikuchi K, Kubo M, et al. Serum concentrations of basic fibroblast growth factor in collagen diseases. *J Am Acad Dermatol* 1996; 35: 392–397.
14. Kubo M, Kikuchi K, Fujimoto M, et al. Serum concentrations of carboxyterminal propeptide of type 1 procollagen and tissue inhibitor of metalloproteinase 1 in patients with dermatomyositis. *Arch Dermatol Res* 1998; 290: 253–257.
15. Kikuchi K, Kubo M, Kadono T, et al. Serum concentrations of vascular endothelial growth factor in collagen diseases. *Br J Dermatol* 1998; 139: 1049–1051.
16. Kubo M, Ihn H, Yamane K, et al. Increased serum levels of soluble vascular cell adhesion molecules-1 and soluble E-selectin in patients with polymyositis/dermatomyositis. *Br J Dermatol* 2000; 143: 392–398.
17. Sontheimer RD, Racila D. Blood levels of soluble vascular adhesion molecules, VCAM-1 and E-selectin, are increased in clinically amyopathic dermatomyositis [abstract]. *J Invest Dermatol* 2001; 117: 440.
18. Kumamoto T, Abe T, Ueyama H, et al. Elevated soluble intercellular adhesion molecules-1 in inflammatory myopathy. *Acta Neurol Scand* 1997; 95: 34–37.
19. De Bleecker JL, Engel AG. Expression of cell adhesion molecules in inflammatory myopathies and Duchenne dystrophy. *J Neuropathol Exp Neurol* 1994; 53(4): 369–376.
20. Tews DS, Goebel HH. Cytokine expression profiles in idiopathic inflammatory myopathies. *J Neuropathol Exp Neurol* 1996; 55: 342–347.
21. Hausmann G, Mascaro JM Jr, Herrero H, et al. Cell adhesion molecule expression in cutaneous lesions of dermatomyositis. *Acta Derm Venereol (Stockh)* 1996; 76: 222–225.

22. Carota A, Pizzolato GP, Redard M, et al. Adhesion molecules in HIV-related and idiopathic polymyositis: immunohistochemical studies. *Clin Neuropathol* 1997; 16: 312–318.
23. Hirakata M, Nagai S. Interstitial lung disease in polymyositis and dermatomyositis [review]. *Curr Opin Rheumatol* 2000; 12: 501–508.
24. Bandoh S, Fujita J, Ohtsuki Y, et al. Sequential changes of KL-6 in sera of patients with interstitial pneumonia associated with polymyositis/dermatomyositis. *Ann Rheum Dis* 2000; 59: 257–262.
25. Kubo M, Ihn H, Yamane K, et al. Serum Kl-6 in adult patients with polymyositis and dermatomyositis. *Rheumatology (Oxford)* 2000; 39: 632–636.
26. Kobayashi I, Ono S, Kawamura N, et al. Kl-6 is a potential marker for interstitial lung disease associated with juvenile dermatomyositis. *J Pediatr* 2001; 138: 274–276.
27. Takubo T, Kumura T, Nakao T, et al. Serum Kl-6 levels in haematologic malignancy and their clinical application. *Haematologia (Budap)* 2001; 31: 61–67.
28. Takahashi M, Lee L, Shi Q, et al. Use of enzyme immunoassay for measurement of skeletal troponin I utilizing isoform specific monoclonal antibodies. *Clin Biochem* 1996; 29: 301–308.
29. Rama D, Margaritis I, Orsetti A, et al. Troponin I immunoenzymometric assays for detection of muscle damage applied to monitoring a triathlon. *Clin Chem* 1996; 42: 2033–2035.
30. Kiely PD, Bruckner FE, Nisbet JA, et al. Serum skeletal troponin I in inflammatory muscle disease: relation to creatine kinase, CKMB and cardiac troponin I. *Ann Rheum Dis* 2000; 59: 750–752.
31. Kobayashi S, Tanaka M, Tamura N, et al. Serum cardiac troponin T in polymyositis/dermatomyositis. *Lancet* 1992; 340: 726.
32. Erlacher P, Lercher A, Falkensammer J, et al. Cardiac troponin and beta-type myosin heavy chain concentrations in patients with polymyositis or dermatomyositis. *Clin Chim Acta* 2001; 306: 27–33.
33. White GH, Tideman PA. Increased troponin T in a patient with dermatomyositis. *Clin Chem* 2001; 47: 1130–1131.
34. Hamilton JS, Sharpe PC. Two cases of inflammatory muscle disease presenting with raised serum concentrations of troponin T. *J Clin Pathol* 2005; 58: 1323–1324.
35. Hammerer-Lercher A, Erlacher P, Bittner R, et al. Clinical and experimental results on cardiac troponin expression in Duchenne muscular dystrophy. *Clin Chem* 2001; 47: 451–458.
36. Bodor GS, Porterfield D, Voss EM, et al. Cardiac troponin I is not expressed in fetal and healthy or diseased adult human skeletal muscle. *Clin Chem* 1995; 41: 1710–1715.
37. Kagen LJ. Myoglobinemia in inflammatory myopathies. *JAMA* 1977; 237: 1448–1452.
38. Dalakas M. Polymyositis, dermatomyositis and inclusion body myositis. *N Engl J Med* 1991; 325(21): 1487–1498.
39. Wu AH, Laios I, Green S, et al. Immunoassays for serum and urine myoglobin: myoglobin clearance assessed as a risk factor for acute renal failure. *Clin Chem* 1994; 40: 796–802.
40. Rowell NR. Urinary creatine excretion and the management of dermatomyositis. *Dermatol Monatsschr* 1984; 170: 34.
41. Rowell NR, Fairris GM. Biochemical markers of myositis in dermatomyositis. *Clin Exp Dermatol* 1986; 11: 69–72.
42. Lian J, Pacman L, Gunberg C, et al. Gamma carboxyglutamate excretion and calcinosis in juvenile dermatomyositis. *Arthritis Rheum* 1982; 25: 1094–1100.
43. Mantegazza R, Bernasconi P. Cellular aspects of myositis. *Curr Opin Rheumatol* 1994; 6: 568–574.
44. Eisenstein DM, O'Gorman MR, Pachman LM. Correlations between change in disease activity and changes in peripheral blood lymphocyte subsets in patients with juvenile dermatomyositis. *J Rheumatol* 1997; 24: 1830–1832.

32

45. O'Gorman MR, Bianchi L, Zaas D, et al. Decreased levels of CD54 (ICAM-1) — positive lymphocytes in the peripheral blood in untreated patients with active juvenile dermatomyositis. *Clin Diagn Lab Immunol* 2000; 7: 693–697.
46. Kikuchi Y, Koarada S, Tada Y, et al. Difference in B cell activation between dermatomyositis and polymyositis: analysis of the expression of RP105 on peripheral blood B cells. *Ann Rheum Dis* 2001; 60: 1137–1140.
47. Iannone F, Cauli A, Yanni G, et al. T-Lymphocyte immunophenotyping in polymyositis and dermatomyositis. *Br J Rheumatol* 1996; 35: 839–845.
48. Miller FW, Love LA, Barbieri SA, et al. Lymphocyte activation markers in idiopathic myositis: changes with disease activity and differences among clinical and autoantibody subgroups. *Clin Exp Immunol* 1990; 81: 373–379.
49. Götterfied I, Seeber A, Anegg B, et al. High dose intravenous immunoglobulin (IVIG) in dermatomyositis: clinical responses and effect on sIL-2R levels. *Eur J Dermatol* 2000; 10: 29–35.
50. Wolf RE, Baethige BA. Interleukin-1 α, interleukin-2, and soluble interleukin-2 receptors in polymyositis. *Arthritis Rheum* 1990; 33: 1007–1014.
51. Barkhaus PE, Nandedkar SD, Sanders DB. Quantitative EMG in inflammatory myopathy. *Muscle Nerve* 1990; 13: 247–253.
52. Uncini A, Lange DJ, Hayes AP, et al. Long-duration polyphasic motor unit potentials in myopathies: a quantitative study with pathological correlation. *Muscle Nerve* 1990; 13: 263–267.
53. Sultan SM, Ioannou Y, Moss K, et al. Outcome in patients with idiopathic inflammatory myositis: morbidity and mortality. *Rheumatology* 2002; 41: 22–26.
54. Robinson LR. AAEM case report#22 Polymyositis. *Muscle Nerve* 1991; 14: 310–315.
55. Oester YT, Rodriguez AA, Fudema JJ. Electromyographic findings in dermatomyositis. *Arch Dermatol* 1957; 76: 91–95.
56. Hernandez RJ, Sullivan DB, Chenevert TL, et al. MR imaging in children with dermatomyositis: musculoskeletal findings and correlation with clinical and laboratory findings. *AJR Am J Roentgenol* 1993; 161: 359–366.
57. Kimball AB, Summers RM, Turner M, et al. Magnetic resonance imaging detection of occult skin and subcutaneous abnormalities in juvenile dermatomyositis. Implications for diagnosis and therapy. *Arthritis Rheum* 2000; 43: 1866–1873.
58. May DA, Disler DG, Jones EA, et al. Abnormal signal intensity in skeletal muscle at MR imaging: patterns, pearls, and pitfalls. *Radiographics* 2000; 20: 295–315.
59. Chapman S, Southwood TR, Fowler J, et al. Rapid changes in magnetic resonance imaging of muscle during the treatment of juvenile dermatomyositis. *Br J Rheumatol* 1994; 33: 184–186.
60. Kaufman LD, Gruber BL, Gerstman DP, et al. Preliminary observations on the role of magnetic resonance imaging for polymyositis and dermatomyositis. *Ann Rheum Dis* 1987; 46(8): 569–572.
61. Reimers CD, Schedel H, Fleckenstein JL, et al. Magnetic resonance imaging of skeletal muscles in idiopathic inflammatory myopathies of adults. *J Neurol* 1994; 241: 306–314.
62. Park JH, Vansant JP, Kumar NG, et al. Dermatomyositis: correlative MR imaging and P-31 MR spectroscopy for quantitative characterization of inflammatory disease. *Radiology* 1990; 177: 473–479.
63. Fujino H, Kobayashi T, Goto I, et al. Magnetic resonance imaging of the muscles in patients with polymyositis and dermatomyositis. *Muscle Nerve* 1991; 14: 716–720.
64. Fleckenstein JL, Reimers CD. Inflammatory myopathies: radiologic evaluation. *Radiol Clin North Am* 1996; 34: 427–439.
65. Stonecipher MR, Jorizzo JL, Monu J, et al. Dermatomyositis with normal muscle enzyme concentrations. A single-blind study of the diagnostic value of magnetic resonance imaging and ultrasound. *Arch Dermatol* 1994; 130: 1294–1299.

66. Lam W, Chan H, Chan YL, et al. MR imaging in amyopathic dermatomyositis. *Acta Radiol* 1999; 40: 69–72.
67. Sayers ME, Chou SM, Calabrese LH. Inclusion body myositis: analysis of 32 cases. *J Rheumatol* 1992; 19(9): 1385–1389.
68. Calabrese LH, Chou SM. Inclusion body myositis. *Rheum Dis Clin North Am* 1994; 20(4): 955–972.
69. Shintani S, Shiigai T. Repeat MRI in acute rhabdomyolysis: correlation with clinicopathological findings. *J Comput Assist Tomogr* 1993; 17: 786–791.
70. Disler DG, Cohen MS, Krebs DE, et al. Dynamic evaluation of exercising leg muscle in healthy subjects with echoplanar MR imaging: work rate and total work determine rate of T2 change. *J Magn Reson Imaging* 1995; 5: 588–593.
71. Maillard SM, Jones R, Owens C, et al. Quantitative assessment of MRI T2 relaxation time of thigh muscles in juvenile dermatomyositis. *Rheumatology* 2004; 43 (5): 603–608.
72. Summers RM, Brune AM, Choyke PL, et al. Juvenile idiopathic inflammatory myopathy: exercise-induced changes in muscle at short inversion time inversion MR imaging. *Radiology* 1998; 209: 191–196.
73. Park JH, Niermann KJ, Ryder NM, et al. Muscle abnormalities in juvenile dermatomyositis patients: P-31 magnetic resonance spectroscopy studies. *Arthritis Rheum* 2000; 43: 2359–2367.
74. Chung YI, Smith EC, Williams SC, et al. In vivo proton magnetic resonance spectroscopy in polymyositis and dermatomyositis. A preliminary study. *Eur J Med Res* 1997; 2: 483–487.
75. Lundberg I, Chung Y-L. Treatment and investigation of idiopathic inflammatory myopathies. *Rheumatology* 2000; 39: 7–17.
76. Park JH, Olsen NJ, King LE, et al. Use of magnetic resonance imaging and P-31 magnetic resonance spectroscopy to detect and quantify muscle dysfunction in the amyopathic and myopathic variant of dermatomyositis. *Arthritis Rheum* 1995; 38: 68–77.
77. Niermann KJ, Olsen NJ, Park JH. Magnesium abnormalities of skeletal muscle in dermatomyositis and juvenile dermatomyositis. *Arthritis Rheum* 2002; 46: 475–488.
78. Stopis JM, Jackson EF, Narayana PA, et al. Proton magnetic resonance imaging and spectroscopic studies of the pathogenesis and treatment of juvenile dermatomyositis. *J Child Neurol* 1993; 8: 242–249.
79. Chung YL, Wassif WS, Bell JD, et al. Urinary levels of creatine and other metabolites in the assessment of polymyositis and dermatomyositis. *Rheumatology (Oxford)* 2003; 42(2): 298–303.
80. Chung YL, Rider LG, Bell JD, et al. Muscle metabolites, detected in urine by proton spectroscopy, correlate with disease damage in juvenile idiopathic inflammatory myopathies. *Arthritis Rheum* 2005; 53(4): 565–570.
81. Olsen NJ, Park JH. Inflammatory myopathies: issues in diagnosis and management. *Arthritis Care Res* 1997; 10: 200–207.
82. Keim DR, Hernandez RJ, Sulivan DB. Serial MRI in juvenile dermatomyositis. *Arthritis Rheum* 1991; 34: 1580–1584.
83. Owen NJ, Owens CM, Bose S, et al. The role of musculoskeletal ultrasound at diagnosis and follow-up in patients with juvenile dermatomyositis. *Radiology* 2002; 217: S495.
84. Weber MA, Jappe U, Essig M, et al. Contrast-enhanced ultrasound in dermatomyositis and polymyositis. *J Neurol* 2006; 253(12): 1625–1632.
85. Meng C, Adler R, Peterson M, et al. Combined use of power Doppler and gray-scale ultrasonography: a new technique for assessment of inflammatory myopathy. *J Phycol* 2001; 28: 1271–1282.
86. Löfberg M, Liewendahl K, Lamminen A, et al. Antimyosin scintigraphy compared with magnetic resonance imaging in inflammatory myopathies. *Arch Neurol* 1998; 55(7): 987–993.

87. Daniels L, Worthingham C. *Muscle Testing*. 4th ed. W.B. Saunders, Philadelphia, 1972.
88. Florence JM, Pandya S, King WM, et al. Intrarater reliability of manual muscle test (Medical Research Council scale) grades in Duchenne's muscular dystrophy. *Phys Ther* 1992; 72: 115–122.
89. Helewa A, Goldsmith CH, Smythe HA. The modified sphygmomanometer – an instrument to measure muscle strength: a validation study. *J Chron Dis* 1981; 34: 353–361.
90. Stroll T, Brühlmann P, Stucki G, et al. Muscle strength assessment in polymyositis and dermatomyositis: evaluation of the reliability and clinical use of a new, quantitative, easily applicable method. *J Rheumatol* 1995; 22: 473–477.
91. Josefson A, Romanus E, Carlson J. A functional index in myositis. *J Rheumatol* 1996; 23: 1380–1384.
92. Alexanderson H, Stenström C, Lundberg I. Safety of a home exercise programme in patients with polymyositis and dermatomyositis: a pilot study. *Rheumatology* 1999; 38: 608–611.
93. Feldman BM, Ayling-Campos A, Luy L, et al. Measuring disability in juvenile dermatomyositis: validity of the childhood health assessment questionnaire. *J Rheumatol* 1995; 22: 326–331.
94. Lennon SM, Ashburn A. Use of myometry in the assessment of neuropathic weakness testing for reliability in clinical practice. *Clin Rehab* 1993; 7: 125–133.
95. Rose AL, Walton JN. Polymyositis: a survey of 89 cases with particular reference to treatment and prognosis. *Brain* 1966; 89: 747–768.
96. Maricq HR, Spencer-Green G, LeRoy EC. Skin capillary abnormalities as indicators of organ involvement in scleroderma (systemic sclerosis), Raynaud's syndrome and dermatomyositis. *Am J Med* 1976; 61: 862–870.
97. Maricq HR, LeRoy EC, D'Angelo WA, et al. Diagnostic potential of in vivo capillary microscopy in scleroderma and related disorders. *Arthritis Rheum* 1980; 23: 183–189.
98. Maricq HR, Maize JC. Nailfold capillary abnormalities. *Clin Rheum Dis* 1982; 8: 455–478.
99. Ganczarczyk ML, Lee P, Armstrong SK. Nailfold capillary microscopy in polymyositis and dermatomyositis. *Arthritis Rheum* 1988; 31: 116–119.
100. Spencer-Green G, Crowe WE, Levinson JE. Nailfold capillary abnormalities and clinical outcome in childhood dermatomyositis. *Arthritis Rheum* 1982; 25: 954–958.
101. Nussbaum AI, Silver RM, Maricq HR. Serial changes in nailfold capillary morphology in childhood dermatomyositis. *Arthritis Rheum* 1983; 26: 1169–1172.
102. Silver RM, Maricq HR. Childhood dermatomyositis: serial microvascular studies. *Pediatrics* 1989; 83: 278–283.
103. Scheja A, Elborgh R, Wildt M. Decreased capillary density in juvenile dermatomyositis and in mixed connective tissue disease. *J Rheumatol* 1999; 26: 1377–1381.
104. Miller OF, Newman ED. Dermatomyositis and polymyositis. In: *Cutaneous Medicine and Surgery*, Arndt KA, Leboit PC, Robinson JK, et al. (eds), W.B. Saunders, Philadelphia, 1996; 283–290.
105. Ganczarczyk ML, Lee P, Armstrong SK. Nailfold capillary microscopy in polymyositis and dermatomyositis. *Arthritis Rheum* 1988; 31(1): 116–119.
106. Blockmans D, Beyens G, Verhaeghe R. Predictive value of nailfold capillaroscopy in the diagnosis of connective tissue diseases. *Clin Rheumatol* 1996; 15: 148–153.
107. Nagy Z, Czirják L. Nailfold digital capillaroscopy in 447 patients with connective tissue disease and Raynaud's disease. *JEADV* 2004; 18: 62–68.
108. Ohtsuka T. The relation between nailfold bleeding and capillary microscopy abnormality in patients with connective tissue diseases. *Int J Dermatol* 1998; 37: 23–26.
109. Dolezalova P, Young SP, Bacon PA, et al. Nailfold capillary microscopy in healthy children and in childhood rheumatic diseases: a prospective single blind observational study. *Ann Rheum Dis* 2003; 62: 444–449.

110. Sontheimer RD. Photoimmunology of lupus erythematosus and dermatomyositis: a speculative review. *Photochem Photobiol* 1996; 63: 583–594.
111. Roelands R. The diagnosis of photosensitivity. *Arch Dermatol* 2000; 136: 1152–1157.
112. Bohan A, Petter JB, Bowman RL, et al. Computer-assisted analysis of 153 patients with polymyositis and dermatomyositis. *Medicine* 1977; 56: 255–286.
113. Everett MA, Curtis AC. Dermatomyositis: a review of 19 cases in adolescents and children. *Arch Intern Med* 1957; 100: 70–76.
114. Euwer R, Sontheimer R. Amyopathic dermatomyositis (dermatomyositis sine myositis). Presentation of six new cases and review of the literature. *J Am Acad Dermatol* 1991; 24: 959–966.
115. Cheong WK, Hughes GR, Norris PG, et al. Cutaneous photosensitivity in dermatomyositis. *Br J Dermatol* 1994; 131: 205–208.
116. Hengstman GD, van Venrooij WJ, Vencovsky J, et al. The relative prevalence of dermatomyositis and polymyositis in Europe exhibits a latitudinal gradient. *Ann Rheum Dis* 2000; 59: 141–142.
117. Okada S, Weatherhead E, Targoff IN. Global surface ultraviolet radiation intensity may modulate the clinical and immunologic expression of autoimmune muscle disease. *Arthritis Rheum* 2003; 48: 2285–2293.
118. Dourmishev L, Meffert H, Piazena H. Dermatomyositis: comparative studies of cutaneous photosensitivity in lupus erythematosus and normal subjects. *Photoderm Photoimmun Photomed* 2004; 20 (5): 230–234.
119. Harber LC, Bickers DR. Photosensitivity Diseases: Principles of Diagnosis and Treatment. BC Decker, Philadelphia, 1989; 295–296.
120. Woo TR, Rasmussen J, Callen JP. Recurrent photosensitive dermatitis preceding juvenile dermatomyositis. *Pediatr Dermatol* 1985; 2: 207–212.
121. Badawy Abdel-Nasser M, Chun SC, Gollnick H, et al. Amyopathic dermatomyositis (dermatomyositis sine myositis) in a male patient and possible induction by UV light. *Eur J Dermatol* 1993; 3: 367–370.
122. Kivanc MT, Klaus MV, Nashel DJ. Reversible polymyositis occurring during psoralen and ultraviolet A (PUVA) therapy. *J Rheumatol* 2000; 27(7): 1823–1824.
123. Nesbitt Jr LT. Cutaneous immunofluorescence in dermatomyositis. *Int J Dermatol* 1980; 19: 270–273.
124. Bilsland D, Diffey BL, Farr PM, et al. Diagnostic phototesting in the United Kingdom. British photodermatology group. *Br J Dermatol* 1992; 127: 297–299.
125. Garzon MC, DeLeo VA. Photosensitivity in the pediatric patient. *Curr Opin Pediatr* 1997; 9: 377–387.
126. Werth VP, Callen JP, Ang G, et al. Associations of tumor necrosis factor and HLA polymorphism with adult dermatomyositis: implications for a unique pathogenesis. *J Invest Dermatol* 2002; 119: 617–620.
127. Chung JH, Kwon OS, Eun HC, et al. Apoptosis in the pathogenesis of cutaneous lupus erythematosus. *Am J Dermatopathol* 1998; 20: 233–241.
128. Pablos JL, Santiago B, Galindo M, et al. Keratinocyte apoptosis and p53 expression in cutaneous lupus and dermatomyositis. *J Pathol* 1999; 188: 63–68.
129. Rider LG, Lachenbruch P, Rennebohm R, et al. Identifying skin lesions in dermatomyositis: interrater reliability of a new cutaneous assessment tool. *Arthritis Rheum* 1996, 38(Suppl): S168.
130. Santmyire-Rosenberger B, Dugan EM. Skin involvement in dermatomyositis. *Curr Opin Rheumatol* 2003; 15(6): 714–722.
131. Feldman BM, Rider LG, Dugan EM, et al. Nailfold capillaries as indicators of disease activity in juvenile idiopathic inflammatory myopathies. *Arthritis Rheum* 1999; 42 (Suppl): S664.
132. Pachman LM, Mendez E, Lechman T, et al. The rash of juvenile dermatomyositis is associated with derangement of capillaries. *Arthritis Rheum* 2000; 43 (Suppl): S380.

32

133. Miller FW, Rider LG, Chung Y-L, et al. Proposed preliminary core set measures for disease outcome assessment in adult and juvenile idiopathic inflammatory myopathies. *Rheumatology* 2001; 40: 1262–1273.
134. Rider LG. Outcome assessment in the adult and juvenile idiopathic inflammatory myopathies. *Rheum Dis Clin North Am* 2002; 28: 935–977.
135. Bode RK, Klein-Gitelman MS, Miller ML, et al. Disease activity score for children with juvenile dermatomyositis: reliability and validity evidence. *Arthritis Rheum* 2003; 49(1): 7–15.

Pathology and Immunopathology of Dermatomyositis

33

33.1 Histopathology and Immunopathology of Myositis in DM Patients

The definitive diagnosis of myositis requires a muscle biopsy. A biopsy should be performed on every patient in whom the diagnosis of an IIM is considered, in order not only to confirm the diagnosis, but also to rule out the conditions that clinically resemble myositis. Previous data suggest that ultrasound imaging could be useful for detecting needle biopsy in the diagnosis of selective involvement in muscle disease, since the muscle changes are often focal rather than diffuse [1]. Later, it was found that muscle ultrasound had sensitivity in detecting histopathologically proven disease not significantly different from electromyography or serum creatine kinase activity [2].

Pathological examination of muscle in DM usually reveals characteristic myopathic findings, including (i) perifascicular atrophy of muscle fibers, (ii) a predominantly perivascular or interfascicular lymphocyte infiltration, and (iii) evidence of vascular damage involving the small vessels. DM is characterized by myosinolysis, floccular degeneration, and capillary loss in the perifascicular regions of the muscle fasciculi [3]. Perifascicular atrophy and inflammatory cells have been also observed in these regions and in the adjacent interstitial connective tissue.

Abnormal perifascicular class I MHC expression is of diagnostic value in patients presenting with clinical features of DM, especially when muscle biopsy fails to show typical features such as inflammatory infiltrates and/or perifascicular atrophy [4]. Normal muscle fibers do not express class I MHC. Abnormal class I MHC expression always occurs in muscle biopsies showing features of IIMs [4].

Perifascicular atrophy, which is reported in 50% of adults and 90% of juvenile DM, is considered as diagnostic [5]. Perifascicular atrophy and an expression of endofascicular hyperperfusion are found only in DM [5]. Muscles that are actively involved show degenerative changes and signs of regeneration. Necrosis occurs at the periphery of the muscle bundle. Muscle fibers in areas of degeneration show loss of their transverse striation and hyalinization of sarcoplasm. Inflammatory myopathies showed distinct patterns of up-regulation of matrix metalloproteinases (MMP) [6]. MMP-9 was strongly expressed in atrophic myofibers in all inflammatory myopathies. In DM, the perifascicular atrophy showed a strong sarcolemmal expression of MMP-9 in atrophic myofibers and some CD4-positive lymphocytes in areas of perifascicular atrophy, probably reflecting denervated patterns of myofibers [6]. Perifascicular myopathic muscle fibers have reduced or absent cytochrome oxidase activity [7]. Two different patterns of myofiber damage were observed in biopsies of juvenile DM: zones with necrosis, and zones where an apoptotic process was dominant [8]. In severe cases, fragmentation and granular and vacuolar degeneration, as well as phagocytosis of degenerated muscle fragments by macrophages, may also be present [9]. The myofibers appear necrotic as a result of microinfarcts [5] and phagocytosis grouped together in an ischemic pattern. Regenerating muscle fibers characterized by basophilia and a reduction in diameter may also present [10]. Moderately abundant IL-1-positive inflammatory cells were observed in muscle fibers in DM, and rarely in PM and IBM [11]. IL-1 is a pleiotropic molecule, implicated in the inflammatory process, but also in tissue protection and remodeling. IL-1-positive muscle fibers were observed mainly in DM, usually remote from inflammatory infiltrates. Positive immunostaining for IL-1 was observed in fibers showing ischemic punched-out vacuoles that correspond to areas of myosinolysis in atrophic perifascicular fibers, and in fibers located within healing microinfarcts. Authier et al. [11] concluded that (i) IL-1 is expressed by muscle fibers undergoing ischemic damage, and (ii) IL-1 expression by muscle fibers is associated with myofibrillar protein breakdown and regeneration.

Chronic lymphocytic and macrophagic infiltration of muscle parenchyma is the hallmark of myositis. The mononuclear inflammatory infiltrate is patchy, perivascular, and perifascicular. Features found more commonly in DM are the accumulations of inflammatory cells selectively around vessels (62%), alkaline phosphatase staining of small vessels (58%), and reduced capillary index [7]. DM muscle infiltrates show mostly CD4+ and B lymphocytes in perimysium and in perifascicular area [12]. Various studies have demonstrated accumulation of CD4 and CD8 lymphocytes and up-regulation of their respective ligands, the MHC antigen classes I and II, at sites of muscle inflammation [13–15]. Both in patients with PM and DM, muscle contains mixed infiltrates of mononuclear cells [16], but the immunological mechanisms of tissue injury are strikingly different [17]. In muscles of PM patients, autoaggressive CD8+ T cells contact and invade muscle fibers, while in DM in contrast, the humoral effector mechanism prevails [16]. Similar levels of perforin mRNA, however, were expressed in PM and DM patients [17]. An abundance of the CD8+ and CD4+ T cells expressing CD45RO antigen in perivascular muscle infiltrates of DM patients has been observed, and the accumulation of the CD45RO+ memory T cells was predominant [18]. The enrichment of perivascular memory T cells in DM is supposedly the result of the enhanced transendothelian migratory capacity of these cells [18]. The perforin in the cytoplasm of DM was distributed randomly in the cytoplasm of muscle-infiltrating T cells, while in PM 43% of the CD8+ T cells were contacted with muscle fiber, and perforin is located vectorially toward the muscle fiber [17]. It has been found that T-cell inflammation in PM and DM patients is not cleared by apoptosis, and the affected muscle fiber does not die by apoptosis [19]. Recently, Mizuno et al. [20] determined peripheral blood T-cell phenotypes, and analyzed distribution of lymphocytes infiltrating the muscle tissues in two patients with juvenile DM. In both of the patients examined, a unique combination of TCR Vβ repertoires was increased within the CD8+ T cells. These subpopulations expressed a characteristic phenotype, indicating that they are memory/effector T cells with killer functions. At the same time, immunohistological and molecular biological examinations of the biopsied muscle samples revealed that identical CD8+ T cell clones with identical-TCR Vβ phenotypes infiltrated within the inflammatory tissue, in particular around vessels.

Immunohistochemical staining has revealed that CD40 was expressed on muscle cells of both PM and DM patients, which suggests that the interaction between T cells and muscle cells was performed by augmenting inflammation via cytokine production by the muscle cells. [21].

Histopathologic observations on juvenile DM from the mid-1960s suggest that the disease may represent a systemic angiopathy [22]. It has been proposed that degenerative changes in muscle represent infarctions resulting from a necrotizing vasculitis, with subsequent occlusion of small perimysial and endomysial vessels by intimal hyperplasia and fibrin thrombi [22]. Muscle damage in DM patients is currently understood to be a complement-mediated injury directed against the intramuscular microvasculature [16]. One of the earliest changes in DM is the focal depletion of muscle capillaries [23]. The primary antigenic target in DM is the endothelium of both the endomysial and skin capillaries [24]. An early reduction of capillary density due to deposit of immunoglobulin and the complement membrane attack complex (MAC) on muscle vessels has been reported [25, 26]. Several immunofluorescence studies have identified MAC deposit in the blood vessels of skeletal muscle biopsy specimens obtained from DM patients [23, 27]. A primary role of complement-induced vessel injury in DM is established, providing consistent evidence of complement cascade activation [23, 27]. The association between MAC microvascular deposits with early histological changes of muscle fiber ischemia in juvenile DM has also been described [27]. Furthermore, morphological evidence for cell-mediated attack against muscle fibers is absent [17], suggesting a primary role of the complement system in the pathogenesis of DM. An inversible relation was found between MAC deposition and presence of CD59 (a complement regulatory protein *Protectin*) in vessels in juvenile DM [28]. The strongest immunochemical staining for protectin was observed in endothelia of blood vessels, and in regenerating muscle cells — myoblasts, myotubes, and regenerating muscle fibers in PM and DM [29].

Overexpression of matrix metalloproteinases MMP-2 and -9 in inflammatory myopathies has been reported [30]. Quantitative PCR analysis revealed significantly elevated mRNA expression of MMP-1 and MMP-9 in DM and PM, and to a lower extent in IBM, whereas the levels of expression of the metalloproteinase tissue inhibitors remained unchanged [31]. Myeloid-related proteins MRP8/MRP14, a proinflammatory subtype of macrophages in DM, inhibited proliferation and differentiation of myoblasts and induced apoptosis via activation of caspase-3 in a time- and dose-dependent manner [32]

Old lesions usually show a rather nonspecific picture of atrophy of the muscle fibers and diffuse interstitial fibrosis, without or with a low level of inflammation [9].

The earliest changes seen by electron microscopy seem to consist of focal disintegration of myofilaments and myofibrils, resulting in areas of vacuolization and in the accumulation of lipid globules and lysosomes within muscle fibers [33, 34]. Intracytoplasmatic tubuloreticular inclusions resembling paramyxovirus are frequently present in endothelial cells of blood vessels [26], in the skin and muscle lesions of DM [34, 35].

33

33.2 Histopathology and Immunopathology of Skin Lesions in DM

The cutaneous histopathologic features of DM are not pathognomonic [36], but certain of them are compatible with the disease [37] and when present, skin biopsy is useful for differentiation from other skin diseases such as psoriasis, lichen planus, cutaneous T-cell lymphoma, atopic dermatitis, and SSc. Skin histopathologic features of DM are not distinguishable from those in lupus erythematosus. Immunofluorescent findings, with the exception of MAC deposit of complement in skin, are also not specific and not secure in diagnosing DM alone, but may help rule out lupus erythematosus.

Histology of the skin biopsy specimen reveals a compact orthokeratosis in the cornified layer, epidermal hyperplasia with focal areas of atrophy, vacuolar degeneration and necrotic keratinocytes along the basal membrane, and superficial perivascular lymphocytic infiltrate [10, 38]. Salient features of DM on skin biopsy include vacuolar alteration of the basal cell layer of the epidermis, necrotic keratinocytes (apoptosis), vascular dilatation, and a sparse, superficial, perivascular lymphocytic infiltrate [39, 40].

More studies of the histopathologic changes in DM skin lesions have been emphasized as nonspecific, with cell-poor interface dermatitis and dermal mucinosis indistinguishable from cutaneous lupus erythematosus [10, 22, 41, 42]. The histopathologic examination of DM skin lesions demonstrates an interface dermatitis characterized by liquefaction degeneration at the dermal epidermal junction and a patchy mononuclear inflammatory infiltrate high in the reticular and papillary dermis [42]. Characteristic light microscopic findings of DM cutaneous lesions included:

(i) Orthokeratotic hypekeratosis
(ii) Epidermal changes including partly atrophic epidermis (57%)
(iii) Focal liquefaction degeneration of basal cells (69%), and vacuolization of the keratinocytes
(iv) Melanin incontinence
(v) Papillary edema
(vi) Mucin deposit
(vii) Discrete perivascular lymphocytic infiltration [22, 41, 42]

These features are similar to those seen in LE and cannot be differentiated; moreover, they closely resemble the findings seen in acute or chronic graft-versus-host reaction [43]. A feature frequently seen in DM is the presence of massive dermal edema and increased quantities of alcian blue-positive glucosaminglycans within the dermis. In the Wong type of DM, biopsies of hyperkeratotic, follicular papules demonstrate hyperkeratosis, follicular plugging, a perifollicular lymphocytic infiltrate, and interface dermatitis [44]. Clinical and histopathological findings similar to the Wong type of DM have been described for follicular graft-versus-host reaction [45].

Recent studies have focused on characteristic microvascular changes found in both adult and juvenile DM skin biopsies, and the role of a vasculopathy in skin lesions. These changes consist of prominent dilatation of blood vessels, intimal hyperplasia, endothelial injury, and occlusive thrombosis and fibrinoid necrosis of dermal capillaries [46].

Microvascular injury plays an important role in the pathogenesis of cutaneous lesions of DM [47, 48]. Immunofluorescence examination of cutaneous lesions in DM demonstrates the deposition of the MAC of complement (C5b-C9) in dermal blood vessels [47]. The complement MAC deposits were found along the dermoepidermal junction and on the vessel walls of the dermis from the lesional skin [47]. One of the earliest changes in DM is the focal depletion of muscle capillaries [48]. Cutaneous lesions in DM showed a greater degree of endothelial injury, vascular ectasia, and vascular fibrin deposition compared with samples of LE lesions [48]. MAC deposits were found along the dermoepidermal junction in around 90% of DM cases and on the vessel walls of the dermis in 80% of biopsy specimens [47, 48]. Discrete cellular interface dermatitis associated with complement-mediated microvascular injury and resultant vessel dropouts are the key histologic features of DM distinguishable from findings in LE [49]. Factors responsible for the initiating vascular damage, antibody deposit and complement activation have not been elucidated, and the target antigen in endothelial cells remains unknown.

In a study of 35 DM patients, direct immunofluorescence showed a positive lupus band test at the basal membrane zone in 19 skin samples (54%). Colloid bodies in sun-exposed skin were found in seven samples [50].

Dourmishev and Wolina [51] reported that cell proliferation indicated with the presence of anti-Ki-67 antibody in skin lesions of DM patients is diminished in areas with epidermal affection. The number of apoptotic keratinocytes was significantly increased in epidermis compared with normal skin in the disrupted basal zone of DM patients [51–53]. It was also reported that DM's skin lesions showed perivascular location of activated CD3+ and CD 45 RO+ lymphocytes [51]. Peripheral blood T cells in adults consist mainly of CD45RO antigens that are associated with antigen-primed memory CD8+ and CD4+ T cells [54].

Recent studies of skin biopsy specimens showed that the majority of cells in inflammatory dermal infiltrates were T lymphocytes and macrophages [41, 42]. The inflammatory infiltrates in DM patients consisted predominantly of T lymphocytes (especially CD4 subset), usually sparse and focal in perivascular and subepidermal locations, and HLA-DR-expressing macrophages scattered through the papillary dermis, surrounding perivascular infiltrates, or in subepidermal accumulations [41]. Dermal infiltrates were found to consist predominantly of T lymphocytes with perivascular location, or have a lichenoid or periadnexal/perifollicular pattern in the dermis and septal hypodermis. In the majority of specimens, CD 45 RO+ cells were more abundant than CD3+ cells [51]. The enrichment of perivascular T cells in dermal compartment of DM patients in memory cells supports the thesis that they are a result of the enhanced transendothelial migratory capacity of these cells [18]. The microvascular injury in the dermis allows transendothelial migration of activated T lymphocytes from blood in perivascular infiltrates or in infiltrates with periadnexal or perifollicular location.

There have been only two reports on immunophenotypic characterization in the cutaneous lesions of DM that emphasize the importance of the infiltrating CD4+ T lymphocytes [41, 55]. Skin biopsy specimens derived from Gottron's papules of patients with DM show that activated CD4+ Th lymphocytes (HLA-DR+ CD40L+) were the principal infiltrating cells in the lesional skin of DM [56]. A mixed Th1/Th2 profile and higher Th1 (IFN-γ, TNF-α, and IL-2) cytokine production, together with significant staining for receptor 3 for CXC chemokines (CXCR3), were detected [56]. Activated CD4+ T cells presumably

33

mediate the main pathogenetic mechanisms in pathognomonic skin lesions. The interaction between CD40 and CD40L could be an important mechanism of cellular activation in cutaneous immune-mediated inflammation, by induction of secretion of proinflammatory cytokines and chemokines. There was a significant quantity of myeloperoxidase positive cells (neutrophil granulocytes) in the inflamed tissue, and they might have a role in sustaining the chronic inflammation. CD4+ Th cells can be classified into different types based on their cytokine profile, type 1 (Th1) and type 2 (Th2). According to a recent definition, Th2 lymphocytes can produce interleukin (IL-4), while Th1 lymphocytes cannot [57]. Furthermore, Th1 lymphocytes preferentially express certain specific receptors, such as CXCR3, while Th2 lymphocytes express receptor 3 for CC chemokines (CCR3) [58, 59]. The prominence of such Th1 cytokines, particularly in Gottron's papules, supports their potential role in the pathogenesis of skin lesions by accelerating cell-mediated immunity and by inducing abnormal keratinization [60]. Hydropic degeneration of basal keratinocytes could be caused by the deposition of C5b-9 and MAC that were found as a keratinocyte decoration of IgG and C5b-9 with direct immunofluorescence [49].

Recent studies focusing on the pathogenic mechanisms of pathognomonic cutaneous lesions (Gottron's papules and sign) indicate that Th1 lymphocyte-mediated inflammation, microvascular injury, and apoptotic dysregulation of basal keratinocytes might play a significant role in their formation [56]. The results have demonstrated Th lymphocytes (CD3+ CD4+) in the lesional skin, with signs of activation (HLA-DR+ CD40L+) and superficial perivascular and periadnexal distribution [41, 55, 56].

Most typical are the histopathologic changes in *poikiloderma atrophicans vasculare* [9]. In the early stage, a slight hyperkeratosis and moderate thinning of the stratum malpighii, effacement of the rete ridges and hydropic degeneration of the basal cells with rare cytoid bodies were observed. In the upper dermis, a bandlike infiltrate mainly consisting of lymphocytes, melanophages, and a few histiocytes was found. The edema in the upper dermis is prominent, and the superficial capillaries are often dilated [9, 10, 61]. In the late stage, the epidermis is markedly thinned and flattened and basal cell liquefactive degeneration is typical. Edema of the upper dermis, melanophages, and telangiectasia could be pronounced [10, 62].

References

1. Heckmatt LZ, Dubovitz V. Ultrasound imaging and detected needle biopsy in the diagnosis of selective involvement in muscle disease. *J Child Neurol* 1987; 2: 205–213.
2. Reimers CD, Fleckenstein JL, Witt TN, et al. Muscular ultrasound in idiopathic inflammatory myopathies of adults. *J Neurol Sci* 1993; 116: 82–92.
3. Buchbinder R, Forbes A, Hall S, et al. Incidence of malignant disease in biopsy-proven inflammatory myopathy. A population-based cohort study. *Ann Intern Med* 2001; 134: 1087–1095.
4. Civatte M, Schleinitz N, Krammer P, et al. Class I MHC detection as a diagnostic tool in non-informative muscle biopsies of patients suffering from dermatomyositis (DM). *Neuropathol Appl Neurobiol* 2003; 29: 546–552.
5. Dalakas M. Polymyositis, dermatomyositis and inclusion body myositis. *N Engl J Med* 1991; 325(21): 1487–1498.

6. Schoser BH, Blottner D, Stuerenburg HJ. Matrix metalloproteinases in inflammatory myopathies: enhanced immunoreactivity nearby atrophic myofibers. *Acta Neurol Scand* 2002: 105: 309–313.
7. Mozaffar T, Pestronk A. Myopathy with anti-Jo-1 antibodies: pathology in perimyium and neighbouring muscle fibres. *J Neurol Neurosurg Psychiatry* 2000; 68: 472–478.
8. Falcini F, Calzolari A, Generini S, et al. Bcl-2, p53 and c-myc expression in juvenile dermatomyositis. *Clin Exp Rheumatol* 2000; 18: 643–646.
9. Lever WF, Schaumburg-Lever G. Dermatomyositis. In: *Histopathology of the Skin*, JB Lippincott, Philadelphia, 1983; 458–461.
10. Janis JF, Winkelmann RK. Histopathology of the skin in dermatomyositis. *Arch Dermatol* 1968; 97: 640–650.
11. Authier FJ, Mhiri C, Chazaud B, et al. Interleukin-1 expression in inflammatory myopathies: evidence of marked immunoreactivity in sarcoid granulomas and muscle fibres showing ischaemic and regenerative changes. *Neuropathol Appl Neurobiol* 1997; 23: 132–140.
12. Engel AG, Arahata K. Mononuclear cells in myopathies: quantitation of functionally distinct subsets, recognition of antigen-specific cell-mediated cytotoxicity in some diseases and implications for the pathogenesis of the different inflammatory myopathies. *Hum Pathol* 1986; 17: 704–721.
13. Arahata K, Engel AG. Monoclonal antibody analysis of mononuclear cells in myopathies. I. Quantification of subsets according to diagnosis and sites of accumulation and demonstration and counts of muscle fibers invaded by T cells. *Ann Neurol* 1984; 16: 193–208.
14. Bartoccioni E, Galluccoci S, Scuderi F, et al. MHC class I, MHC class II and intercellular adhesion molecule-1 (ICAM-1) expression in inflammatory myopathies. *Clin Exp Immunol* 1994; 95: 166–172.
15. Dalakas MC. Molecular immunology and genetics of inflammatory muscle diseases. *Arch Neurol* 1998; 55: 1509–1512.
16. Hohfeld R, Engel AG. The immunology of muscle. *Immunol Today* 1994; 15: 269–274.
17. Goebels N, Michaelis D, Engelhardt M, et al. Differential expression of perforin in muscle-infiltrating T cells in polymyositis and dermatomyositis. *J Clin Invest* 1996; 12: 2905–2910.
18. De Bleecker JL, Engel AG. Immunocytochemical study of CD45 T cell isoforms in inflammatory myopathies. *Am J. Pathol* 1995; 146: 1178–1187.
19. Schneider C, Gold R, Dalakas MC, et al. MHC class I-mediated cytotoxicity does not induce apoptosis in muscle fibers nor in inflammatory T cells: studies in patients with polymyositis, dermatomyositis and inclusion body myositis. *J Neuropathol Exp Neurol* 1996; 55: 1205–1209.
20. Mizuno K, Yachie A, Nagaoki S, et al. Oligoclonal expansion of circulating and tissue-infiltrating CD8+ T Cells with killer/effector phenotypes in juvenile dermatomyositis syndrome. *Clin Exp Immunol* 2004; 137: 187–194.
21. Sugiura T, Kawaguchi Y, Harigai M, et al. Increased CD40 expression on muscle cells of polymyositis and dermatomyositis: role of CD40-CD40 ligand interaction in IL-6, IL-8, IL-15, and monocyte chemoattractant protein-1 production. *J Immunol* 2000; 164: 6593–6600.
22. Banker BQ, Victor M. Dermatomyositis (systemic angiopathy) of childhood. *Medicine (Baltimore)* 1966; 45(4): 261–289.
23. Emslie-Smith AM, Engel AG. Microvascular changes in early and advanced dermatomyositis: a quantitative study. *Ann Neurol* 1990; 48: 26–30.
24. Dalakas MC, Hohlfeld R. Polymyositis and dermatomyositis. *Lancet* 2003; 362(9388): 971–982.
25. Whitaker JN, Engel WK. Vascular deposits of immunoglobulin and complement in idiopathic inflammatory myopathy. *N Engl J Med* 1972; 286: 333–338.

26. De Visser M, Emslie-Smith AM, Engel AG. Early ultrastructural alterations in adult dermatomyositis. Capillary abnormalities precede other structural changes in muscle. *J Neurol Sci* 1989; 94: 181–192.
27. Kissel JT, Mendell JR, Rammohan KW. Microvascular deposition of complement membrane attack complex in dermatomyositis. *N Engl J Med* 1986; 314: 329–334.
28. Goncalves FGP, Chimelli L, Sallim AME, et al. Immunohistological analysis of CD59 and membrane attack complex of complement in muscle in juvenile dermatomyositis. *J Rheumatol* 2002; 29: 1301–1307.
29. Gendek-Kubiaka H, Gendek EG. Immunolocalization of protectin (CD59) and macrophages in polymyositis and dermatomyositis. *J Neuroimmunol* 2004; 149: 187–194.
30. Choi YC, Dalakas MC. Expression of matrix metalloproteinases in the muscle of patients with inflammatory myopathies. *Neurology* 2000; 54: 65–71.
31. Kiesier BC, Schneider C, Clements JM, et al. Expression of specific matrix metalloproteinases in inflammatory myopathies. *Brain* 2001; 124: 341–351.
32. Seeliger S, Vogl T, Engels IH, et al. Expression of calcium-binding proteins MRP8 and MRP14 in inflammatory muscle diseases. *Am J Pathol* 2003; 163: 947–956.
33. Gonzalez-Anagulo A, Fraga A, Mintz G. Submicroscopic alterations in capillaries of muscles in polymyositis. *Am J Med* 1968; 45: 873–879.
34. Hashimoto K, Robinson L, Velayos E, et al. Dermatomyositis. Electron microscopic, immunologic, and tissue culture studies of paramyxovirus-like inclusions. *Arch Dermatol* 1971; 103: 120–135.
35. Landry M, Winkelmann RK. Tubular cytoplasmic inclusions in dermatomyositis. *Proc Mayo Clin* 1972; 47: 479–492.
36. Euwer R, Sontheimer R. Amyopathic dermatomyositis (dermatomyositis sine myositis). Presentation of six new cases and review of the literature. *J Am Acad Dermatol* 1991; 24: 959–966.
37. Kasper CS, White CL 3rd, Freeman RG. Pathology and immunopathology of polymyositis/dermatomyositis. *Clin Dermatol* 1988; 6(2): 64–75.
38. Ackerman AB. Dermatomyositis. In: *Diagnosis of Inflammatory Skin Diseases. An Algorithmic Method Based on Pattern Analysis*, Williams & Wilkins, Baltimore, MD, 1997; 289–293.
39. Mitra D, Lovell CL, Macleod TI, et al. Clinical and histological features of 'mechanic's hands' in a patient with antibodies to Jo-1 — a case report. *Clin Exp Dermatol* 1994; 19(2): 146–148.
40. Callen JP. Dermatomyositis. *Lancet* 2000; 355: 53–57.
41. Hausmann G, Mascarò JM Jr, Herrero C, et al. Cell adhesion molecule expression in cutaneous lesions of dermatomyositis. *Acta Derm Venereol (Stockh)* 1996; 76: 222–225.
42. Dourmishev L, Obreshkova E. Histopathologic changes in skin of dermatomyositis patients. *Dermatol Venereol (Sofia)* 2001; 50(1): 18–22 [Bulgarian].
43. Santmyire-Rosenberger B, Dugan EM. Skin involvement in dermatomyositis. *Curr Opin Rheumatol* 2003; 15(6): 714–722.
44. Lupton JR, Figueroa P, Berberian BJ, et al. An unusual presentation of dermatomyositis: the type Wong variant revisited. *J Am Acad Dermatol* 2000; 43: 908–912.
45. Freidman KJ, LeBoit PE, Farmer ER. Acute follicular graft versus host reaction. A distinct clinicopathologic presentation. *Arch Dermatol* 1988; 124: 688–691.
46. Bowyer SL, Clark RA, Ragsdale CG, et al. Juvenile dermatomyositis: Histological findings and pathogenetic hypothesis for the associated skin changes. *J Rheumatol* 1986; 13(4): 753–759.
47. Mascaro JM, Hausmann G, Herrero C, et al. Membrane attack complex deposits in cutaneous lesions of dermatomyositis. *Arch Dermatol* 1995; 131: 1386–1392.
48. Crowson AN, Magro CM. The role of microvascular injury in the pathogenesis of cutaneous lesions of dermatomyositis. *Hum Pathol* 1996; 27(1): 15–19.
49. Magro CM, Crowson AN. The immunofluorescent profile of dermatomyositis: a comparative study with lupus erythematosus. *J Cutan Pathol* 1997; 24: 543–552.

50. Vaughan-Jones SA, Black MM. The value of direct immunofluorescence as a diagnostic aid in dermatomyositis — a study of 35 cases. *Clin Exp Dermatol* 1997; 22: 77–81.
51. Dourmishev L, Wolina U. Dermatomyositis: immunopathologic study of skin lesions. *Acta Dermatoven APN* 2006; 15: 45–51.
52. Chung JH, Kwon OS, Eun HC, et al. Apoptosis in the pathogenesis of cutaneous lupus erythematosus. *Am J Dermatopathol* 1998; 20: 233–241.
53. Pablos JL, Santiago B, Galindo M, et al. Keratinocyte apoptosis and p53 expression in cutaneous lupus and dermatomyositis. *J Pathol* 1999; 188: 63–68.
54. Mason M. Subsets of CD+ T cells defined by their expression of different isoforms of the leucocyte-common antigen, CD45. *Biochem Soc Trans* 1992; 20: 188–190.
55. Hausmann G, Herrero C, Cid MC, et al. Immunopathologic study of skin lesions in dermatomyositis. *J Am Acad Dermatol* 1991; 25: 225–230.
56. Carponi M, Torchia D, Cardinali C, et al. Infiltrating cells, related cytokines and chemokine receptors in lesional skin of patients with dermatomyositis. *Br J Dermatol* 2004; 151: 784–791.
57. Romagnani S. The Th2 hypothesis in allergy — "Eppur si muove!". *ACI Int* 1998; 10: 158–165.
58. Hu-Li J, Huang H, Ryan J, et al. In differentiated CD4+ T cells, interleukin 4 production is cytokine-autonomous, while interferon gamma production is cytokine-dependent. *Proc Natl Acad Sci USA* 1997; 94: 3189–3194.
59. Liblau RS, Singer SM, McDevitt HO. Th1 and Th2 CD4+ T cells in the pathogenesis of organ-specific autoimmune diseases. *Immunol Today* 1995; 1: 34–38.
60. Arany I, Brysk MM, Brysk H, et al. Regulation of inducible nitric oxide synthase mRNA levels by differentiation and cytokines in human keratinocytes. *Biochem Biophys Res Commun* 1996; 220: 618–622.
61. Bonvalet D, Colan-Gohm K, Belaich S, et al. Les différentes formes du parapsoriasis en plaques. *Ann Dermatol Venereol* 1977; 104: 18–25.
62. Horn RC Jr. Poikilodermatomyositis. *Arch Dermatol Syph* 1941; 44: 1086–1097.

Diagnosis and Differential Diagnosis of DM

Medical Evolution of Dermatomyositis 34

The wide spectrum of cutaneous manifestations of DM: (i) complicate developing the diagnosis, (ii) make difficult differential diagnosis with other skin diseases, such as LE, psoriasis, pityriasis rubra pilaris, lichen ruber, sebborrhoic dermatitis, or SSc, and (iii) hamper classification of amyopathic DM.

DM can usually be diagnosed by a complete history, physical examination, laboratory studies (complete blood cell count, biochemical screen, muscle enzymes, MSAs, muscle biopsy), EMG, and other noninvasive imaging techniques. Several features are important to discern [1]:

(i) **Characteristic of the muscle weakness**: is the weakness proximal or distal, progressive or intermittent, fatigable, exercise-related, or sudden or gradual in onset?
(ii) **Other origin of clinical features**: are there CTD or neurologic signs?
(iii) **Genetic background of disease**: is there a familial component?
(iv) **Inducing factors**: is there a drug or toxic history?

The diagnosis of DM is often missed, even by dermatologists [2]. This can lead to delay in diagnosing the muscle disease and in carefully investigating the patients for a occult malignancy. Patients with the typical cutaneous involvement of DM should be assessed for myositis and other organ involvement. The diagnosis of muscle involvement can be determined by physical examination demonstrating muscle weakness or loss of power, as well as by serum muscle enzyme studies (AST, ALT, aldolase, and CK) and electromyography (EMG). EMG studies detect evidence of muscle irritability and myopathy. A definitive diagnosis, however, should be established by muscle biopsy, since other clinical conditions can produce muscle weakness and mimic an inflammatory muscle disease. It is necessary to obtain a muscle biopsy in all cases, to establish a diagnosis of muscle involvement. Some studies showed that MRI studies detecting T2-weighted images and phosphorus 31 MR spectroscopy or muscle ultrasound examination are sensitive techniques for detecting of muscle inflammation. These techniques, coupled with needle muscle biopsies, could become standards of practice, replacing EMG and open muscle biopsy techniques.

L.A. Dourmishev and A.L. Dourmishev, *Dermatomyositis: Advances in Recognition, Understanding and Management*,

Upon determining the extent of muscle disease, it is essential to evaluate internal involvement. Generally this can be done by clinical evaluation. Pulmonary involvement occurring as ILD can be evaluated radiographically, as well as with pulmonary function studies (spirometry and single-breath CO_2 diffusion studies). Patients can also develop esophageal dysmotility, which can lead to significant dysphagia or aspiration. If clinical symptoms are suggestive, then further evaluation with a cine-esophagram study is indicated.

The other issue of great importance is to determine if there is a coexisting malignancy. Numerous studies have demonstrated that DM can be a paraneoplastic syndrome, especially after the age of 40. It is necessary to provide individualized and age-appropriate screening for evidence of lung, breast, colonic, ovarian, and pelvic neoplasia. The patients are evaluated with a mammogram, urinalysis, chest radiograph, and screening for occult gastrointestinal blood loss. Female patients are also evaluated for possible ovarian or cervical tumors, using a pelvic and intravaginal ultrasound examination at least once a year and a cancer antigen (CA 125) examination for at least 5 years.

Because DM is the classic example of systemic disease with cutaneous manifestations, the skin and myositis features become of equal value in developing the diagnosis (Table 34.1). The table contains a combined set of hallmark cutaneous manifestations of DM proposed by authors based on their own experience and on analysis of most published dermatologic series [3, 4], associated with criteria for myositis suggested by Bohan and Peter [5] and Tanimoto et al. [6], in addition to new noninvasive diagnostic imaging techniques [7] and various MSAs [8]. Absence of cutaneous manifestations is indicative of PM; the presence of skin and muscle involvement is characteristic of classic DM; availability of pathognomic skin rash and lacking of myositis is typical for amyopathic DM.

Finally, we have included a patient evolution algorithm for diagnosis of DM (Fig. 34.1) [9].

Table 34.1 Diagnostic steps in diagnosis of dermatomyositis

History of disease	1. General medical history	
	2. Onset, duration, and characterization of cutaneous manifestations	
	3. Evaluation of weakness in proximal muscle groups	
	4. Absence of multisystem disease	
	5. Association of malignancy	
	6. History of toxins (e.g., alcohol), infections, travel, or drug intake	
	7. Familial history	
	I. Evolution of muscle strength	1. Assessment of strength in shoulder and hip muscle groups
		2. Proximal muscle weakness
		3. Respiratory muscle weakness
		4. Muscle atrophy
		5. Muscle calcification
	II. Neurological evolution	1. Ruling out a neurological cause for the weakness

(continued)

Table 34.1 (continued)

Physical examination	**III. Dermatologic evaluation**	1. Pathognomonic cutaneous manifestations of DM: (a) Heliotrope rash (periorbital violaceous erythema) (b) Gottron's papules (c) Gottron's sign 2. Characteristic cutaneous manifestations of DM: (a) Shawl sign or V-sign (symmetrical macular violaceous erythema) (b) Nailfold changes (periungual erythema, telangiectases, cuticular hypertrophy, hemorrhagic infarcts) (c) Scalp scaly dermatosis 3. Compatible cutaneous manifestations of DM: (a) Periorbital edema (facial swelling) (b) Poikilodermia vascularis atrophicans (photosensitive poikiloderma) (c) Pruritus 4. Less common manifestations of DM: (a) Cutaneous vasculitis (b) Panniculitis (c) Calcinosis 5. Rare cutaneous manifestations of DM: (a) Mechanic's hands (b) Follicular hyperkeratosis (type Wong) (c) Centripetal linear or flagellate erythema (d) Erythroderma (erythrodermic dermatomyositis) (e) Vesicular and subepidermal bullous lesions (f) Epidermal necrosis
Laboratory examinations	**I. Evaluation of muscle disease**	1. Biochemical: CK, aldolase, creatine 2. EMG 3. Muscle biopsy 4. Imaging techniques: MRI, muscle ultrasound 5. MSAs: (a) Mi 2 antibody: photosensitive features (shawl sign), cuticular overgrowth (b) Jo-1: antisynthetase syndrome (c) EJ: antisynthetase syndrome, increased frequency of skin changes (d) SRP: fulminant disease, cardiac involvement

(continued)

34

Table 34.1 (continued)

Laboratory examinations	**II. Skin disease evaluation**	1. Skin biopsy for routine histopathologic evaluation
		2. Direct immunofluorescence
		3. Nailfold microscopy
		4. Photo test
	III. Evaluation for organ involvement	1. Chest radiograph
		2. Pulmonary function tests: CO diffusion capacity
		3. Esophageal studies: manometry or cineradiography
Evaluation for malignancy	**I. Comprehensive medical history**	
	II. Physical examination	1. Review of systems
		2. Manual touching (rectal, vaginal)
		3. Laryngoscopy assessment of ears, nose, and throat (in Asian patients for nasopharyngeal cancer), and the checking of serum IgA-Epstein-Barr virus antibody
	III. Baseline laboratory screen	1. Complete blood count
		2. Blood chemistries
		3. Stool occult blood examination
		4. Prostate-specific antigen in man
	IV. Imaging techniques	1. Endoscopy (esophagogastroduodenoscopy, sigmoidoscopy, colonoscopy)
		2. Barium swallow and esophageal motility studies
		3. Radiography (chest radiograph, mammogram, bone)
		4. Computer axial tomography (CAT, abdominal/pelvis computed tomography scan, positron emitting tomography)
		5. Ultrasonography (ovarian ultrasound, transvaginal ultrasonography)
	V. Tumor markers	CEA, CA-125, CA 15-3, MUC-1, and TPS

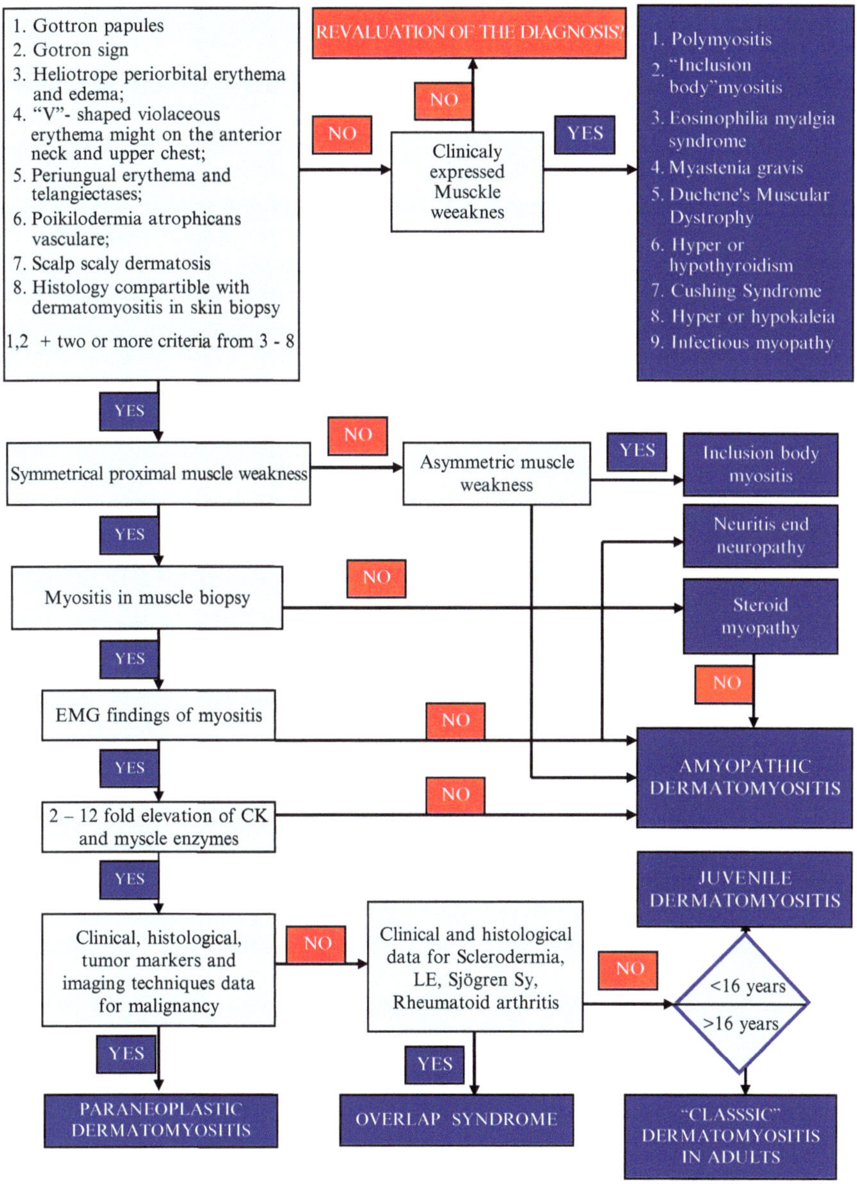

Fig. 34.1 Algorithm for diagnostic of DM [9]

34

References

1. Plotz PH, Dalakas M, Leff RL, et al. Current concepts in the idiopathic inflammatory myopathies: polymyositis, dermatomyositis, and related disorders. *Ann Intern Med* 1989; 111(2): 143–157.
2. Jorizzo JL. Dermatomyositis: practical aspects. *Arch Dermatol* 2002; 138: 114–116.
3. Euwer R, Sontheimer R. Amyopathic dermatomyositis (dermatomyositis sine myositis). Presentation of six new cases and review of the literature. *J Am Acad Dermatol* 1991; 24: 959–966.
4. Sontheimer RD. Dermatomyositis: an overview of recent progress with emphasis on dermatologic aspects. *Dermatol Clin* 2002; 20: 387–408.
5. Bohan A, Peter JB. Polymyositis and dermatomyositis. *N Engl J Med* 1975; 292 (Part I): 344–347.
6. Tanimoto K, Nakano K, Kano S, et al. Classification criteria for polymyositis and dermatomyositis. *J Rheumatol* 1995; 22: 668–674.
7. Stonecipher MR, Jorizzo JR, Monu J, et al. Dermatomyositis with normal muscle enzyme concentration. A single-blind study of the diagnostic value of magnetic resonance imaging and ultrasound. *Arch Dermatol* 1994; 130: 1294–1299.
8. Targoff IN, Miller FW, Medsger TA Jr, et al. Classification criteria for the idiopathic inflammatory myopathies. *Curr Opin Rheumatol* 1997; 9(6): 527–535.
9. Dourmishev LA. Dermatomyositis: Current aspects. Ph.D. thesis, Sofia, January 2002; 140.

Differential Diagnosis of Dermatomyositis

35

There is a wide differential diagnosis for the clinical symptoms of cutaneous manifestations and muscle weakness in DM patients. Differential diagnoses of early skin manifestations of DM include acute allergic contact dermatitis, photodermatitis, polymorphic light eruption, systemic LE, subacute cutaneous LE (SCLE), seborrhoic dermatitis, lichen planus, psoriasis, orbital cellulites, cutaneous T-cell lymphoma, and atopic dermatitis [1].

The heliotrope eyelid eruption in DM is considered as a hallmark of the disease. The associated periorbital redness and edema producing ptosis, chemosis, and exophthalmos may initially be mistaken for infective orbital cellulitis.

Edematous erythematous facial rash in juvenile DM has to be distinguished from cellulitis and acute allergic contact dermatitis by the presence of closely spaced telangiectases. If the poikiloderma is noticed, but the photodistribution is missed, clinical misdiagnosis of cutaneous T-cell lymphoma might be made. Poikilodermatomyositis can usually be distinguished from other causes of atrophic patches by its distribution and by clinical history.

The characteristic violaceous poikiloderma of DM is distinguished from that seen in patients with LE. The lesions of DM differ slightly in their distribution, occurring exclusively over bone prominences, and they are frequently accompanied by severe pruritus [2]. The eruption in patients with DM has a violaceous color and a distribution around the eyes and extensor surfaces, and is often accompanied by nailfold telangiectasias and cuticular dystrophy [3]. In contrast, in subacute cutaneous lupus erythematosus the erythematous papulosquamous eruption is less pruritic, and is distributed over the malar eminences sparing the periorbital skin; and when the hands and feet are involved, it typically spares the skin between the joints instead of the surface overlying the joints [4]. The lesions of LE, however, are usually more red or pink, generally occur between the knuckles and seldom have accompanying symptoms [2]. To distinguish LE from DM by taking routine skin biopsy is not helpful. Clues to a specific histopathologic diagnosis are an exceedingly thinned epidermis associated with abundant mucin in the reticular dermis, in concert with perivascular lymphocytic infiltrates [5]. Direct immunofluorescence (lupus band test), which assesses for immunoglobulin deposition along the dermoepidermal junction of either involved or uninvolved skin, has been used to distinguish LE from DM [6]. Immunofluorescent microscopy is positive in LE patients and should be negative in patients with DM, but approximately 50% of SCLE patients have positive fluorescence, and sun-exposed lesions may be falsely positive. The lupus band test cannot always be considered as a reliable diagnostic tool, since there are cases of LBT-positive DM [7] and LBT-negative LE [8], and it has no diagnostic value in amyopathic DM [9]. However, the combination of a negative LBT, vascular MAC deposition and negative Ro, La, and RNP serology has been proposed as a predictor of DM versus LE with a sensitivity of 90.5% and a specificity of 96.8% [9]. Serological tests are also not secure in differentiating of DM from SCLE, since only 25% of DM patients are Mi-2 positive, and 60–70% of SCLE patients are Ro(SS-A) antibody positive [2].

Patients with DM may have a similar clinical presentation to those with SLE, along with positive ANA, but their anti-dsDNA antibodies are negative [10]. Amyopathic DM can be difficult to distinguish from SCLE [2], when histopathological lesions are formed of sparse superficial perivascular infiltrates of lymphocytes in combination with an epidermis which is focally thinned, and a cornified layer is normal or mostly compactly orthokeratotic [5]. If the photodistribution and poikiloderma are correctly diagnosed, but only the diagnosis of LE is considered, than a misdiagnosis can be made [3].

Poikiloderma atrophicans vasculare has been observed, seen in three different groups of dermatoses [11]:

(i) In association with genodermatoses as

  (a) Poikiloderma congenitale of Rothmund–Thompson
  (b) Bloom's syndrome
  (c) Congenital dyskeratosis

(ii) As an early stage of cutaneous T-cell lymphoma (mycosis fungoides), or as skin involvement in chronic graft-versus-host disease (GVHD)
(iii) As cutaneous manifestation of DM, and less commonly in LE

The association of poikiloderma with DM is often referred to as poikilodermatomyositis [12, 13]. In contrast to DM, the amount of inflammatory infiltrate seen in poikilodermatous mycosis fungoides increases with time; so-called "mycosis cells," the cells with large, hyperchromic nuclei appear, and the epidermotropism of the infiltrate is often marked [14].

Several dermatoses cause lesions on the fingers that can mimic Gottron's papules and signs. In lichen planus, LE and psoriasis, red scaly lesions do not occur only on the skin overlying knuckles as do Gottron's papules. When the photodistribution of the eruption is not detected, a misdiagnosis of psoriasis can occur, because of the secondary psoriasiforme scale than accumulates on the poikilodermatous patches [3]. Clinical distinction from psoriasis is occasionally difficult, but histopathological assessment is helpful [2].

When cutaneous lesions are not present or are not characteristic, differential diagnosis of PM is much more extensive.

Differential diagnoses of muscle weakness include metabolic, neurologic, endocrine disorders, CTDs, prolonged use of drugs, inflammatory myopathy from virus, bacterial, or protozoa origin, paraneoplastic syndromes and miscellaneous myopathy.

Drugs are a common cause of muscle weakness (see also the Chapter 24). Corticosteroids may induce muscle weakness by symptomatic hypokalemia or by causing steroid myopathy. Hypokalemia, hypocalcemia, and hypophosphatemia are observed rarely in patients with prolonged treatment with diuretics. High levels of CK or aldolase above normal limits are rarely seen in myopathies other than DM or PM, except rhabdomyolysis secondary to trauma or metabolitic disorders.

The presence of elevated AST, ALT, or LDH serum levels in a patient with an early stage of disease who has fatigue and minimal weakness often directs attention toward the diagnosis of liver disease and unnecessary liver biopsy [15]. Since thyroid abnormalities such as hypothyroidism with raised CK levels or hyperthyroidism are common, thyroid-stimulating hormone serum levels should be determined in patients with weakness. Feebleness can be observed also in patients with other endocrine diseases such as Cushing's disease, Addison's disease, and hypoparathyroidism.

Neurologic diseases such as myasthenia gravis, amyotrophic lateral sclerosis, Guillain–Barré syndrome or neuropathy from diabetes mellitus have to be distinguished from DM by the clinical picture, lack of raised CK and urinary creatine excretion, and often by EMG. In the absence of a rash, the family history may suggest a diagnosis of muscular dystrophy or a metabolic myopathy. The detection of atypical myopathic, short-duration, low-amplitude action potentials with normal interference pattern in EMG helps to exclude most metabolic myopathies and neuromuscular disease [16].

Some remote neuromuscular paraneoplastic syndromes have been reported, including cachectic myopathy, Lambert–Eaton myasthenic syndrome, and necrotizing myopathy [17].

Connective tissue diseases are distinguished from IIMs clinically and serologically. Myositis is a feature of so-called MCTD, LE, SSc, and many overlap syndromes, However, in contradistinction to DM and PM patients, muscle enzyme abnormalities are generally much less prominent [18].

DM might be confused with SSc, and the two conditions can occur together in scleromyositis overlap syndrome. Occasionally, patients with SSc show dilatation of the nailfold capillaries and cuticular changes. Polymyalgia rheumatica presents as abrupt onset of proximal stiffness, but not true weakness.

Pain and fever are rarely prominent in patients with DM, and when present they implicate infectious myopathy such as trichinosis or viral myositis. The patients with trichinosis have painful muscles and periorbital swelling and edema, but not other features of DM [19]. Therefore the first cases of DM were described as pseudo-trichinosis [20, 21].

Trichinosis or trichinellosis is a cosmopolitan zoonose. It is caused by ingestion of raw or undercooked meat infected with larvae of the tissue nematode *Trichinella*. Approximately 150 *Trichinella* species are known (often *Trichinella spiralis* is the cause agent). In the USA, the main sources for infection are meat from pork (60%), bear (23%), walrus (10%), and cougar (7%); in Africa, meat from wild canids and felids, and in Europe meat from wild boar and horse [22]. Humans are incidental hosts. The diagnosis is based on associations of the main clinical symptoms such as: fever up to 39°C in ~90% of cases, myalgia (~90%), facial (periorbital) edema (~80%), headache (50%), skin rash (20%) and laboratory features of eosinophilia, and positive serological tests or muscle biopsy for trichinosis. Muscles become stiff, hard, and edematous. Myalgias and pain of muscles upon exertion engage mostly the muscles of the eyes (with photophobia), masseters (with pseudotrismus), tongue, diaphragm, intercostal muscles, flexural muscle of extremities, etc. Myalgias and fatigue persist for a long time (in 90% of patients up to 2 years, and in 25% of patients even after 10 years). Muscle tenderness and weakness are also frequent [22]. Palpebral (orbital or facial) edema, often associated with chemosis and proptosis

35

[23] is symmetrical and makes the patient unrecognizable. The usual incubation period of trichinosis is 8–15 days [24] The disease progresses from an enteric (or intestinal) phase of 2–7 days to a invasive phase lasting from a week to several months and finally to a period of convalescence [22]. Conjunctivitis with subconjunctival hemorrhages is frequent and resolves slowly. Cutaneous rash may occurs in several forms such as urticaria (most common), petechiae, splinter and nailbed hemorrhages, peripheral plantar and volar edema, and erythema with desquamation [24, 25]. Eosinophilia and leukocytosis are earliest laboratory findings. Levels of muscle enzymes CK and LDH are also elevated.

The main clinical and laboratory findings of trichinellosis in children are fever, abdominal pain, myalgia, facial and/or eyelid edema, rash, eosinophilia, and increased muscular enzymes [26]. The incubation period is similar in children and adults, but myalgia (66% versus 96%, $p < 0.01$), facial and/or eyelid edema (57% versus 86%, $p < 0.05$), eosinophilia (52% versus 96%, $p < 0.01$), and increased serum CK (38% versus 79%, $p < 0.01$) are less common in children than in adults.

Eosinophilia–myalgia syndrome and toxic oil syndrome are diseases associated with an ingestion of products containing L-tryptophan or its derivatives [27]. A pain in proximal muscles, stiffness, muscular weakness primarily of the extremities resemble the clinical features of PM; however, the distinguishable symptom is a prominent eosinophilia, with no evidence of parasitic disease. Cutaneous manifestations resemble a sclerodermatous disease (50%) and peripheral or truncal edema [28].

References

1. Winkelmann RK. The cutaneous diagnosis of dermatomyositis, lupus erythematosus, and scleroderma. *N Y State J Med* 1963; 63: 3080.
2. Callen JP. Dermatomyositis. *Lancet* 2000; 355: 53–57.
3. Jorizzo JL. Dermatomyositis: practical aspects. *Arch Dermatol* 2002; 138: 114–116.
4. Kovacs SO, Kovacs SC. Dermatomyositis. *J Am Acad Dermatol* 1998; 39(6): 899–920.
5. Ackerman AB. Dermatomyositis. In: *Diagnosis of Inflammatory Skin Diseases. An Algorithmic Method Based on Pattern Analysis*, Williams & Wilkins, Baltimore, MD, 1997; 289–293.
6. Kasper CS, White CL 3rd, Freeman RG. Pathology and immunopathology of polymyositis/dermatomyositis. *Clin Dermatol* 1988; 6(2): 64–75.
7. Nesbitt LT Jr. Cutaneous immunofluorescence in dermatomyositis. *Int J Dermatol* 1980; 19: 270–273.
8. Chen Z, Maize JC, Silver RM, et al. Direct and indirect immunofluorescence findings in dermatomyositis. *J Cutan Pathol* 1985; 12: 18–27.
9. Magro CM, Crowson AN. The immunofluorescent profile of dermatomyositis: a comparative study with lupus erythematosus. *J Cutan Pathol* 1997; 24(9): 543–552.
10. Ghate J, Katsambas A, Augerinou G, Jorizzo JL. A therapeutic update on dermatomyositis/polymyositis. *Int J Dermatol* 2000; 39: 81–87.
11. Lever W, Schaumburg-Lever G. Dermatomyositis. In: *Histopathology of the Skin*. 6th ed. JB Lippincott, Philadelphia, 1983; 458–461.
12. Guy WH, Grauer RC, Jacob FM. Poikilodermatomyositis. *Arch Dermatol Syph* 1939; 40: 867–878.
13. Horn RC Jr. Poikilodermatomyositis. *Arch Dermatol Syph* 1941; 44: 1086–1097.

14. Vella Briffa D, Warin AP, Calnan CD. Parakeratosis variegata: a report of two cases and their treatment with PUVA. *Clin Exp Dermatol* 1979; 4(4): 537–541.
15. Dalakas M. Polymyositis, dermatomyositis and inclusion body myositis. *N Engl J Med* 1991; 325(21): 1487–1498.
16. Mills JA. Dermatomyositis. In: *Dermatology in General Medicine*, Fitzpatrick TB, Eisen AZ, Wolff K, et al. (eds), McGraw-Hill, New York, 1993; 2148–2155.
17. Fam AG. Paraneoplastic rheumatic syndromes. *Baillieres Best Pract Res Clin Rheumatol* 2000; 14(3): 515–533.
18. Provost TT, Flynn JA. Dermatomyositis. In: *Cutaneous Medicine: Cutaneous Manifestations of Systemic Disease*, Provost TT, Flynn JA (eds), BC Decker, Hamilton, Ontario, Canada, 2000: 82–104.
19. Herrera R, Varela E, Morales G, et al. Dermatomyositis-like syndrome caused by trichinose: report of two cases. *J Rheumatol* 1985; 12: 782.
20. Unverricht H. Über eine eigenthümliche Form von akuter Muskelentzündung mit einem der Trichinose ähnelnden Krankheitsbilde. *Münchner Med Wochenschr* 1887; 34: 488–492.
21. Hepp P. Über Pseudo-trichinose, eine besondere Form von acuter parenchymatose Polymyositis. *Berl Klin Wochenschr* 1887; 24: 297, 332.
22. Murray C. Trichinosis. In: *eMedicine, Infectious Diseases*, Chandrasekar, FT Pharm, et al. (eds), eMedicine Corp, St. Petersburg, 1996–2008/*eMedicine Dermatology* [journal serial online] 2007. Available at: http://www.emedicine.com/med/TOPIC2306.HTM
23. Astudillo LM, Arlet PM. Images in clinical medicine. The chemosis in trichinosis. *N Engl J Med* 2004; 351: 487.
24. Arnold LK. Trichinosis. In: *eMedicine, Emergency Medicine*, Gaeta T, Talavera F, et al. (eds), eMedicine Corp, St. Petersburg, 1996–2008/*eMedicine Dermatology* [journal serial online] 2005. Available at: http://www.emedicine.com/emerg/TOPIC612.HTM
25. Walsh DS, Jongsakul K, Watt G. Hand rash in trichinellosis. *Clin Exp Dermatol* 2001; 26(3): 272–273.
26. Ozdemir D, Ozkan H, Akkoc N, et al. Acute trichinellosis in children compared with adults. *Pediatr Infect Dis J* 2005; 24(10): 897–900.
27. Hertzman PA, Blevins WL, Mayer J, et al. Association of the eosinophilia–myalgia syndrome with the ingestion of tryptophan. *N Engl J Med* 1990; 322: 869–873.
28. Kaufman LD, Seidman RJ, Philips ME, et al. Cutaneous manifestations of the l-tryptophan-associated eosinophilia–myalgia syndrome: a spectrum of sclerodermatous skin disease. *J Am Acad Dermatol* 1990; 23: 1063–1069.

Etiology and Pathogenesis

Etiology of Dermatomyositis 36

The etiology of DM remains unknown. Many genetic and environmental factors could be significant in the development of DM.

36.1 Environmental Factors

The role of the environment on the evolution of DM, whether in regard to climate or geographic latitude, has not been fully identified, and may vary by the time and the location. The first environmental factor that has recently been suggested as playing a role as a causative factor in DM is ultraviolet (UV) light. DM patients show high cutaneous photosensitivity [1] and disease prevalence depending on the geographical latitude [2]. A recent report showed that the relative prevalence of DM increased significantly from northern Europe (latitude 64°) to southern Europe (latitude 38°) [2]. A latitudinal gradient similar to the DM prevalence was found for the MSAs (anti-synthetase, anti-M2, and anti-SPR autoantibodies) that occur more commonly in the southern countries [3]. In contrast, the myositis-associated autoantibodies (MAAs), with the exception of the anti-Ro52 and anti-U1 sn RNP autoantibodies, were more commonly detected in patients from northern countries [3]. Similarly, a preliminary analysis of the juvenile DM new-onset registry data identified geographic clusters of newly diagnosed children in the USA [4]. An earlier review of data on disease onset in 286 newly diagnosed juvenile DM patients did not show seasonal predilection [5]. However, epidemiological data in USA encompassing the period from 1989 to 1992 revealed an increased frequency of disease onset in spring and summer months in all geographic regions of the country [6]. Sun exposure and especially the exposure to UVB light, which may induce cellular production of TNF-α [7], possibly precipitates juvenile DM in some children who have the TNF-α-308A allele [8]. The incidence of increased cutaneous photosensitivity in DM patients has been documented in some case reports [9–11], and photosensitivity has been tested in a small number of patients [1, 12, 13].

A few case reports have suggested an association between DM/PM and silicon breast implants [14, 15]. Two thousand six hundred and twenty two women who underwent a treatment with injectable bovine collagen implants were observed for a 4-year period [15]. Seven patients were confirmed with DM after bovine collagen treatment, rather than the 30.2 cases which would have been expected according to the 5-year incidence rate [15]. In a retrospective cohort study of 7,442 women who underwent breast implantation for cosmetic reasons or after breast cancer surgery reconstruction, and 3,353 women with breast reduction surgery in the Swedish national inpatient registry during 1964–93, 29 women with implants were hospitalized for definite CTD, compared with the 25.5 cases which would have been expected based on the general population rates (standardized hospitalization ratio 1.1; 95% confidence interval (CI) 0.8–1.6) [16]. This large nationwide cohort study shows no evidence of the association between breast implants and CTD or DM [16]. Women with extracapsular silicone (silicone gel outside of the fibrous scar that forms around breast implants) were more likely to report having fibromyalgia (FM) ($p = 0.004$) or other CTD, including DM, PM, MCTD, eosinophilic fasciitis, and polymyalgia ($p = 0.008$) than other women in a study by Brown et al. [17]. The odds ratios were 2.8 (95% CI 1.2–6.3) for FM, and 2.6 (95% CI 0.8–8.5) for other CTD. These data suggest an association between extracapsular silicone from ruptured silicone breast implants and FM. Recently, a case of DM following the rupture of a silicon gel breast implant has been reported [18].

Other noninfectious agents and exposures currently suspect in the pathogenesis of DM are vaccines: influenza [19, 20], hepatitis B [21], mumps–measles–rubella vaccine, typhoid, and cholera [22], BCG [23] and drugs such as the cholesterol-lowering drugs, some NSAIDs, antineoplastic drugs, anti-infectious drugs, and other unrelated medicines [8, 24, 25] (Table 36.1) (see also Chapter 24).

36.2 Infectious Agents

In addition to the climate, there are many regional differences in DM occurrence due to exposure to certain infectious agents. Some epidemiological studies have documented an antecedent illness in the 3-month period before the onset of symptoms of juvenile DM, and suggest that disease pathophysiology is indeed antigen-driven and that onset may be the result of molecular mimicry [26].

Infectious organisms that have been implicated in the etiology of DM include viruses, bacteria, and parasites. A viral etiology for inflammatory myopathies has been suspected for many years. Viral infections often precede attacks of rhabdomyolysis.

Although several viruses, particularly influenza [27], parainfluenza, hepatitis B [28] and C [29, 30], Epstein–Barr virus [31], RNA picornaviruses (i.e., coxsackie B) [8, 32, 33] and most recently parvovirus B19 [34–37] have been indirectly associated with chronic and acute myositis [38]; sensitive PCR studies have not amplified the viral genome from muscle of these patients [39, 40].

Table 36.1 Drug's activity in inducing of PM, DM, and amyopathic DM [25]

Features	Polymyositis	Dermatomyositis	Amyopathic DM
1. Myositis	+	+	–
2. Cutaneous rash	–	+	+
3. Muscle enzymes	+	+	–
4. rugs with adverse reactions as:	d-Penicillamine, Sulfasalazine, Simvastatin, Pravastatin, Lovastatine, Gemfibrozil, Fenofibrate, Zidovudine	d-Penicillamine, Diclofenac Sulfasalazine, Simvastatin, Pravastatin, Phenylbutazone, Chlorpromazine, Isoniazid, Benzylpenicillin, Antazoline, Clemizole, Tamoxifen	Hydroxyurea, Cyclophosphamid Etoposid
5. Drug's activity	Contained oxygen atom from a carbonyl and hydroxyl group in an interval $-0.350 < Q_o < -0.320$ a.u.	Contained reduced sulfur ($0.07 < Q_s < 0.450$ a.u.) and a nitrogen atom (in a cyclical fragment and anticyclical in a sp3-hybridization) in an interval of charge: $-0.390 < Q_N < -0.140$ a.u.	Contained nitrogen and require additional condition for the nitrogen atoms participating in the structures of these active compounds like N atom in a sp3-hybridization which changed its charge as compared to the charge of N

The acute onset of myositis as a viral-like syndrome in some patients is one of the reasons for suspecting infectious agent involvement in DM. A 48-year-old woman suffering from DM associated with the presence of parvovirus B19 DNA in two muscle biopsy has been reported [36]. Parvovirus B19 DNA was detected by primers for VP1 and NS1 as well as IgG, but non-IgM-specific antibodies were detected in patient serum [36]. One child with recent onset of juvenile DM showed serological evidence of acute parvovirus B19 infection [34]. Amplification of viral DNA by PCR was positive in an early simple serum, but was negative in muscle biopsy and peripheral blood leucocytes drawn at the time of biopsy [34]. Another 7-year-old girl exposed to parvovirus B19 infection developed acute hepatitis and myositis followed by the life-threatening ILD [41]. Parvovirus B19 DNA in bone marrow, lung, and serum, and elevated IgM and IgG antibody titers in serum, were detected. Muscle biopsy showed type II fiber atrophy without significant inflammation, but parvovirus B19 DNA detection was not performed [41]. It was hypothesized that a host response to coxsackie B virus could be related to juvenile DM, since there was a statistically significant prevalence of complement-fixing coxsackie B viral antibody relative to hospitalized patients with juvenile rheumatoid arthritis, and this antibody correlated with the course of the disease [33, 42]. The discovery of a number of MSAs against tRNA synthetase has increased interest in a possible role of picornavirus in the etiology of inflammatory myopathies. Because specific regions of the RNA of picornavirus are homologous to surface proteins of histidyl-tRNA synthetase (Jo-1 antigen), against which anti-Jo-1-antibodies are generated [43], and in situ hybridization with RNA probes for a murine picornavirus revealed an evidence of infection in the muscle of adult DM [44], picornaviruses are thought to be possible causes of myositis in PM/DM patients [43–47]. However, a proposed molecular mimicry based on a structural homology between coxsackie viruses and Jo-1 synthetase has not been proved yet [39, 40, 48]. The best evidence of a viral connection of PM is found with retroviruses [48]. The retroviruses, however, are found only in occasional endomysial macrophages [49–52] and do not replicate within the muscle fibers or cause persistent infection [50–52].

Bacterial pathogens linked with the onset of juvenile and adult DM include *Borrelia burgdorferi* [53] and *Group A α-hemolytic streptococci* [54]. Additionally, *Streptococcus pyogenes* has been associated with recurrences or exacerbations of juvenile DM [55]. In a case-controlled study of patients with IIMs in the USA, in which sex-matched siblings were used as controls, no support for a preceding infection has been found [56]. No evidence for viral RNA or bacterial DNA has been detected in muscle biopsies from patients with active untreated juvenile DM [57]. Viral antibody analyses of sera were also negative.

Parasites, such as *Toxoplasma gondii*, also have been linked with DM [58, 59]. Increased frequency of antitoxoplasma Ig M antibodies was reported in PM/DM patients [60]. Several patients with a rash and myositis similar to those found in DM have been reported [61–64]. These patients have had evidence of the disease, and responded to antitoxoplasma medications such as pyramethamine and sulfadiazine [60, 63].

Long-term-acting infectious agents have been suggested as possible causative or trigger factors for DM. This hypothesis is based on case reports with DM in which different types of virus-like particles, bacteria, or protozoa have been identified from the muscle tissue, or antibodies against infectious agents have been isolated in the serum of these patients. However, no definite evidence that these agents are causative factors in DM has been found.

References

1. Dourmishev L, Meffert H, Piazena H. Dermatomyositis: comparative studies of cutaneous photosensitivity in lupus erythematosus and normal subjects. *Photodermatol Photoimmunol Photomed* 2004; 20: 230–234.
2. Hengstman GJ, van Venrooij WJ, Vencovsky J, et al. The relative prevalence of dermatomyositis and polymyositis in Europe exhibits a latitudinal gradient. *Ann Rheum Dis* 2000; 59: 141–142.
3. Brouwer R, Hengstman GJD, Vree Egberts W, et al. Autoantibody profiles in the sera of European patients with myositis. *Ann Rheum Dis* 2001; 60: 116–123.
4. Reed AM, Mendez EP, Pachman LM. Geographical and environmental exposures in the development of juvenile dermatomyositis. *Arthritis Rheum* 2000; 43:1880.
5. Rider LG, Miller FW. Classification and treatment of the juvenile idiopathic inflammatory myopathies. *Rheum Dis Clin N Am* 1997; 23: 619–655.
6. Pachman LM, Hayford JR, Chung A, et al. Juvenile dermatomyositis at diagnosis: clinical characteristics of 79 children. *J Rheumatol* 1998; 25: 1198–1204.
7. Schwarz A, Bhardwaj R, Arganc Y, et al. Ultraviolet B induced apoptosis of keratinocytes: evidence for partial involvement of tumor necrosis factor-alpha in the formation of sunburn cells. *J Invest Dermatol* 1995; 104: 922–927.
8. Pachman LM. Juvenile dermatomyositis: immunogenetics, pathophysiology, and disease expression. *Rheum Dis Clin North Am* 2002; 28: 579–602.
9. Woo TR, Rasmussen J, Callen JP. Recurrent photosensitive dermatitis preceding juvenile dermatomyositis. *Pediatr Dermatol* 1985; 2: 207–212.
10. Badawy Abdel-Nasser M, Chun SC, Gollnick H, et al. Amyopathic dermatomyositis (dermatomyositis sine myositis) in a male patient and possible induction by UV light. *Eur J Dermatol* 1993; 3: 367–370.
11. Kivanc MT, Klaus MV, Nashel DJ. Reversible polymyositis occurring during psoralen and ultraviolet A (PUVA) therapy. *J Rheumatol* 2000; 27: 1823–1824.
12. Everett MA, Curtis AC. Dermatomyositis: a review of 19 cases in adolescents and children. *Arch Intern Med* 1957; 100: 70–76.
13. Cheong WK, Hughes GR, Norris PG, et al. Cutaneous photosensitivity in dermatomyositis. *Br J Dermatol* 1994; 131: 205–208.
14. Houpt KR, Sontheimer RD. Autoimmune connective tissues disease and connective tissue disease-like illnesses after silicon gel augmentation mammoplasty. *J Am Acad Dermatol* 1994; 31: 626–642.
15. Hanke CW, Thomas JA, Lee WT, et al. Risk assessment of polymyositis/dermatomyositis after treatment with injectable bovine collagen implants. *J Am Acad Dermatol* 1996; 34: 450–454.
16. Nyren O, Yin L, Josefsson S, et al. Risk of connective tissue disease and related disorders among women with breast implants: a nationwide retrospective cohort study in Sweden. *BMJ* 1998; 316: 417–422.
17. Brown SL, Pennello G, Berg WA, et al. Silicone gel breast implant rupture, extracapsular silicone, and health status in a population of women. *J Rheumatol* 2001; 28: 996–1003.
18. Caramaschi P, Biasi D, Volpe A, et al. A new case of dermatomyositis following the rupture of a silicone gel breast implant. *Clin Exp Rheumatol* 2005; 23: 430–431.

36

19. Winkelmann RK. Influenza vaccine and dermatomyositis. *Lancet* 1982; 2(8296): 495.
20. Jani FM, Gray JP, Lanham J. Influenza vaccine and dermatomyositis. *Vaccine* 1994; 12(15): 640–650.
21. Altman A, Szyper-Kravitz M, Shoenfeld Y. HBV vaccine and dermatomyositis: is there an association? *Rheumatol Int* 2008; 28(6): 609–612.
22. Cotterill JA, Shapiro H. Dermatomyositis after immunization. *Lancet* 1978; 2(8100): 1158–1159.
23. Kass F, Straume S, Mellbaye OJ, et al. Dermatomyositis associated with BCG vaccination. *Scand J Rheumatol* 1979; 8: 187–191.
24. Dourmishev A, Dourmishev L. Dermatomyositis and drugs. *Adv Exp Med Biol* 1999; 455: 187–191.
25. Kamenska V, Dourmishev L, Dourmishev A, et al. Quantitative structure–activity relationship modeling of dermatomyositis activity of drug chemicals. *Arzneimittelforschung* 2006; 56(12): 856–865.
26. Pachman LM, Hayford JR, Hochberg MC, et al. New-onset juvenile dermatomyositis: comparisons with a healthy cohort and children with juvenile rheumatoid arthritis. *Arthritis Rheum* 1997; 40(8): 1526–1533.
27. Dietzman DE, Schaller AP, Ray CG et al. Acute myositis associated with influenza B infection. *Pediatrics* 1976; 57: 255–258.
28. Pittsley RA, Shearn MA, Kaufman L. Acute hepatitis B simulating dermatomyositis. *JAMA* 1978; 239: 959.
29. McMurray RW, Elbourne K. Hepatitis C virus infection and autoimmunity. *Semin Arthritis Rheum* 1997; 26: 689–701.
30. Gomes A, Solans R, Simeon CP, et al. Dermatomyositis, hepatocarcinoma, and hepatitis C: comment on the article by Weidensul et al. [letter]. *Arthritis Rheum* 1997; 40: 394–395.
31. Yamashita K, Hosokawa M, Hirohashi S, et al. Epstein–Barr virus-associated gastric cancer in a patient with dermatomyositis. *Intern Med* 2001; 40: 96–99.
32. Traver RL, Hughes GR. Coxsackie B neutralization titers in polymyositis/dermatomyositis. *Lancet* 1977; 1: 1268.
33. Christiansen ML, Pachman LM, Schneiderman R, et al. Prevalence of coxsackie B virus antibodies in patients with juvenile dermatomyositis. *Arthritis Rheum* 1986; 29: 1365–1370.
34. Lewkonia RM, Horne D, Dawood MR. Juvenile dermatomyositis in child infected with human parvovirus B19. *Clin Infect Dis* 1995; 21: 430–432.
35. Crowson AN, Magro CM, Dawood MR. A causal role for parvovirus B19 infection in adult dermatomyositis and other autoimmune syndromes. *J Cutan Pathol* 2000; 27: 505–515.
36. Chevrel G, Calvet A, Belin V, et al. Dermatomyositis associated with the presence of parvovirus B19 DNA in muscle. *Rheumatol* 2000; 39: 1037–1039.
37. Lehmann H, Kuhner L, Beckenlehner K, et al. Chronic human parvovirus B19 infection in rheumatic disease of childhood and adolescence. *J Clin Virol* 2002; 25: 135.
38. Reed AM, Ytterberg SR. Genetic and environmental risk factors for idiopathic inflammatory myopathies. *Rheum Dis Clin N Am* 2002; 28: 891–916.
39. Leff RL, Love LA, Miller FW, et al. Viruses in the idiopathic inflammatory myopathies: absence of candidate viral genomes in muscle. *Lancet* 1992; 339: 1192–1195.
40. Leon-Monzon M, Dalakas MC. Absence of persistent infection with enteroviruses in muscles of patients with inflammatory myopathies. *Ann Neurol* 1992; 32: 219–222.
41. Bousvaros A, Sundel R, Thorne GM, et al. Parvovirus B19-associated interstitial lung disease, hepatitis and myositis. *Pediatr Pulmonol* 1998; 26: 365–369.
42. Bowles NE, Dubowitz V, Sewry CA, et al. Dermatomyositis, polymyositis and Coxsackie B-virus infection. *Lancet* 1987; 1: 1004–1007.
43. Walker EJ, Jeffery PD. Sequence homology between encephalomyocarditis virus protein VPI and histidyl-tRNA synthetase supports a hypothesis of molecular mimicry in polymyositis. *Med Hypotheses* 1988; 25: 21–26.

44. Rosenberg NL, Rothbar HA, Abzug MJ, et al. Evidence for a novel picornavirus in human dermatomyositis. *Am Neurol* 1989; 26: 204–209.
45. Targoff IN. Immunologic aspects of myositis. *Curr Opin Rheumatol* 1989; 1: 432–442.
46. Targoff IN. Immune mechanisms in myositis. *Curr Opin Rheumatol* 1990; 2: 882–888.
47. Dalakas M. Polymyositis, dermatomyositis and inclusion body myositis. *N Engl J Med* 1991; 325(21): 1487–1498.
48. Dalakas MC, Hohfeld R. Polymyositis and dermatomyositis. *Lancet* 2003; 362: 971–982.
49. Morgan OS, Rodgers-Johnson P, Mora C, et al. HTLV-I and polymyositis in Jamaica. *Lancet* 1989; 2: 1184–1187.
50. Illa I, Nath A, Dalakas MC. Immunocytochemical and virological characteristics of HIV-associated inflammatory myopathies: similarities with seronegative polymyositis. *Ann Neurol* 1991; 29: 474–481.
51. Leon-Monzon M, Illa I, Dalakas MC. Polymyositis in patients infected with HTLV-I: the role of the virus in the cause of the disease. *Ann Neurol* 1994; 36: 643–649.
52. Cupler EJ, Leon-Monzon M, Miller J, et al. Inclusion body myositis in HIV-I and HTLV-I infected patients. *Brain* 1996; 119: 1887–1893.
53. Hoffman JC, Stichtenoth DO, Zeidler H, et al. Lyme disease in a 74-year old forest owner with symptoms of dermatomyositis. *Arthritis Rheum* 1995; 38: 1157–1160.
54. Albani S, Costouros N, Massa M, et al. Identification of cross-reactive epitopes on human skeletal myosin and streptococcal M5 protein in patients with juvenile dermatomyositis (JDM). *Arthritis Rheum* 1997, 40: S140.
55. Martini A, Ravelli A, Albani S, et al. Recurrent juvenile dermatomyositis and cutaneous necrotizing arthritis with molecular mimicry between streptococcal type M5 protein and human skeletal myosin. *J Pediatr* 1992; 121: 739–742.
56. Lyon MG, Bloch DA, Hollak B, et al. Predisposing factors in polymyositis–dermatomyositis: results of a nationwide survey. *J Rheumatol* 1989; 16: 1218–1224.
57. Pachman LM, Litt DL, Rowley AH, et al. Lack of detection of enteroviral RNA or bacterial DNA in magnetic resonance imaging-directed muscle biopsies from twenty children with active untreated juvenile dermatomyositis. *Arthritis Rheum* 1995; 38: 1513–1518.
58. Schroter HM, Sarnet HB, Matheson DS, et al. Juvenile dermatomyositis induced by toxoplasmosis. *J Child Neurol* 1987; 2: 101–104.
59. Martinez-Cordero E, Martinez-Marinada E, Aguilar Leon DE. Autoantibodies in juvenile dermatomyositis. *Clin Rheum* 1993; 12: 426–428.
60. Magit SK, Kagen LJ. Serologic evidence for acute toxoplasmosis in polymyositis/dermatomyositis: increased frequency of specific anti-toxoplasma Ig M antibodies. *Am J Med* 1983; 75: 313–320.
61. Pollock JL. Toxoplasmosis appearing to be dermatomyositis. *Arch Dermatol* 1979; 115: 736–737.
62. Topi GC, D'Alessandro L, Carticala C, et al. Dermatomyositis-like syndrome due to toxoplasmosis. *Br J Dermatol* 1979; 101: 589–591.
63. Harland CC, Marsden JR, Vernon SA, et al. Dermatomyositis responding to treatment of associated toxoplasmosis. *Br J Dermatol* 1991;125:76–78.
64. Saberin A, Lutgen C, Humbel RL, et al. Dermatomyositis-like syndrome following acute toxoplasmosis. *Bull Soc Sci Med Grand Duche Luxemb* 2004; (2): 109–119.

Pathogenesis of Dermatomyositis 37

Over the past 25 years, much has been learned about the cellular and humoral immune-mediated mechanisms involved in the pathogenesis of DM. More recently, the role of complement, specifically the MAC, in immune-mediated vascular injury has been further elucidated. Additionally, susceptibility to develop juvenile DM has been linked with the class II major histocompatibility complex HLA-DQA1*0501 allele, and disease course and various complications have been associated with polymorphisms at the TNF-α-308 locus. In this way, the genetic background of children with DM is integrally entwined with the type of elicited inflammatory response. More recently, data has become available regarding the molecular genetics of children affected with juvenile DM and the impact these genes have on disease expression and clinical course [1].

37.1 Genetic Data

Familial occurrences of juvenile and adult DM [2–4], and investigations of the genes involved in the pathogenesis of IIM, such as HLA DQA1 0501 for juvenile DM [5], has shown that the genetic background of affected patients plays a role in their susceptibility to developing DM and also in their clinical course. In earlier studies, it has been shown that children with DM of Caucasian race are very often carriers of HLA-B8 [6] and HLA-DR3 alleles, while adult DM patients have HLA-B14, HLA-Cw7, HLA-DR3, HLA-DRw52, and HLA-DQA1 alleles [7]. Patients of Caucasian race with "antisynthetase syndrome" are in 90% of cases carriers of HLA-DR3 gene [8], and drug-induced DM is associated with HLA-B18, HLA-B35, and HLA-DR4 alleles [9].

L.A. Dourmishev and A.L. Dourmishev, *Dermatomyositis: Advances in Recognition, Understanding and Management,*

37.2 The HLA-DQA1*0501 Allele

Among the identified genes, the class II major histocompatibility complex allele HLA-DQA1*0501 has emerged as a risk factor for all of the major clinical forms of sporadic and familial IIM in both white adults and children in the USA and Europe [10]. HLA-DQA1*0501 has also been found to be an important predisposing factor for juvenile DM in children of African-American and Hispanic ethnicity [11]. The association of DQA1*0501 with DM has not been confirmed in all ethnic backgrounds. In Korean patients with IIM, no HLA allele has been found as a risk factor, suggesting that the genetic risk factors for inflammatory myopathies in children and adults are multifactorial, and may be due to regional factors [12]. Additionally, the presence of the DQA1*0501 allele has not been associated with a chronic disease course [13], defined as requiring immunosuppressive therapy for 36 months or longer to bring disease activity under control.

37.3 Gene Expression Profiling

A group of interferon-inducible genes being overexpressed in DM and relative to PM and IBM has been reported [14]. This was confirmed comparing gene expression profile data from untreated juvenile DM patients, positive for the DQA1*0501 allele, with data from children with Duchenne muscular dystrophy and healthy controls [15]. Profound dysregulation was found in muscle biopsies from the children with juvenile DM; most of the dysregulated genes were found to be interferon-inducible genes [15, 16]. This pattern of gene expression supports the hypothesis that the pathogenesis of juvenile DM is a response to an infectious agent, particularly since transcription of IFN-inducible genes is a hallmark of the host defense mechanism against infection [16]. The investigators hypothesized a model of disease pathogenesis that involves a repetitive cycle of muscle injury, and in which both IFN-αβ and IFN-cascades lead to muscle ischemia and increased production of TNF-α and nitric oxide. Later, TNF-α and nitric oxide interact with the immune response cascades in the endothelium and with infiltrating T and natural killer cells, thus exacerbating the IFN-induced processes. The IFN-induced response cascades, which inhibit mitosis and protein synthesis cascades, thereby inhibit regeneration of necrotic muscle fibers. TNF-α is an important mediator of the inflammatory response, and may be one of the critical interpathway communicating proteins that in conjunction with the effects of the IFN-induced cascades induce muscle cell injury [16].

37.4 The TNF-α-308A Allele

The TNF-α-308A allele is located in the class III region of the major histocompatibility complex on the short arm of chromosome 6, a region that is involved with the regulation of TNF-α transcription [12]. The secretion of TNF-α is strongly influenced by a promoter polymorphism at position-308, which is either a G (wild-type) or an A [17], and high transcription rates are found, possibly through increased binding of specific transcription factors to the area of the polymorphism [18]. The G-A amino acid substitution at the NcoI restriction site has been noted to occur at a higher frequency in white children with untreated juvenile DM than in age-matched controls [13]. Associated with increased production of TNF-α by peripheral blood mononuclear cells as well as by muscle fibers themselves from juvenile DM, [13, 19], the TNF-α-308A allele has been connected with a chronic disease course. It also has been associated with capillary occlusion and vascular compromise in the untreated muscle [20]. The TNF-α-308A allele has been associated with increased plasma thrombospondin-1 (TSP-1) levels in juvenile DM [21]. TSP-1 plays an important role in vascular smooth muscle cell proliferation, which leads to intimal hyperplasia and blood vessel lumen narrowing, thus contributing to vascular occlusion [22]. The increased circulating levels of TSP-1 in children with the TNF-α-308A allele may be linked to the augmented vascular occlusion seen in juvenile DM patients with this genetic marker [21, 22]. The TNF-α-308A allele has been associated with a chronic disease course, more resistant to immunosuppressive therapy and often complicated with an increased frequency of pathologic calcifications [13]. An association of the overproducing TNF-α-308A variant with adult DM has been found, and also with subacute cutaneous LE [23]. The TNF-α-308A polymorphism suggests a pathophysiologic contribution from UV-induced production of TNF-α, similar to those in SCLE. Adult DM patients with one variant TNF-α-308A allele had at least two mannose binding lectin (MBL) polymorphisms versus controls [24]; thus, low-producing MBL genes are strongly associated with adult DM [23, 24].

37.5 The Role of Complement

Earlier studies have established a primary role of complement-induced vessel injury in DM, and evidence of activation of the complement cascade resulting in MAC (C5b-9) mediated capillary damage [25]. One of the earliest histologic abnormalities was the detection of MAC deposited in small arterioles and capillaries of affected muscle [25, 26], and its presence correlated with the duration of clinical disease [27]. Deposition of MAC in small vessels is partially regulated by CD59, a protective regulatory membrane protein expressed in numerous cells and tissues throughout the body, including endothelium from several tissues as skin, skeletal muscle, lung, and myocardium. CD59 regulates MAC activity by binding to C8 and C9 molecules already incorporated into MAC, blocking further C9 recruitment and polymerization, thereby preventing full assemblage of MAC [28]. The sarcolemma of normal skeletal muscle fibers has been found strongly stained by immunohistochemistry using a monoclonal antibody to CD59 [29]. In a recent study, the presence of CD59 and deposition of MAC in skeletal muscle of patients with untreated juvenile DM in comparison with patients with muscular dystrophy and children biopsied for other diagnostic purposes has been reported [30]. The investigators found: (1) immunohistochemical staining for CD59 was weak and irregularly distributed on the muscle fibers of all juvenile DM patients, while strong, uniformly distributed immunoreactivity to CD59 was detected on the sarcolemma and in the intramuscular endothelium of all muscle samples from children without myositis and from those affected with muscular dystrophy, (2) immunostaining for MAC was present in the majority (67%) of vessels of the juvenile DM patients, with intense staining present in two thirds of those positive for MAC; no intense staining for MAC was found in vessels from children without myositis or from those with muscular dystrophy, and (3) an inverse relation existed between MAC deposition and the presence of CD59 in the vessels of the juvenile DM muscle biopsies and in all normal and muscular dystrophy samples. It has been shown that neutralization of CD59 renders cells susceptible to complement killing [31]. Goncalves et al. hypothesize that decreased CD59 expression in the muscle fibers and vessels of children with juvenile DM may be associated with the onset and perpetuation of inflammation and muscle cell damage due to excessive activation of complement, mediated by deposition of MAC [30]. A theory for the mechanism of CD59 depletion is cleavage of the CD59 glycolipid anchor by phospholipases activated in the inflammatory process, rendering the endothelial cells susceptible to MAC activity. Deposition of MAC in the small vessels then leads to muscle ischemia, and renders muscle cells incapable of maintaining synthesis of normal amounts of CD59, constituting another means for decreased protection against MAC activity [30].

37.6 The Role of Cytokines

Various cytokines and their mRNA, including interleukins 1, 2, 6, and 10, TNF-α, IFN-γ, and TGF-β, are amplified in DM and PM [32–35]. Some of them, such as INF-γ and IL-1b, may have a myocytotoxic effect [36, 37], whereas others, such as TGF-β, may promote chronic inflammation and fibrosis [38]. A major immunoregulatory mechanism is the control of the balance of cytokines secreted by two subpopulations of helper T cells, termed type 1 (Th1) and type 2 (Th2). Th1 cells secrete IFN-γ and Il-2, while Th2 produce IL-4 [39]. Th1 but not Th2 cytokines were found in IIMs, with production of pro-inflammatory cytokines [40]. No specific cytokine profile, however, was found in any of the myositis subtypes [40]. In the muscles of patients with PM or DM, there is an overexpression of the signal transduction and activation of transducers type I [41], indicating cytokine upregulation. After successful immunotherapy, there is downregulation of cytokines with reduction of inflammation and fibrosis [42]. Chemokines, a class of small cytokines [43], including interleukin 8 (CXCL8), RANTES (CCL9), MCP-1 (CCL2), Mig CXCL9), and IP-10 (CXCL10), are also overexpressed in the endomysial inflammatory cells, the extracellular matrix, and the muscle fibers [33], and may facilitate trafficking of activated T cells to the muscle or promote tissue fibrosis. The matrix metalloproteinases MMP-2 and MMP-9, which promote the migration of lymphocytes through extracellular matrix, are also overexpressed on the muscle fibers and the autoinvasive CD8-positive cells [44, 45]. The degree of clinically present muscle weakness or fatigue in patients with classic DM does not always exactly correlate with the degree of inflammation on muscle biopsy and the elevation of serum enzymes [46]. It is supposed that inflammatory cytokines might be capable of mediating metabolitic disturbances within muscle that can exacerbate muscle weakness and fatigue [46, 47].

37.7 Soluble Adhesion Molecules

The role of soluble adhesion molecules in the inflammatory process has been studied in adult patients and children with DM [48–50]. Specifically, serum levels of five soluble adhesion molecules: (i) intercellular adhesion molecule 1 (ICAM-1), (ii) ICAM-3, (iii) vascular cell adhesion molecule 1 (VCAM-1), (iv) L-selectin, and (v) E-selectin, which are critical to leukocyte adhesion to and migration across the endothelium to sites of inflammation, have been measured and correlated with various rheumatic disease states [51]. Recently, measurement of serum levels of soluble adhesion molecules in children with a variety of pediatric rheumatic diseases, including juvenile DM, was undertaken [50]. Levels were compared among patients with active versus inactive disease with the following results: (1) ICAM-1 and L-selectin levels were significantly elevated in juvenile DM, compared with normal children, (2) VCAM-1 was significantly elevated in juvenile DM patients, when compared with normal controls, and (3) ICAM-1 was significantly higher in patients with active disease compared with inactive disease, suggesting that ICAM-1 may be a useful marker for monitoring disease activity. The elevated serum VCAM-1 levels in classic DM correlated with elevated ESR and elevated serum hyaluronate concentrations [48]. High serum E-selectin levels in DM in adults were correlated with enhanced CK activity [48]. Additionally, in active juvenile DM, ICAM-1-positive lymphocytes are adherent to endothelial cells in the lumen of blood vessels in muscle. Upregulation of ICAM-1 on lymphocytes, coupled with vascular smooth muscle cell proliferation, may perpetuate the small vessel occlusion that occurs in juvenile DM [21]. The upregulation of adhesion molecules has been reported in muscle biopsy specimens in IIMs and in cutaneous biopsy specimens [52–54]. VCAM-1 and E-selectin are secreted mainly from activated endothelian cells [55, 56], and are expressed on the activated endothelial cells after stimulation with IL-1, TNF-α, and IFN-γ [57, 58]. The elevated serum levels of VCAM-1 and E-selectin may be a consequence of chronic exposure to these cytokines in DM patients [48].

References

1. Wargula JC. Update on juvenile dermatomyositis: new advances in understanding its etiopathogenesis. *Curr Opin Rheumatol* 2003; 15(5): 595–601.
2. Rider LG, Gurley RC, Randey JP, et al. Clinical, serologic, and immunogenetic features of familial idiopathic inflammatory myopathy. *Arthritis Rheum* 1998; 41: 710–719.
3. Plamondon S, Dent PB, Reed AM. Familial dermatomyositis. *J Rheumatol* 1999; 26: 2691–2692.
4. Davies MG, Hickling P. Familial adult dermatomyositis. *Br J Dermatol* 2001; 144: 415–416.
5. Reed AM, Ytterberg SR. Genetic and environmental risk factors for idiopathic inflammatory myopathies. *Rheum Dis Clin N Am* 2002; 28: 891–916.
6. Pachman LM, Cook N. Juvenile dermatomyositis: a clinical and immunological study. *J Pediatr* 1980; 96: 226.
7. Adams-Gandhi LB, Boyd AS, King LE. Diagnosis and management of dermatomyositis. *Compr Ther* 1996; 22: 156–164.

8. Goldstein R, Duvic M, Targoff I, et al. HLA-D region genes associated with autoantibody responses to Jo-1 (histidyl-tRNA synthetase) and other translation-related factors in myositis. *Arthritis Rheum* 1990; 33: 657–665.
9. Wilson CL, Bradlow A, Wonjarowska F. Cutaneous problems with drug therapy in rheumatoid arthritis. *Int J Dermatol* 1991; 30: 148–149.
10. Shamim EA, Rider LG, Miller FW. Update on the genetics of the idiopathic inflammatory myopathies. *Curr Opin Rheumatol* 2000; 12: 482–491.
11. Reed AM, Stirling JD. Association of the HLA-DQA1*0501 allele in multiple racial groups with juvenile dermatomyositis. *Human Immunol* 1995; 44: 131–135.
12. Pachman LM. Juvenile dermatomyositis: immunogenetics, pathophysiology, and disease expression. *Rheum Dis Clin North Am* 2002; 28: 579–602.
13. Pachman LM, Liotta-Davis MR, Hong DK, et al. TNF alpha-308A allele in juvenile dermatomyositis — associations with increased TNF alpha production, disease duration and pathological calcifications. *Arthritis Rheum* 2000; 43: 2368–2377.
14. Greenberg SA, Sanoudou D, Haslett JN, et al. Molecular profiles of inflammatory myopathies. *Neurology* 2002; 59: 1170–1182.
15. Tezak Z, Hoffman EP, Lutz JL, et al. Gene expression profiling in DQA1*0501 + children with untreated dermatomyositis: a novel model of pathogenesis. *J Immunol* 2002; 168: 4154–4163.
16. Hoffman EP, Rao D, Pachman LM. Clarifying the boundaries between the inflammatory and dystrophic myopathies: insights from molecular diagnostics and microarrays. *Rheum Dis Clin N Am* 2002; 28: 743–757.
17. Pociot F, Briant L, Jongeneel CV, et al. Association of tumor necrosis factor (TNF) and class II major histocompatibility complex alleles with the secretion of TNF-alpha and TNF-beta by human mononuclear cells: a possible link to insulin-dependent diabetes mellitus. *Eur J Immunol* 1993; 23: 224–231.
18. Kroeger KM, Carville KS, Abraham LJ. The -308 tumor necrosis factor-alpha promoter polymorphism effects transcription. *Mol Immunol* 1997; 34: 391–399.
19. Pachman LM, Fedczyna TO, Lutz JL, et al. Juvenile dermatomyositis: the association of the TNFα-308A allele and disease chronicity. *Curr Rheumatol Rep* 2001; 5: 379–386.
20. Pachman LM, Lingen M, Caliendo J, et al. Muscle biopsy findings in 38 untreated children with juvenile dermatomyositis (JDM): capillary occlusion is associated with the TNFα allele. *Arthritis Rheum* 1999; 42: S403.
21. Lutz J, Huwiler KG, Fedczyna T, et al. Increased plasma thrombospondin-1 (TSP-1) levels are associated with the TNF alpha-308A allele in children with juvenile dermatomyositis. *Clin Immunol* 2002; 103: 260–263.
22. Jimenez B, Volpert OV, Crawford SE, et al. Signals leading to apoptosis-dependent inhibition of neovascularization by thrombospondin-1. *Nature Med* 2000; 6: 41–48.
23. Werth VP, Callen JP, Ang G, et al. Associations of tumor necrosis factor α and HLA polymorphism with adult dermatomyositis: implications for a unique pathogenesis. *J Invest Dermatol* 2002; 119: 617–620.
24. Werth VP, Berlin JA, Callen JP, et al. Mannose binding lectin (MBL) polymorphisms associated with low MBL production in patients with dermatomyositis. *J Invest Dermatol* 2002; 119: 1394–1399.
25. Kissel JT, Mendell JR, Rammohan KW. Microvascular deposition of complement membrane attack complex in dermatomyositis. *N Engl J Med* 1986; 314: 329–334.
26. Emslie-Smith AM, Engel AG. Microvascular changes in early and advanced dermatomyositis: a quantitative study. *Ann Neurol* 1990; 27: 343–356.

27. Kissel JT, Halterman RK, Rammohan KW, et al. The relationship of complement-mediated microvasculopathy to the histologic features and clinical duration of disease in dermatomyositis. *Arch Neurol* 1991; 48: 26–30.
28. Rollins SA, Sims PJ. The complement-inhibitory activity of CD59 resides in its capacity to block incorporation of CD59 into C5b-9. *J Immunol* 1990; 144: 3478–3483.
29. Navenot JM, Villanova M, Lucas-Heron B, et al. Expression of CD59, a regulator of the membrane attack complex of complement, on human skeletal muscle fibers. *Muscle Nerve* 1997; 20: 92–96.
30. Goncalves FG, Chimelli L, Sallum AM, et al. Immunohistological analysis of CD59 and membrane attack complex of complement in muscle in juvenile dermatomyositis. *J Rheumatol* 2002; 29: 1301–1307.
31. Gasque P, Morgan BP, Legoedec J, et al. Human skeletal myoblasts spontaneously activate allogenic complement but are resistant to killing. *J Immunol* 1996; 156: 3402–3411.
32. Tews DS, Goebel HH. Cytokine expression profiles in idiopathic inflammatory myopathies. *J Neuropathol Exp Neurol* 1996; 55: 342–347.
33. De Bleecker JL, De Paepe B, Vanwalleghem IE, et al. Differential expression of chemokines in inflammatory myopathies. *Neurology* 2002; 58: 1779–1785.
34. Kuru S, Inukai A, Liang Y, et al. Tumor necrosis factor-α expression in muscles of polymyositis and dermatomyositis. *Acta Neuropathol* 2000; 99: 585–588.
35. Dalakas MC, Hohfeld R. Polymyositis and dermatomyositis. *Lancet* 2003; 362: 971–982.
36. Leon-Monzon M, Dalakas MC. Interleukin-1 (IL-1) is toxic to human muscle. *Neurology* 1994; 44 (Suppl): 132.
37. Kalovidouris AE, Plotkin Z. Synergistic cytotoxic effect of interferon γ and tumor necrosis factor α on cultured human muscle cells. *J Rheumatol* 1995; 22: 1698–1703.
38. Murakami N, McLennan IS, Nonaka I, et al. Transforming growth factor-β2 is elevated in skeletal muscle disorders. *Muscle Nerve* 1999; 22: 889–898.
39. Del Prete G, Maggi E, Romagnani S. Human Th1 and Th2 cells: functional properties, mechanisms of regulation, and role in diseases. *Lab Invest* 1994; 70: 299–306.
40. Lepidi H, Frances V, Figarella-Branger D, et al. Local expression of cytokines in idiopathic inflammatory myopathies. *Neuropathol Appl Biol* 1998; 24: 73–79.
41. Illa I, Gallardo E, Gimeno R, et al. Signal transducer and activator of transcription 1 in human muscle: implications in inflammatory myopathies. *Am J Pathol* 1997; 151: 81–88.
42. Dalakas MC, Illa I, Dambrosia JM, et al. A controlled trial of high dose intravenous immunoglobulin infusions as treatment for dermatomyositis. *N Engl J Med* 1993; 329: 1993–2000.
43. Kunkel EJ, Butcher EC. Chemokines and the tissue-specific migration of lymphocytes. *Immunity* 2002; 16: 1–4.
44. Choi YC, Dalakas MC. Expression of matrix metalloproteinases in the muscle of patients with inflammatory myopathies. *Neurology* 2000; 54: 65–71.
45. Kieseier BC, Schneider C, Clements JM, et al. Expression of specific matrix metalloproteinases in inflammatory myopathies. *Brain* 2001; 124: 341–351.
46. Sontheimer RD. Dermatomyositis: an overview of recent progress with emphasis on dermatologic aspects. *Dermatol Clin* 2002; 20(3): 387–408.
47. Lundberg IE. Idiopathic inflammatory myopathies: why do the muscles become weak? *Curr Opin Rheumatol* 2001; 13: 457–460.
48. Kubo M, Ihn H, Yamane K, et al. Increased serum levels of soluble vascular cell adhesion molecules-1 and soluble E-selectin in patients with polymyositis/dermatomyositis. *Br J Dermatol* 2000; 143: 392–398.

49. Sontheimer RD, Racila D. Blood levels of soluble vascular adhesion molecules, VCAM-1 and E-selectin, are increased in clinically amyopathic dermatomyositis [abstract]. *J Invest Dermatol* 2001; 117: 440.
50. Bloom BJ, Miller LC, Blier PR. Soluble adhesion molecules in pediatric rheumatic diseases. *J Rheumatol* 2002; 29: 832–836.
51. Mojcik CF, Shevach EM. Adhesion molecules: a rheumatologic perspective. *Arthritis Rheum* 1997; 40: 991–1004.
52. Hausmann G, Mascaro JM, Herrero C. Cell adhesion molecule expression in cutaneous lesions of dermatomyositis. *Acta Derm Venereol* 1996; 76(3): 222–225.
53. Kumamoto T, Abe T, Ueyama H, et al. Elevated soluble intercellular adhesion molecules-1 in inflammatory myopathy. *Acta Neurol Scand* 1997; 95: 34–37.
54. Twes DS, Goebels HH. Expression of cell adhesion molecules in inflammatory myopathies. *J Neuroimmunol* 1995; 59: 185–194.
55. Newman W, Beall LD, Carson CW, et al. Soluble E-selectin is found in supernatans of activated endothelian cells and is elevated in the serum of patients with septic shock. *J Immunol* 1993; 150: 644–654.
56. Leca G, Mansur SE, Bensussan A. Expression of VCAM 1 (CD106) by a subset of TCTγδ-bearing lymphocyte clones. Involvement of a metalloproteinase in the specific hydrolytic release of the soluble isoform. *J Immunol* 1995; 154: 1069–1077.
57. Thornhil MH, Haskard DO. Il-4 regulates endothelial cell activation by IL-1, tumor necrosis factor, or IFN-γ. *J Immunol* 1990; 145: 865–872.
58. Wellicome SM, Thornhill MH, Pitzalis C, et al. A monoclonal antibody that detects a novel antigen on endothelial cells that is induced by tumor necrosis factor, IL-1, or lipopolysaccharide. *J Immunol* 1990; 144: 2558–2565.

Pathophysiology, Hypotheses for Pathogenesis and Animal Models of DM

38

Dermatomyositis is thought to be autoimmune in origin, based on: (i) an increased incidence of HLA DR3 phenotype, (ii) association with other autoimmune diseases, (iii) the frequent presence of autoantibodies, (iv) inducing of tissue damage mediated by either complement or cytotoxic T cells, and (v) response to immunosuppressive therapy [1]; however, its pathogenesis remains unclear. While the exact triggers of the immune response in DM patients have not been identified, recent studies have endeavored, with some success, to uncover the targets of such abnormal immune responses.

Dermatomyositis is an autoimmune disease where muscle and skin incur ischemic damage from an immune-mediated microvasculopathy [2]. Various studies of immunologic mechanisms by which DM could be induced have yielded conflicting results.

The **first hypothesis** of pathogenesis of DM proposes a ***molecular mimicry*** based on structural homology between picornaviruses and tRNA synthetase [3–7] and homology between microbial antigens (Streptococcus M5 protein) and myosin heavy chain of T-cell epitope [8, 9].

Abnormal responses to microbial antigens that share homology with self-antigen targets may lead, either directly or indirectly, to the development of disease [9]. Recent research has shown that self epitopes in the human skeletal myosin heavy chain are homologous to specific amino acid sequences in the M5 protein of *Streptococcus pyogenes*. The recognition of these self epitopes in skeletal muscle then triggers activation of disease-specific cytotoxic T cells, which results in chronic autoimmune damage [8, 9]. Amino acid sequences that share homology between skeletal myosin and the *S. pyogenes* M5 protein are identified as targets of cytotoxic T-cell responses [9]. Serum levels of antibodies to streptococcal rM12 protein in DM patients are statistically significantly increased compared with SLE patients and healthy controls [10]. Cross-reactivity between streptococcal M protein surface antigen and human skeletal muscle or skin myosin has also been reported. Other common pathogens, including *Borrelia burgdorferi*, *Mycoplasma hominis*, *Haemophilus influenzae*, *Helicobacter pylori*, *Escherichia coli*, and *Bacillus subtilis* (HSP70), have been determined to share sequence homologies with the Myo (aa114-122) peptide of human skeletal myosin [9]. Taken together, these reports suggest that the etiology and pathogenesis of juvenile DM are antigen-driven, with a role for molecular mimicry. Triggering by infectious agents in genetically susceptible individuals has been regarded to play some role in the pathogenesis of DM [9, 11–14]. However, the precise

38

mechanisms leading to characteristic muscle destruction and vascular damage are largely unknown.

The **second hypothesis** for pathogenesis of DM emphasizes a role for the ***immune complex*** by demonstrating the presence of the MAC of serum complement in the blood vessels of biopsy specimens from muscle [15]. Complement activation is an early pathogenic step, leading to the formation of cytolytic C5b-9 MAC, which deposits in the walls of endomysial capillaries and sometimes in larger perimysial blood vessels [15]. These complexes produce osmotic lysis of endothelial cells, necrosis of capillaries, and eventual muscle ischemia and microinfarcts. Complement activation also induces proinflammatory cytokines and chemotactic factors, which recruit inflammatory cells and upregulate cellular adhesion molecules on leukocytes and endothelial cells in the affected region [16]. According to the immune complex hypothesis, DM appears to be a microangiopathy affecting muscle and skin, where activation and deposition of complement cause lysis of endomysial capillaries and muscle ischemia [16]. The evidence for a humoral pathogenesis, at least with respect to juvenile and "classic" DM in adults, is supported by the fundamental differences from PM in which immune complex deposit in muscle biopsies has not been identified. The primary antigenic target is the endothelium of the endomysial capillaries [16]. The disease begins when putative antibodies are directed against endothelial cells and activate complement C3. Activated C3 leads to formation of C3b, C3bNEO, and C4b fragments and C5b-9 MAC, the lytic component of the complement pathway [15, 17, 18]. MAC, C3b, and C4b are detected early in the patients' serum [19], and these complement complexes are deposited on capillaries before inflammatory or structural changes are seen in the muscle [15, 17, 18]. Later, the complement deposits induce swollen endothelial cells, vacuolization, capillary necrosis, perivascular inflammation, ischemia, and destruction of muscle fibers [7, 16, 20]. At the end, there is a striking reduction in the number of capillaries per muscle fiber, with compensatory dilatation of the lumen of the remaining capillaries [16]. However, the pathogenic importance of complement activation by immune complex is challenged by the fact that DM can occur in patients with hereditary complement deficiency [21, 22]. A case of C2 deficiency [21] and another with C9 deficiency in young adult Japanese woman [22] have been reported. C9 deficiency is a common genetic abnormality in Japan, with an incidence of homozygosity of 1 in 1,000; in contrast, only a few cases of C9 deficiency have been identified in the USA and the Europe. The membrane attack complex comprises the complement components C5b-9 and, when inserted into the cell membrane of nucleated cells, results in cell death by necrosis or apoptosis. MAC deposits have been detected in the intramuscular vassels [15, 17, 23, 24], muscle fibers [23] and dermoepidermal junction [25] of biopsy specimens taken from DM patients, thereby implicating MAC in the pathogenesis of disease.

These observations argue for the primacy of humoral immune mechanisms in the pathogenesis of DM.

The **third hypothesis**: ***auto-reactive T-cell mechanisms*** are thought to be the main component of human IIMs, though the antigen still remains unknown [26]. It is based on the predominantly lymphocytic cellular infiltrate in involved muscle, and has stimulated numerous studies of cell-mediated immunity as a pathogenic mechanism for DM [27]. Mononuclear cells from peripheral blood of DM patients have been reported to be cytotoxic to cultured human or animal myocytes [28]. Autoimmune diseases are characterized by tissue injury caused by autoantibodies or killer T cells reacting with self antigens. Recently, further evidence has been presented supporting the concept that cell-mediated myocytotoxicity plays a important role in the pathogenesis of DM. Both myocytotoxic CD3 + T cell clones and non-HLA-restricted myocytotoxic cells of other lineages have been shown to present in the peripheral blood of patients with inflammatory myopathies [29]. A study by Massa et al. identified a self T-cell epitope (myosin heavy chain) and its homolog (Streptococcus M5 protein) in juvenile DM patients, and indicated T-cell cross-recognition of bacterial and human homologs by analyzing TCR Vβ gene usage of peptide-specific T cells [9]. Specific types of HLA class I or class II molecules are associated with increased risks of certain autoimmune diseases [30].

Organspecific or widespread systemic tissue injury results, depending on the nature of the autoreactive antibodies or T cells.

DM is characterized by a marked decrease in circulating CD8 + T cells and significant increase in CD20 + B cells, suggesting that immune mechanisms are primarily involved in its pathogenesis [31–35]. Muscle biopsy findings also implicate antibodies and T cells reacting with autoantigens in the muscle injury. Immunoglobulins and complement are deposited on vessels and muscle fibers. Both B cells and T cells infiltrate around the vessels and interfascicular areas. In accordance with these findings, it has recently been reported that muscle tissue of juvenile DM patients is infiltrated with T cells containing specific CDR3 Ag-binding region, indicating that oligoclonal expansion of antigen-specific T cells plays significant roles in the pathogenesis of juvenile DM [36]. Mizuno et al. examined TCR structures in the peripheral blood and muscle tissue of two juvenile DM patients [36]. In both cases, abnormal expansion of CD8 + T cells with particular TCR Vβ structures was proved in the peripheral blood. Several pieces of evidence show that the increase of these Vβ repertoires was functionally significant and represents oligoclonal expansion of antigen-specific killer/effector T cells. Most of these antigens are closely associated with cytotoxic/effector phenotypes of T cells, suggesting that these T cells proliferate in response to certain antigens. In performing CDR3 analysis of the infiltrating cells in muscle, CDR3 nucleotide sequences of predominant clones in the patient's peripheral CD8 + T cells are identical to those of the infiltrating T cells. So most of the infiltrating T cells in the muscle and predominantly CD8 + T cell clone in the peripheral blood are thought to be of the same origin. The analysis of muscle biopsy samples in both patients revealed that CD8 + T cells infiltrated within the interfascicular muscle tissue and around the blood vessels. In contrast, CD20 + B cells were concentrated around the small vessels, but absent within the interfascicular region. These findings indicate that CD8 + T cells with killer/effector functions proliferated in response to precipitating antigens, and triggered muscle injury in juvenile DM [36].

The **fourth hypothesis** for pathogenesis of DM presents a malignancy-provoked speculation about the role of ***tumor immunity*** in the pathogenesis of such cases [37]. Some patients exhibit delayed skin sensitivity to injection of aqueous extracts of their tumors [38]. The immediate cutaneous reaction and passive transfer tests established the humoral nature of immunological reaction [39]; however, the significance of these observations is uncertain. The facts supporting this hypothesis are: (1) the simultaneous occurrence of malignancy and DM (s.c. paraneoplastic phenomenon), (2) the beginning of DM during the treatment with medicines or ionizing therapy for cancer, and (3) the appearance of reversible leukemia and lymphoma during the treatment of DM with immunosuppressive drugs. However, given the time-course in paraneoplastic DM patients, malignancy seems more likely to be a consequence of DM; the iatrogenic immunosuppression may simply be been unmasked by immunosuppressive drug therapy. Based on this background, Kamel et al. [40] have described that a proportion of lymphoid neoplasms in patients with DM exhibited features similar to those of immunosuppression-related lymphomas, suggesting that this phenomenon might be partly attributable to the treatment received, especially of methotrexate or azathioprine administration. Conversely, Kojima et al. [41], conducting a clinicopathologic study of five patients with malignant lymphoma complicating rheumatic diseases other than Sjögren's syndrome, found that two of their patients fulfilled the diagnostic criteria for DM and the use of immunosuppressive drugs for DM before the onset of malignant lymphoma was recorded in both (the first case with vincristine, cyclophosphamide, prednnine, adriamycin (VEPA), and the second with predonine). Kojima et al. found no evidence for a causative association between iatrogenic immunosuppression and the development of EBV-related lymphoma [41].

The **fifth hypothesis** for pathogenesis of DM is based on the accumulating evidence that **TNF-α** could play a role in the pathogenesis of muscle injury in DM and in photosensitivity experienced by many DM patients. Several evidences have suggested a pathogenic role for TNF-α:

(i) UV light is a potential trigger of the skin reaction in DM, and studies in vitro have shown that UV-B triggers release of TNF-α from human skin keratinocytes and fibroblasts [42].
(ii) UV light induces apoptosis in skin cells [43], and the increased keratinocyte apoptosis in the cutaneous lesions of DM [44–46] could possibly be related also to TNF-α induction by UV light [47].
(iii) Immunolocalization of TNF-α in muscle fibers has been observed in biopsies from juvenile DM and inflammatory myopathies [48–51].

The pathophysiology of photosensitive autoimmune skin diseases may include the photoinduction of TNF-α secretion, which leads to keratinocyte apoptosis and translocation of previously sequestered cellular antigens and subsequent activation of immune system [52, 53]. An association of the overproducing of the TNF-α-308A variant is found in adult DM and in subacute cutaneous LE patients [53]. The TNF-α-308A polymorphism is associated with DM, which suggests a pathophysiologic contribution from UV-induced production of TNF-α, similar to subacute cutaneous LE. The differences in linkage with HLA-DR3, as well as several divergent clinical features, indicate that there are also fundamental pathophysiological differences between DM and subacute cutaneous LE [53]. In adult DM patients, one TNF-α-308A allele had at least two mannose binding lectin (MBL) polymorphisms with low serum levels of MBL versus controls [53]. Thus, low-producing MBL genes are very strongly associated with adult DM. This model shows that genetic polymorphisms leading to overproduction of apoptotic keratinocytes, and then impaired clearance of these cells, contribute to the pathogenesis of photoinduced autoimmune skin disease as adult DM [53]. It has been suggested that low serum MBL levels can exacerbate photoinduced autoimmune diseases through at least four mechanisms [53]:

(i) In the first one, the low MBL levels have been associated with increased levels of TNF-α and raised proinflammatory cytokine production by monocytes (IL-6 and IL-1b) [54].

(ii) As MBL plays a role in clearing immune complexes [55], the deficiency of MBL contributes to the greater numbers of immune complexes seen in muscles and skin of DM patients.
(iii) MBL levels affect adhesion molecule expression by inflammatory cells [54], and the deficiency of MBL increases monocyte adhesion to the vascular system.
(iv) The incidence of atypical and bacterial infections is increased in patients with MBL deficiencies [56], and it is tempting to speculate that this protein deficiency accounts for both increased infections and autoimmunity.

Immunohistochemical investigations have demonstrated that the number of apoptotic keratinocytes in the disrupted basal zone was significantly increased in patients with DM and cutaneous LE compared with normal skin [44, 45]. Unlike normal skin, a large number of keratinocytes, particularly those morphologically apoptotic, expressed p53 protein. The MBL is present in irradiated, but not in non-irradiated skin, and in irradiated skin it is bound to apoptotic keratinocytes [57]. MBL comes from an exogenous source, bound to apoptotic keratinocytes, and increases the uptake of these cells by dendritic cells and thus facilitates non-inflammatory clearance of apoptotic debris in patients with photosensitive forms of DM [57].

The **sixth hypothesis** suggests as a possible mechanism ***fetal microchimerism*** as an etiological factor for the onset of DM during the postpartum period. During the course of pregnancy, fetal cells (predominantly lymphocytes) pass routinely into the maternal circulation [58, 59]. Production of antibodies to fetal (paternal) HLA antigens has also been confirmed. Such immunological changes in the mother may be potentially relevant to the development of autoimmune disease [60]. It has also been shown that fetal cells can persist after delivery [61]. Persistent fetal microchimerism has been suggested to be one of the causes of elevated susceptibility to the disease, or a trigger factor of subclinical DM during pregnancy provoked by another factor as the puerperium [62]. Persistent fetal microchimerism have been suggested to be one of the cause of DM in parous women [60, 62, 63]. As with other CTD such as SSc [60], maternal microchimerism has been observed in juvenile DM patients [59]. An increased number of maternal chimeric cells have been determined in peripheral blood as well as in muscle tissue of patients with juvenile DM compared to controls, suggesting that microchimerism could play an important role in the pathogenesis of disease [58, 59]. Moreover, the pathogenic significance of aloreactive maternal lymphoid cells in the circulation of children with DM remains known.

The **seventh hypothesis** implicates some ***drugs*** applied for treatment of other chronic disorders in inducing DM features. The symptoms usually begin within months or years of medication intake, and patients and physicians do not pay attention to the relation between treatment and disease.

38.1 Animal Models of Dermatomyositis

Dermatomyositis has previously been described in the Shetland sheepdog and rough collie dog breeds. It is of interest that familial canine DM has been described in collie dogs, and it resembles human juvenile DM [64, 65]. Canine DM is characterized by a cicatricial

38

alopecia and hypopigmentation of the face, limbs, and extremities, preceded by erythema, papules, and vesicules. Some affected animals have a concurrent myositis [66].

The initial characterization of canine DM indicates that there is definite familial autosomal dominant tendency, at least in the rough collie dog [67].

The typical age of the onset in these breeds is between 7 weeks and 6 months of age, although the initiation of disease in adulthood has also been recognized. In the Shetland sheepdog and rough collie dog, DM is typically a disease of the juvenile dog [68].

The cutaneous signs are characterized by erythema, transient vesicules, ulceration progressing to cicatricial alopecia, and hypopigmentation. Lesions are distributed over the bony prominences of limbs, distal extremities, lips, periocular and facial skin, and the concave aspect of the pinnae [66]. The severity of the skin manifestations and accompanying myositis can vary among individuals. Sunlight may exacerbate existing cutaneous lesions. Myositis is a common, but not consistent, development.

There are no specific clinicopathological features associated with canine DM. ANA titers and rheumatoid factors are negative. However, high levels of CH50, C4, C2, and C3 as well as circulating IgG immune complexes have been demonstrated in severely affected dogs [67, 69].

The pathogenesis of the disease includes viral or autoimmune pathophysiology, although the possibility of both mechanisms being involved must be entertained [70, 71]. On histopathological examination a subtle vasculitis is noted, causing the presumption that the follicular atrophy is a consequence of an ischemic vasculopathy [72].

Recently, a controllable muscle-specific promoter system to upregulate MHC class I in the skeletal muscles of young transgenic mice has been reported [73]. These mice develop clinical, biochemical, histological, and immunological features very similar to human myositis. The disease is inflammatory, limited to skeletal muscles, self-sustaining, more severe in females, and often accompanied by autoantibodies, most often to histidyl-tRNA synthetase. The muscle weakness and wasting starts at about 3 months of age, and becomes severe by 5–7 months. At 6 months of age, female mice had a 40–50% reduction in body weight. It was accompanied by increased serum levels of CK and glutamic-oxaloacetic transaminase. The skeletal muscles of the treated mice at 5.5 months showed centralized nuclei, significant variation in muscle fiber diameter, muscle fiber degeneration and regeneration, atrophy, obliteration of the striations of the contractile apparatus, mononuclear cell infiltration, and the invasion of some muscle fibers by phagocytes [73].

In conclusion, the precise immunologic mechanisms by which DM could be induced in human as well as animals have not yet been determined.

References

1. Plotz PH, Dalakas M, Leff RL, et al. Current concepts in the idiopathic inflammatory myopathies: polymyositis, dermatomyositis, and related disorders. *Ann Intern Med* 1989; 111(2): 143–157.
2. Greenberg SA, Amato AA. Uncertainties in the pathogenesis of adult dermatomyositis. *Curr Opin Neurol* 2004; 17: 359–364.

3. Walker EJ, Jeffery PD. Sequence homology between encephalomyocarditis virus protein VPI and histidyl-tRNA synthetase supports a hypothesis of molecular mimicry in polymyositis. *Med Hypotheses* 1988; 25: 21–26.
4. Rosenberg NL, Rothbar HA, Abzug MJ, et al. Evidence for a novel picornavirus in human dermatomyositis. *Am Neurol* 1989; 26: 204–209.
5. Targoff IN. Immunologic aspects of myositis. *Curr Opin Rheumatol* 1989; 1: 432–442.
6. Targoff IN. Immune mechanisms in myositis. *Curr Opin Rheumatol* 1990; 2: 882–888.
7. Dalakas M. Polymyositis, dermatomyositis and inclusion body myositis. *N Engl J Med* 1991; 325(21): 1487–1498.
8. Rider LG, Miller FW. Laboratory evaluation of the inflammatory myopathies. *Clin Diagn Lab Immunol* 1995; 2: 1–9.
9. Massa M, Costouros N, Mazzoli F, et al. Self epitopes shared between human skeletal myosin and *Streptococcus pyogenes* M5 protein are targets of immune responses in active juvenile dermatomyositis. *Arthritis Rheum* 2002; 46(11): 3015–3025.
10. Ichimiya M, Yasui H, Hirota Y, et al. Association between elevated serum antibody levels to streptococcal M12 protein and susceptibility to dermatomyositis. *Arch Dermatol Res* 1998; 290(4): 229–230.
11. Bardelas JA, Winkelstein JA, Seto DS, et al. Fatal ECHO 24 infection in a patient with hypogammaglobulinemia: relationship to dermatomyositis-like syndrome. *J Pediatr* 1977; 90: 396–399.
12. Lewkonia RM, Horne D, Dawood MR. Juvenile dermatomyositis in a child infected with human parvovirus B19. *Clin Infect Dis* 1995; 21: 430–432.
13. McMurray RW, Elbourne K. Hepatitis C virus infection and autoimmunity. *Semin Arthritis Rheum* 1997; 26: 689–701.
14. Lehmann H, Kuhner L, Beckenlehner K, et al. Chronic human parvovirus B19 infection in rheumatic disease of childhood and adolescence. *J Clin Virol* 2002; 25: 135.
15. Kissel JT, Mendell JR, Rammohan KW. Microvascular deposition of complement membrane attack complex in dermatomyositis. *N Engl J Med* 1986; 314: 329–334.
16. Dalakas MC, Hohlfeld R. Polymyositis and dermatomyositis. *Lancet* 2003; 362: 971–982.
17. Emslie-Smith AM, Engel AG. Microvascular changes in early and advanced dermatomyositis: a quantitative study. *Ann Neurol* 1990; 27: 343–356.
18. Kissel JT, Halterman RK, Rammohan KW, et al. The relationship of complement-mediated microvasculopathy to the histologic features and clinical duration of disease in dermatomyositis. *Arch Neurol* 1991; 48: 26–30.
19. Basta M, Dalakas MC. High-dose intravenous immunoglobulin exerts its beneficial effect in patients with dermatomyositis by blocking endomysial deposition of activated complement fragments. *J Clin Invest* 1994; 94: 1729–1735.
20. Crowson AN, Magro CM. The role of microvascular injury in the pathogenesis of cutaneous lesions of dermatomyositis. *Hum Pathol* 1996; 27(1): 15–19.
21. Leddy JP, Griggs RC, Klemperer MR, et al. Hereditary complement (C2) deficiency with dermatomyositis. *Am J Med* 1975; 58: 83–91.
22. Ichikawa E, Furuta J, Kawachi Y, et al. Hereditary complement (C9) deficiency associated with dermatomyositis. *Br J Dermatol* 2001; 144: 1080–1083.
23. Sewry CA, Dubowitz V, Abraha A, et al. Immunocytochemical localisation of complement components C8 and C9 in human diseased muscle. *J Neurol Sci* 1987; 81: 141–153.
24. Griggs RC, Karpati G. The pathogenesis of dermatomyositis. *Arch Neurol* 1991; 48: 21–22.
25. Mascaro JM Jr, Hausmann G, Herrero C, et al. Membrane attack complex deposits in cutaneous lesions of dermatomyositis. *Arch Dermatol* 1995; 131: 1386–1392.
26. O'Hanlon T, Miller F. T cell-mediated immune mechanisms in myositis. *Curr Opin Rheumatol* 1995; 7: 503–509.

27. Ytterberg S. Cellular immunity in polymyositis/dermatomyositis. *Mt Sinai J Med* 1988; 55: 494–500.
28. Hayashi Y, Kikuchi-Tada A, Jitsukawa K, et al. Muscle regeneration and cell-mediated cytotoxicity in the autologous muscle culture of dermatomyositis. *Acta Derm Venereol* 1990; 70(1): 53–55.
29. Bank I, Miranda AF, Chess L. Mechanism of cell-mediated myocytotoxicity in the peripheral blood of patients with inflammatory myopathies. *J Clin Immunol* 2001; 21: 328–334.
30. Tezak Z, Hoffman EP, Lutz JL, et al. Gene expression profiling in DQA1*0501 + children with untreated dermatomyositis: a novel model of pathogenesis. *J Immunol* 2002; 168: 4154–4163.
31. Mantegazza R, Bernasconi P. Cellular aspects of myositis. *Curr Opin Rheumatol* 1994; 6: 568–574.
32. Eisenstein DM, O'Gorman MR, Pachman LM. Correlations between change in disease activity and changes in peripheral blood lymphocyte subsets in patients with juvenile dermatomyositis. *J Rheumatol* 1997; 24: 1830–1832.
33. Dalakas MC. Molecular immunology and genetics of inflammatory muscle diseases. *Arch Neurol* 1998; 55: 1509–1512.
34. O'Gorman MR, Bianchi L, Zaas D, et al. Decreased levels of CD54 (ICAM-1)-positive lymphocytes in the peripheral blood in untreated patients with active juvenile dermatomyositis. *Clin Diagn Lab Immunol* 2000; 7: 693–697.
35. Kikuchi Y, Koarada S, Tada Y, et al. Difference in B cell activation between dermatomyositis and polymyositis: analysis of the expression of RP105 on peripheral blood B cells. *Ann Rheum Dis* 2001; 60: 1137–1140.
36. Mizuno K, Yachie A, Nagaoki S, et al. Oligoclonal expansion of circulating and tissue-infiltrating CD8 + T Cells with killer/effector phenotypes in juvenile dermatomyositis syndrome. *Clin Exp Immunol* 2004; 137: 187–194.
37. Lakhanpal S, Bunch TW, Ilstrup DM, et al. Polymyositis–dermatomyositis and malignant lesions: Does an association exist? *Mayo Clin Proc* 1986; 61: 645–653.
38. Grace JT Jr, Dao TL. Dermatomyositis in cancer: a possible etiological mechanism. *Cancer* 1959; 12(4): 648–650.
39. Curtis AG, Heckmann JH, Wheeler AK. Study of the autoimmune reaction in dermatomyositis. *JAMA* 1961; 178: 571.
40. Kamel OW, van de Rijn M, Le Brun DP, et al. Lymphoid neoplasms in patients with rheumatoid arthritis and dermatomyositis: frequency of Epstein–Barr virus and other features associated with immunosuppression. *Hum Pathol* 1994; 25: 638–643.
41. Kojima M, Nakamura S, Futamura N, et al. Malignant lymphoma in patients with rheumatic diseases other than Sjögren's syndrome: a clinicopathologic study of five cases and a review of the Japanese literature. *Jpn J Clin Oncol* 1997; 27(2): 84–90.
42. Werth VP, Zhang W. Wavelength-specific synergy between ultraviolet radiation and interleukin-1 alpha in the regulation of matrix-related genes: mechanistic role for tumor necrosis factor-alpha. *J Invest Dermatol* 1999; 113(2): 196–201.
43. Zhuang L, Wang B, Sauder DN. Molecular mechanism of ultraviolet-induced keratinocyte apoptosis. *J Interferon Cytokine Res* 2000; 20(5): 445–454.
44. Chung JH, Kwon OS, Eun HC, et al. Apoptosis in the pathogenesis of cutaneous lupus erythematosus. *Am J Dermatopathol* 1998; 20: 233–241.
45. Pablos JL, Santiago B, Galindo M, et al. Keratinocyte apoptosis and p53 expression in cutaneous lupus and dermatomyositis. *J Pathol* 1999; 188: 63–68.
46. Dourmishev L, Wolina U. Dermatomyositis: immunopathologic study of skin lesions. *Acta Dermatoven APN* 2006; 15: 45–51.

47. Schwarz A, Bhardwaj R, Arganc Y, et al. Ultraviolet B induced apoptosis of keratinocytes: evidence for partial involvement of tumor necrosis factor-alpha in the formation of sunburn cells. *J Invest Dermatol* 1995; 104: 922–927.
48. De Bleecker JL, Meire VI, Declercq W, et al. Immunolocalization of tumor necrosis factor-alpha and its receptors in inflammatory myopathies. *Neuromuscul Disord* 1999; 9(4): 239–246.
49. Pachman LM, Liotta-Davis MR, Hong DK, et al. TNF alpha-308A allele in juvenile dermatomyositis: association with increased production of tumor necrosis factor alpha, disease duration, and pathologic calcifications. *Arthritis Rheum* 2000; 43: 2368–2377.
50. Fedczyna TO, Lutz J, Pachman LM. Expression of TNF alpha by muscle fibers in biopsies from children with untreated juvenile dermatomyositis: association with the TNF alpha-308A allele. *Clin Immunol* 2001; 100(2): 236–239.
51. Kuru S, Inukai A, Kato T, et al. Expression of tumor necrosis factor-alpha in regenerating muscle fibers in inflammatory and non-inflammatory myopathies. *Acta Neuropathol* 2003; 105(3): 217–224.
52. Sontheimer RD. Photoimmunology of lupus erythematosus and dermatomyositis: a speculative review. *Photochem Photobiol* 1996; 63: 583–594.
53. Werth VP, Callen JP, Ang G, et al. Associations of tumor necrosis factor α and HLA polymorphism with adult dermatomyositis: implications for a unique pathogenesis. *J. Invest Dermatol* 2002; 119: 617–620.
54. Jack DL, Read RC, Tenner AJ, et al. Mannose-binding lectin regulates the inflammatory response of human professional phagocytes to *Neisseria meningitidis* Serogroup B. *J Infect Dis* 2001; 84: 1152–1162.
55. Walport MJ. Complement. *N Engl JMed* 2001; 344: 1140–1144.
56. Turner MW, Hamvas RM. Mannose-binding lectin: structure, function, genetics and disease associations. *Rev Immunogenet* 2000; 2: 305–322.
57. Lokitz ML, Zhang W, Bashir M, et al. Ultraviolet-B recruits mannose-binding lectin into skin from non-cutaneous sources. *J Invest Dermatol* 2005; 125: 166–173.
58. Artlett CM, Miller FW, Rider LG. Persistent maternally derived peripheral microchimerism is associated with the juvenile idiopathic inflammatory myopathies. *Rheumatology* 2001; 20: 1279–1284.
59. Reed AM, Picornell YJ, Harwood A, et al. Chimerism in children with juvenile dermatomyositis. *Lancet* 2000; 356: 2156–2157.
60. Nelson JL. Microchimerism: implications for autoimmune disease. *Lupus* 1999; 8(5): 370–374.
61. Bianchi DW, Zickwolf GK, Weil GJ, et al. Male fetal progenitor cells persist in maternal blood for as long as 27 years postpartum. *Proc Natl Acad Sci USA* 1996; 93(2): 705–708.
62. Kanoh H, Izumi T, Seishima M, et al. A case of dermatomyositis that developed after delivery: the involvement of pregnancy in the induction of dermatomyositis. *Br J Dermatol* 1999; 141(5): 897–900.
63. Ishii N, Ono H, Kawaguchi T, et al. Dermatomyositis and pregnancy. Case report and review of the literature. *Dermatologica* 1991; 183: 146–149.
64. Hargis AM, Haupt KH, Hegreberg GA, et al. Familial canine dermatomyositis. Initial characterization of the cutaneous and muscular lesions. *Am J Pathol* 1984; 116: 234–244.
65. Hargis AM, Prieur DJ, Haupt KH, et al. Prospective study of familial canine dermatomysitis. Correlation of the severity of dermatomyositis and circulating immune complex levels. *Am J Pathol* 1986; 123: 465–479.
66. Hargis AM, Mundell AC. Familial canine dermatomyositis. In: Compendium of continuing education for practicing veterinarians. *Small Animal Practice* 1992; 14: 855–864.

67. Haupt KH, Prieur DJ, Moore MP, et al. Familial canine dermatomyositis: clinical electrodiagnostic and genetic studies. *Am J Vet Res* 1985; 46: 1861–1869.
68. Jackson HA, Olivry T. Ulcerative dermatosis of the Shetland sheepdog and rough collie dog may represent a novel vesicular variant of cutaneous lupus erythematosus. *Vet Dermatol* 2001; 12: 19–27.
69. Hargis AM, Winkelstein JA, Moore MP, et al. Complement levels in dogs with familial canine dermatomyositis. *Vet Immunol Immunopathol* 1988; 20(1): 95–100.
70. Schmeitzel LP. Dermatomyositis: an immune-mediated disease with a link to canine lupus erythematosus. In: Compendium of continuing education for practicing veterinarians. *Small Animal Practice* 1992; 14: 866–871.
71. Kunkle GA. Canine dermatomyositis: a disease with an infectious origin. In: Compendium of continuing education for practicing veterinarians. *Small Animal Practice* 1992; 14: 866–871.
72. Yager JA, Wilcox BP. Dermatopathology and skin tumors. In: *Colour Atlas and Text of Surgical Pathology of the Dog and Cat.* Mosby Year Book, London, 1994; 90.
73. Nagaraju K, Raben N, Loeffler L, et al. Conditional up-regulation of MHC class I in skeletal muscle leads to self-sustaining autoimmune myositis and myositis-specific autoantibodies. *Proc Natl Acad Sci USA* 2000; 97(16): 9209–9214.

Treatment of Dermatomyositis

The treatment of DM is still a matter of debate. Before adequate treatment regimens had been evaluated, roughly equal numbers of patients lived and died [1]. In some old studies of treatment, a mortality rate of about 50% was reported in DM patients [2, 3]. The therapy course depends on the disease activity, as well as the cutaneous activity of DM, and may develop and respond separately from the inflammatory muscle manifestations. Up to now, only a few well-designed studies have been reported, and only three randomized controlled trials of DM therapy has been published [4–7].

The goals of therapy in DM patients are to improve the function and the ability to carry out activities of daily living by increasing muscle strength, to ameliorate extramuscular manifestations (rash, dysphagia, dyspnea, arthralgia, fever), and to prevent contractures and disability [8, 9]. The treatment regimen must be instituted early, and requires a team approach between dermatologist, rheumatologist, the physical therapist, and family physician. Other subspecialist involvement may be required, depending on the particular manifestations of the disease.

References

1. Sheldon JH, Young F, Dyke SC. Acute dermatomyositis. *Lancet* 1989; 1: 82–84.
2. Steiner WR. Dermatomyositis, with report of a case which presents a rare muscle anomaly but once described in man. *J Exp Med* 1903; 6: 407.
3. O'Leary PA, Waisman M. Dermatomyositis. *Arch Dermatol Syphilol* 1940; 41: 1001–1009.
4. Miller FW, Leitman SF, Cronin ME, et al. Controlled trial of plasma exchange and leucopheresis in polymyositis and dermatomyositis. *N Engl J Med* 1992; 326: 1380–1384.
5. Dalakas MC, Illa I, Dambrosia JM, et al. A controlled trial of high-dose intravenous immune globulin infusions as treatment for dermatomyositis. *N Engl J Med* 1993; 329: 1993–2000.
6. Vencovsky J, Jarosova K, Machacek S, et al. Cyclosporine A versus methotrexate in the treatment of polymyositis and dermatomyositis. *Scand J Rheumatol* 2000; 29: 95–102.
7. Cordeiro AC, Isenberg DA. Treatment of inflammatory myopathies. *Postgrad Med J* 2006; 82(969): 417–424.
8. Callen JP. Dermatomyositis. *Lancet* 2000; 355: 53–57.
9. Dalakas MC, Hohlfeld R. Polymyositis and dermatomyositis. *Lancet* 2003; 362: 971–982.

39 Pharmacologic Agents in the Treatment of DM

The cornerstone of therapy is immunosuppressive medication. Corticosteroids, immunosuppressive agents, high-dose intravenous immunoglobulin (IVIG), and antimalarial drugs are the principal medicines with marked efficacy in the treatment of DM [1–3]. Truly refractory patients may benefit from pulse corticosteroids, followed by tapering of oral prednisone, intravenous immunoglobulin, or cyclosporine A [4].

39.1 Corticosteroids

Systemic corticosteroids are the initial pharmacologic agent for the treatment of DM. The earlier the therapy with corticosteroids is initiated, the better overall prognosis will be achieved [5]. These drugs are accepted as diminishing morbidity and mortality in adult and juvenile disease [6]. Prednisone is the corticosteroid of choice. Treated with prednisone, children had shorter acute outbreak, diminished hospitalization time, and decreased time at home than patients not receiving steroids [7]. This medication is designed to allow patients to remain active and functional while the acute stage of disease is being treated [7]. Treatment of DM with corticosteroids is determined almost exclusively by whether there is muscle disease or involvement of other critical organs, such as the lungs or joints [8]. The justification for steroid usage in DM involves: (i) the probable participation of immune MAC and complement, (ii) the presence of autoantibodies in many patients, and (iii) association of inflammatory myopathies with vascular disease [9]. Patients with an inflammatory myositis, severe ILD, or deforming arthritis require treatment with corticosteroids. Some authorities have believed that in acute disease giving high-dose corticosteroids is essential, and that low-dose therapy offers little chance of improvement [10]. The type of disease may influence the responsiveness to corticosteroids: patients with overlap syndrome respond more poorly than those with a classic DM [11].

Drugs. The most commonly employed medication in the treatment of DM is prednisone. Children with juvenile DM may have an erratic gut absorption pattern resulting in an

L.A. Dourmishev and A.L. Dourmishev, *Dermatomyositis: Advances in Recognition, Understanding and Management,* © Springer-Verlag Berlin Heidelberg 2009

39

extended half-life of the drug [12]. Prednisolone has also been used. Fluorinated steroids are contraindicated in IIM, due to their effects on muscle tissue and electrolytes [13]. Because of their greater propensity to produce myopathy, the more potent fluorinated corticosteroids should not be used to treat DM [14]. Intravenous hydrocortisone has also been used [15]. Children receiving 500 mg hydrocortisone in four doses, every 6 h, demonstrated decreased signs and symptoms of their disease within 24 h.

Regimen. Several regimens are put in practice (Table 39.1) [2]. The standard dose is at least 1 mg of prednisone (or prednisolone) per kg of body weight. In most cases, the initial dose is usually 60 mg/day of oral prednisone, given in one daily dose in the morning at 8.00 a.m., and treatment continues for 3–4 months, provided there is clinical or laboratory response, before tapering of corticosteroids [1, 8]. High-dose prednisone therapy is preferable in early disease [16]. If there is evidence of efficacy and no serious adverse reactions have appeared, it is often necessary to continue this therapeutic regimen even after the muscle enzymes (CK, aldolase) have normalized.

Another regimen involves oral prednisone (prednisolone), 0.5–1.5 mg/kg given in a divided daily dose until myositis has become clinically inactive and serum CK has normalized [24]. As no placebo-controlled trials with the use of corticosteroids have been performed, a starting dose of prednisone of 0.75 mg/kg/day (which corresponds to a dose of 40–60 mg/day) is likely to suffice in most myositis patients [25]. In mild cases, alternate

Table 39.1 Protocols for corticosteroid administration in dermatomyositis (Modified from [10])

Disease type	Initial dose	Regiment	Endpoint	Taper	Maintenance therapy	Reference
Prednisone						
Adult DM	1 mg/kg/day	t.i.d.	Improvement	10% every 2 weeks	–	[17]
Juvenile DM	1–1.5 mg/kg/day	–	Improvement	2.5 mg q. 4th day	–	[18]
Juvenile DM	1–2 mg/kg/day	q.i.d.	4 weeks	50% for 4 weeks, then 1 mg 1–2 weeks	Suppression of clinical/enzymatic parameters	[19]
Juvenile DM	2 mg/kg/day	b.i.d.	4–6 weeks	Monthly	10–15 mg/day	[20]
Methylprednisolone						
Adult DM	500 mg/day	3 days	3–9 weeks	Prednisone 1 mg/kg/day	–	[21]
Adult DM	1 g/day	3 days	3 weeks	Prednisone 1 mg/kg/day	10–15 mg/day	[22]
Juvenile DM	30 mg/kg	3 days	–	–	–	[23]

day therapy with as little as 20 mg of prednisone may be sufficient to control the disease process [1]. Seventy-six percent of patients on an alternate day regimen of prednisone either remained clinically stable or improved after resolution of the acute stage [11]. However, initial treatment with every-other-day steroids in severe DM is not advised because of higher incidence of relapse [26]. One of the most frequent mistakes made in treating DM is initial medication with too low a dose of prednisone or for too short a period of time, causing inadequate control of the disease [8]. Tapering of corticosteroids should be done in a systemic, slow manner, usually by 5 mg/week. Tapering below 20 mg/day is often best achieved by lowering the daily dose by 2.5 mg each week, and below 10 mg/day, tapering the daily dose by 1 mg can fine-tune the lowest tolerated dose, minimizing flares and symptoms of corticosteroid withdrawal [8]. After analysis of a series of studies published in literature as well as our data, Jorizzo [27] suggests that an average patient is best treated after the onset of muscle disease by institution of systemic corticosteroid therapy with a dose of 1 mg/kg prednisone, tapered to half of that dose during a 6-month period, and then tapered to zero during next 24 months. Corticosteroid treatment in consolidation dosages of 5–15 mg/day is often required for several years [25]. The course of prednisone treatment is divided into monocyclic and polycyclic, or chronic polycyclic [6].

Steroid withdrawal symptoms such as fever, headache, nausea, fatigue, malaise, somnolence, anorexia, flulike symptoms, arthralgia, and myalgia can develop if the reduced dosage remains supraphysiologic [28]. These are particularly a problem after a prolonged course of relatively high-dose corticosteroids.

Corticosteroids are preferably administered intravenously. Patients who present with profound and progressive muscle weakness and who do not respond to the intermediate doses of corticosteroids (60 mg/day) for 2–4 months are classified as "steroid-resistant." These patients require more aggressive therapy, or treatment with high-dose corticosteroids in a pulse method with methylprednisolone. Yanagiesawa et al. [29] are the first who reported three adults with fulminant DM in whom 1 g of methylprednisolon sodium succinate was given intravenously for 3 consecutive days per week. This weekly schedule was repeated two or three times, followed by 60 mg of oral prednisone daily. All three patients improved. The regimen of pulse corticosteroids is not standardized, but has ranged from 500 to 1,000 mg of methylprednisolone sodium succinate given slowly infused over a 4-h period daily for 3–5 consecutive days, and repeated three times at an interval of 1 week [21, 22, 30]. Thereafter, patients are generally treated with oral prednisone 1 mg/kg/day. This dosage should be maintained until the patients have achieved and maintained disease stability and levels of CK have normalized for at least 4–8 weeks. The steroid dosage then can be tapered. This can typically be done by a 5 mg increment every 1–2 weeks until a dosage of 20 mg is reached. At that point, tapering is less rapid (i.e., 1 mg/week). Once muscle disease activity is controlled, the prednisone treatment with a single daily dose of 5–10 mg/day will continue over a 12-month period, minimizing the risk of recrudescence [24].

Clinical response. Systemic corticosteroids are the first-line therapy of DM, resulting in an improved lifestyle and prognosis in more than 50% of cases [31]. A treatment "response" from corticosteroids in DM is usually defined as clinical improvement in patient's muscular strength and sense of well being and/or normalization of serum enzymes [10]. Several authors have believed that muscle strength should be the definitive criterion, since it is known that serum enzymes may reach normal values despite the continued clinical weakness [32, 33]. Among the extramuscular feature of diseases, the fever disappeared after the first methylprednisolone pulse therapy [34]. Objective improvement in muscle strength occurs in up to 25% of patients, and is usually seen after the third month of therapy [9, 35, 36]. Eighty-five percent of patients in one prednisone study group had normal muscle strength after 4 months of therapy [37]. Some patients require maintenance on low doses of prednisone for a prolonged course of years to control symptoms. One third of patients with a short delay to diagnosis responded completely to prednisone, whereas no patient with a long delay did [38]. In the past 2 decades, the aggressive use of corticosteroids with or without immunosuppressive agents has markedly reduced mortality and increased functional recovery, even though the total duration of the disease may not have shortened [31, 39].

Katzenstein and Fiorelli [40] reported that some DM/PM patients with ILD represented nonspecific interstitial pneumonia that responded well to corticosteroid therapy.

Corticosteroids do not appear to be helpful for the residual contractures and musculoskeletal deficits, or for inactive disease. About 25% of DM patients not respond to systemic corticosteroid treatment, and 25–50% of them develop substantial steroid-related side effects [3].

Adverse reactions. There is a general agreement about the use of corticosteroids as first-line treatment for patients with newly diagnosed disease, but they are associated with high rates of recurrence and morbidity [38]. About one fifth of all patients with DM either do not respond to treatment with corticosteroids ("steroid resistance") or are unable to tolerate them [17]. Oral corticosteroids have serious toxicities such as gastrointestinal symptoms, adrenal suppression, immunosuppression, retarded growth in children, hypertension, subcapsular cataractas, avascular necrosis, and osteoporosis, which is mostly a problem of prolonged high-dose use. Acute side effects of corticosteroids include psychiatric disorders, insomnia, salt and fluid retention, and hyperglycemia [8].

The long-term use of prednisone may cause progressive weakness associated with a normal or unchanged CK level, but the 24-h urinary creatine excretion is raised [41]. This effect is referred to as a steroid myopathy [16]. Increased weakness as result of steroid myopathy during DM therapy mimics worsening of the disease, or both processes can occur simultaneously [9, 42]. Patients with steroid myopathy involving the respiratory musculature have also been reported [43]. Increased muscle weakness in a patient who previously responded well to high doses of prednisone may be related to an induced myopathy, or to the fact that the disease activity has become resistant to steroids, or that DM can be complicated by other factors such as hypokalemia, infection, or decreased mobility. Regular electrolyte estimations are required. Selective atrophy of muscle fibers type II has been reported in steroid myopathy [44]. Reduction of neck flexor strength is usually seen in the natural progression of disease, and can be used as a hallmark of distinction between these two conditions. In these circumstances, the decision to rise or lower the prednisone dosage depends on the patient's muscle strength, CK levels, other medical conditions, and the evaluation of steroid dosage in previous 2 months [9]. If none of these criteria are informative, the prednisone dosage can be adjusted arbitrarily and judged by the changes in the patient's strength in the next 2–8 weeks [16].

References

1. Drake LA, Dinehart SM, Farmer ER, et al. Guidelines of care for dermatomyositis. *J Am Acad Dermatol* 1996; 34: 824–829.
2. Kovacs SO, Kovacs SC. Dermatomyositis. *J Am Acad Dermatol* 1998; 39: 899–920.
3. Callen JP. Dermatomyositis. *Lancet* 2000; 355: 53–57.
4. Dalakas MC. Controlled studies with high-dose intravenous immunoglobulin in the treatment of dermatomyositis, inclusion body myositis, and polymyositis. *Neurology* 1998; 51: S37–S45.
5. Fafalak RG, Peterson MG, Kagen IJ. Strength in polymyositis and dermatomyositis: best outcome in patients treated early. *J Rheumatol* 1994; 21: 643–648.
6. Spencer CH, Hanson V, Singsen BH, et al. Course of treated juvenile dermatomyositis. *J Pediatr* 1984; 105: 399–408.
7. Rose AL. Childhood polymyositis: a follow-up study with special reference to treatment with corticosteroids. *Am J Dis Child* 1974; 127: 518–522.
8. Werth V. Glucocorticoids in autoimmune connective diseases. *Dermatol Ther* 2001; 14: 134–142.
9. Dalakas MC. Pharmacologic concerns of corticosteroids in the treatment of patients with immune-related neuromuscular diseases. *Neurol Clin* 1990; 8: 93–118.
10. Boyd AS, Neldner KH. Therapeutic options in dermatomyositis/polymyositis. *Int J Dermatol* 1994; 33: 240–250.
11. Bohan A, Peter JB, Bowman RL, Pearson CM. A computer-assisted analysis of 153 patients with polymyositis and dermatomyositis. *Medicine* 1977; 56: 255–286.
12. Pachman LM, Cooke N. Juvenile dermatomyositis: a clinical and immunologic study. *J Pediatr* 1980; 96: 226–234.
13. Winkelmann RK. Dermatomyositis in childhood. *Clin Rheum Dis* 1982; 8: 353–368.
14. Mills JA. Dermatomyositis. In: *Dermatology in General Medicine*, Fitzpatrick TB, Eisen AZ, Wolff K, et al. (eds), McGraw–Hill, New York, 1993; 2148–2155.
15. Miller JJ. Prolonged use of large intravenous steroid pulse in the rheumatic disease in children. *Pediatrics* 1980; 65: 989–994.
16. Dalakas MC. Polymyositis, dermatomyositis and inclusion body myositis. *N Engl J Med* 1991; 325: 1487–1498.
17. Tuffanelli D, Lavole PE. Prognosis and therapy of polymyositis/dermatomyositis. *Clin Dermatol* 1988; 6: 93–104.
18. Dubowitz V. Treatment of dermatomyositis in childhood. *Arch Dis Child* 1976; 51: 494–450.
19. Sullivan DB, Cassidy JT, Petty RE, et al. Prognosis in childhood dermatomyositis. *J Pediatr* 1972; 80: 555–563.
20. Fink CW. Overview of corticosteroid therapy in the treatment of rheumatic diseases of childhood. *Clin Exp Dermatol* 1991; 9(Suppl 6): 9–13.
21. Matsubara S, Sawa Y, Takamori M, et al. Pulsed intravenous methylprednisolone combined with oral steroids as the initial treatment of inflammatory myopathies. *J Neurol Neurosurg Psychiatry* 1994; 57(8): 1008.
22. Matsubara S, Hirai S, Sawa Y. Pulsed intravenous methylprednisolone therapy for inflammatory myopathies: evaluation of the effect by comparing two consecutive biopsies from the same muscle. *J Neuroimmunol* 1997; 76: 621–624.
23. Laxer RM, Stein LD, Petty RD. Intravenous pulse methylprednisolone treatment of juvenile dermatomyositis. *Arthritis Rheum* 1987; 30: 328–334.
24. Oddis CV, Medsger TA. Current management of polymyositis and dermatomyositis. *Drugs* 1989; 37: 382–390.
25. Lundberg I, Chung Y-L. Treatment and investigation of idiopathic inflammatory myopathies. *Rheumatology* 2000; 39: 7–17.

39

26. Hoffman GS, Franck WA, Raddatz DA, et al. Presentation, treatment, and prognosis of idiopathic inflammatory muscle disease in a rural hospital. *Am J Med* 1983; 75(3): 433–438.
27. Jorizzo JL. Dermatomyositis: practical aspects. *Arch Dermatol* 2002; 138: 114–116.
28. Dixon RB, Christy NP. On the various forms of corticosteroid withdrawal syndrome. *Am J Med* 1980; 68: 224–230.
29. Yanagiesawa T, Sueishi M, Nawata Y, et al. Methylprednisolone pulse therapy in dermatomyositis. *Dermatologica* 1983; 167: 47–51.
30. Rougeau J. Pulse glucocorticoid therapy, the big "shot" revised. *Arch Dermatol* 1996; 132: 1499–1502.
31. Trüeb RM. Dermatomyositis. *Dermatol Ther* 2001; 14: 70–80.
32. Fudman EJ, Schnitzer TJ. Dermatomyositis without creatine kinase elevation: a poor prognostic sign. *Am J Med* 1986; 80: 329–332.
33. Gran JT, Myklebast G. Adult idiopathic polymyositis without elevation of creatine kinase: case report and review of the literature. *Scand J Rheumatol* 1993; 22: 94.
34. Bolosiu HD, Man L, Rednie S. The effect of methylprednisolone pulse therapy in polymyositis/dermatomyositis. *Adv Exp Med Biol* 1999; 455: 349–357.
35. Dalakas M. Treatment of polymyositis and dermatomyositis. *Curr Opin Rheumatol* 1989; 1: 443–449.
36. Kaye SA, Isenbery DA. Treatment of polymyositis and dermatomyositis. *Br J Hosp Med* 1994; 52: 463–468.
37. Dawkins MA, Jorizzo JL, Walker FO, et al. Dermatomyositis: a dermatology-based case series. *J Am Acad Dermatol* 1998; 38: 397–404.
38. Joffe MM, Love LA, Leff RL, et al. Drug therapy of the idiopathic inflammatory myopathies: predictors of response to prednisone, azathioprine and methotrexate and a comparison of their efficacy. *Am J Med* 1993; 94: 379–387.
39. Sullivan DB, Cassidy JT, Petty RE. Prognosis in childhood dermatomyositis. *J Pediatr* 1977; 20: 327–331.
40. Katzenstein AL, Fiorelli RF. Nonspecific interstitial pneumonia/fibrosis. Histologic features and clinical significance. *Am J Surg Pathol* 1994; 18: 136–147.
41. Askari A, Vignos PJ, Moskowitz RW. Steroid myopathy in connective tissue disease. *Am J Med* 1976; 61: 485–492.
42. Dalakas MC. Current treatment of the inflammatory myopathies. *Curr Opin Rheumatol* 1994; 6: 595–601.
43. Janssens S, Decramer M. Corticosteroid-induced myopathy and the respiratory muscles. *Chest* 1989; 95: 1160–1162.
44. Oddis CV. Therapy of inflammatory myopathy. *Rheum Dis Clin North Am* 1994; 20: 899–918.

39.2 Immunosuppressive and Steroid-Sparing Drugs

There are circumstances in which corticosteroid therapy is inadequate for DM patients and further immunosuppressant medication is necessary. If a recurrence of muscle disease appears, then immunosuppressive drugs should be initiated as a corticosteroid-sparing agent. Specific instances where this may become necessary include: (i) intolerable side-effects of steroid use, (ii) lack of response to high doses of corticosteroids, (iii) the occurrence of repeated relapses after attempts to lower a high steroid dosage, (iv) ineffectiveness of corticosteroids and development of rapidly progressive disease, and (v) the presence of severe systemic involvement (for example, respiratory failure) [1, 2]. Steroid-sparing treatment is necessary in up to one quarter of patients. Early intervention with immunosuppressive agents, such as methotrexate, azathioprine, cyclosporine A, cyclophosphamide, mycophenolate mofetil, or chlorambucil have been effective in inducing or maintaining a remission of DM patients [3]. No convincing evidence exists that one immunosuppressive drug is superior to another [1]. About 50–75% of patients treated with an immunosuppressive agent respond with increase in muscle strength, decrease in serum enzyme levels, or a decrease in corticosteroid dose [4]. Unfortunately, there are no double-blind, placebo-controlled studies that show the effectiveness of any of these agents and compare different immunosuppressive regimens.

39.2.1 Methotrexate

Methotrexate is the first-line adjuvant therapy in DM recalcitrant to corticosteroids, and clinical improvement has been observed in the majority of patients [5–10]. Methotrexate is an irreversible inhibitor of dihydrofolate reductase. This potent immunosuppressant and cytotoxic medication also has anti-inflammatory properties [11]. The drug was first used in the treatment of corticosteroid-resistant DM by Malaviya et al. in 1968. In four adults with DM, three of whom were resistant to prednisone, a good response to intravenous methotrexate was reported [12]. Successful use of this drug in juvenile DM in four children with steroid-resistant disease has also been reported [13].

Regimen. With increasing understanding of the relative safety of use of methotrexate, this medication has been employed increasingly alone or in combination with prednisone in different regimens:

(i) Once-weekly doses of 25–50 mg given as an intramuscular injection; most authorities favor this regimen for 6–10 weeks [14]
(ii) 7.5–15 mg (2.5–5.0 mg in 3 doses/12h weekly) given orally [10, 15]
(iii) 10 mg given intravenously, increasing by 2.5 mg up to 0.5–0.8 mg/kg body weight [8, 11, 12, 16]

In children, doses of 1 mg/kg body weight or 20 mg/m^2 skin surface have been used successfully [6, 7].

The other regimen that may be of benefit in some patients with refractory myositis is i.v. methotrexate with leucovorin [17, 18].

While the methotrexate dosage is increased, prednisone should be tapered [19]. Low oral doses of methotrexate are the first choice for patients who fail corticosteroid therapy or develop intolerable adverse effects. A pretreatment and periodic liver biopsy is appropriate if the patients are obese, diabetic, or have abnormal liver function tests.

Clinical response. Previous retrospective studies have suggested that intravenous methotrexate is efficacious in improving strength and allows corticosteroid taper in patients with refractory PM/DM [12, 14]. In a study of 16 children with recalcitrant juvenile DM unresponsive to prednisone alone, oral methotrexate in dosage 20 mg/m^2 skin surface plus prednisone for more than 8 months tended to increase the muscle strength in all patients at a median of 35 weeks after initiation of therapy [7]. An excellent therapeutic effect was seen in 12 children, and in 11 of them it was possible to lower the prednisone dose to less than 5 mg/day [7]. The CK level normalized in all patients. Withdrawal of methotrexate in five patients, however, resulted in a recurrence of disease activity. Similar therapeutic responses to methotrexate in adult patients with DM have been observed by Bohan et al. [5]. In uncontrolled, open-label studies, methotrexate in doses of 15–35 mg/week has been reported to be useful in treating DM patients [9, 10, 20]. A combination of oral methotrexate with azathioprine may be of benefit to treat resistant PM/DM cases according a controlled trial [17]. Myositis patients with Jo-1 antibodies with incomplete clinical response to corticosteroids were reported to have an improvement of additional treatment with methotrexate [21].

Adverse reactions. In one third of the patients with DM treated with methotrexate, severe abdominal pain, elevated liver functional tests, decreased pulmonary diffusion capacity, or opportunistic infections have been observed [7]. The less frequently reported side-effects of methotrexate usage include pruritus, fever, nausea, stomatitis, gastrointestinal symptoms, leukopenia, pancytopenia, pneumonitis, hepatic fibrosis, and cirrhosis [6, 8]. Methotrexate can induce pulmonary fibrosis [5], and this complication may be confused with concomitant fibrosing alveolitis in patients with DM. Some authors recommend folic acid, 1–3 mg daily for minimizing adverse reactions without sacrificing efficacy [19]. A case with DM who developed multiple subcutaneous nodules after treatment with methotrexate (methotrexate nodulosis) has been reported [22]. Histopathology revealed septal panniculitis. The nodules regressed gradually after methotrexate cessation and treatment with hydroxychloroquine. A 12-year-old boy with DM who developed a "macrophage activation syndrome" after receiving the second dose of methotrexate was recently reported [23]. The clinical signs included high temperature, hepato- and splenomegaly, and neurological changes (coprolalia, insomnia, and agitation). He also had melena, severe pancytopenia, abnormalities in prothrombin time, and an increased ESR. All these symptoms improved after discontinuation of methotrexate and the initiation of therapy with corticosteroids and cyclosporine A for primary disease. Macrophage activation syndrome occurs most frequently in children with CTD such as systemic LE, juvenile idiopathic arthritis [24, 25] or as platelet-specific hemophagocytosis in juvenile DM [26].

Reversible lymphomas associated with Epstein–Barr virus and lymphoproliferative-disorders primarily involving the skin occurring during methotrexate therapy for DM have been reported [27–29].

39.2.2 Azathioprine

When methotrexate is ineffective, patients with DM are frequently treated with another immunosuppressive agent. Mc Falin and Griggs [30] initially described three patients with DM who improved after adding azathioprine to their prednisone regimen. Azathioprine is one of the few drugs to have been tested in a comparative fashion [31, 32].

Regimen. Based on empirical experience and its relative safety, azathioprine is used in divided doses of 2–3 mg/kg body weight for 4–6 months [33], with a maintenance dose of 0.5–1 mg/kg/once daily, and the concomitant prednisolone is reduced to 15 mg or less per day. The usual dosage of azathioprine is 100–200 mg/day [16]. A beneficial response should be expected after at least 3 months. Monthly reduction in dosage of azathioprine should be done in 25-mg intervals, with the expectation of maintaining the patient on a regimen of 50 mg/day.

Clinical response. Azathioprine (1–2 mg/kg/day) in combination with prednisone has been compared with prednisone alone in PM patients, showing no significant differences in strength after a 3-month period [31]. At 3-year follow-up, the group receiving prednisone and azathioprine had less functional disability and required less corticosteroids than the group receiving prednisone alone [32]. One third of 70 patients with DM/PM who received azathioprine reported increased muscle strength [5]. Some authors preferred to use azathioprine as a first corticosteroid-sparing drug in PM/DM, and if the drug was ineffective, to change it with methotrexate [1].

Adverse reactions. Azathioprine is rapidly metabolized in vivo by three competitive enzyme systems: hypoxanthine–guanine phosphoribosyl transferase (HGPT), thiopurine methyltransferase (TPMT), and xanthine oxidase. Screening patients for homozygous or heterozygous thiopurine methyltransferase deficiency, which occur in 0.3% and 11% of the Caucasian population respectively, can reduce the chance of toxicity associated with the use of the drug [34, 35]. Hematologic monitoring is essential to detect leukopenia and anemia [36]. Side-effects of azathioprine include nausea, vomiting, oral ulcerations, leukopenia from bone marrow suppression, hepatotoxicity, and increased risk of lymphoma [19]. Monitoring for neutropenia is essential in the first 3–4 months. Patients with DM or PM with a complex karyotype, including monosomy 7 and trilineage dysplastic features, treated with azatioprine may develop acute myeloid leukemia [37, 38].

39.2.3 Cyclosporine A

In the early 1980s, T-cell-specific immunosuppressant cyclosporine A, derivative from the fungus *Tolypocladium inflatum*, was first used for refractory DM unresponsive to conventional therapy [39]. A 15-year-old girl with acute fulminant DM who failed to respond to methylprednisolone and azathioprine treatment improved within days of starting a 3.0 mg/kg/day cyclosporine A regimen [39]. Reports of similar successes [40–45] and failures [46, 47] using the drug have been reported subsequently. Two larger studies of patients with "classic" DM in adults [48] and juvenile DM [49] have shown sufficient effect and no serious side-effects. Moreover, cyclosporine A has been found effective in corticosteroid-resistant interstitial pneumonitis [50–52]. Cyclosporine A impairs T-cell proliferation by blocking transcription of cytokine-encoding genes by inhibiting calcium-dependent T-cell activation [53].

Regimen. Many studies and case reports have indicated the efficacy of cyclosporine A in refractory DM at doses between 3 and 10 mg/kg/day, with outcome parameters of clinical improvement, normalization of serum muscle enzymes, and steroid sparing [48, 52, 54,

55–57]. Some studies suggest initial doses about 5 mg/kg, and maintaining a serum concentration of 200–300 ng/mL [58].

Clinical response. In one of the early studies, 14 children with long-standing DM treated with cyclosporine A were able to drastically reduce or stop their prednisone, with a concomitant increase in muscle strength [49]. In an open study of "classic" DM in adults, cyclosporine A but not corticosteroids was reported to be a first-line drug [58]. Cyclosporine A has also been used as a single agent for initial treatment of juvenile DM, with excellent results [43]. Two retrospective studies of respectively ten [48] and 12 [59] DM patients have suggested the efficacy of cyclosporine A as a valid second-line treatment in refractory DM. Two other reports described the efficacy of cyclosporine A in treating ILD in myositis [51, 52]. Only one randomized controlled trial [57] has evaluated the separate use of cyclosporine A and methotrexate in the treatment of PM and DM. The comparison between cyclosporine A and methotrexate did not show any significant difference between the two drugs in efficacy and toxicity over a 6-month period, and confirmed the reliability of both drugs in the treatment of myositis. In one clinical study, 12 patients with "classic" DM in adults and eight PM patients were treated with prednisone and cyclosporine A, alone or associated with IVIG and plasmapheresis [60]. Despite a transient response to prednisone and cyclosporine A in 16/20 cases (80%), this combination alone did not induce full remission in 13/20 cases, which led to the IVIG trial with or without plasmapheresis. Patients receiving prednisone and cyclosporine A plus IVIG had a significantly higher probability of maintaining complete remission at the end of the 4-year follow-up period than those treated with prednisone and cyclosporine A alone ($p < 0.001$). The presence of arthritis significantly correlated with a poorer response to treatment ($p < 0.05$). The combination of cyclosporine A and IVIG (with or without plasmapheresis) seems to assure a longer disease-free period and is more beneficial than cyclosporine A alone, confirming the preliminary report of Saadeh et al. [55]. The trend towards normalization of muscle strength and CK values was more evident from the first months of treatment in the group treated with IVIG, independently of the type of myositis [60].

Adverse reactions. Side-effects of cyclosporine A are generally described in 8–15% of patients, and include fatigue, paresthesias, hyperesthesias, tremor, hypertrichosis, gingival hyperplasia, arterial hypertension, hepatotoxicity, nephrotoxicity, and increased risk of malignancy (lymphoma, squamous cell carcinoma) [19, 59]. Recently, a case of a DM patient who developed interstitial pneumonitis induced by cytomegalovirus (CMV) while receiving immunosuppressive treatment was reported [61]. The manifestations of CMV pneumonitis appeared 30 days after the onset of oral ulcerations, and 40 days after cyclosporine treatment onset.

39.2.4 Cyclophosphamide

Cyclophosphamide has not been as beneficial as other immunosuppressive and steroid-sparing agents in treatment of DM [19]. Its place in the treatment of DM is in cases refractory to the above medications, since alone it does not adequately treat myositis [62, 63], and due to its hematologic and oncogenic potential the use of this drug is limited. Combined with corticosteroids, oral cyclophosphamide can be effective for both PM/DM and ILD [64]. Cyclophosphamide is a "prodrug"; that is converted in the liver to active forms that have chemotherapeutic activity.

Regimen. Cyclophosphamide is used orally at 1–3 mg/kg/day or intermittent intravenous pulse at 2–4 mg/kg/day in conjunction with prednisone [65]. As an alternative, pulse cyclophosphamide, 750 mg/m^2, may also be employed [63].

Clinical response. Some studies have shown benefit of cyclophosphamide in patients with severe and refractory PM [65, 66]. Only two of six adults with DM/PM showed clinical improvement after cyclophosphamide treatment [5]; however, in four patients with juvenile DM, three of whom failed to respond to methotrexate therapy, all four showed improvment [67]. Pulse cyclophosphamide in doses of 500 mg intravenously every few weeks was found helpful in severe PM [65], whereas monthly infusions at 0.75–1.375 g/m^2 were unsuccessful [63]. Cyclophosphamide has been added to prednisone therapy, with much improvement in patients with PM/DM and ILD [64], when is used at an earlier lung disease stage [68]. One patient with PM and Sjögren's syndrome benefited solely from cyclophosphamide [69]. Cyclophosphamide has been used in combination with prednisone and methotrexate in severe PM/DM not responding to the usual therapeutic regiments [70, 71]; however, oral or intravenous cyclophosphamide seems to be less effective than either methotrexate or azathioprine [63].

Adverse reactions. The potential adverse reactions to cyclophosphamide include anorexia, nausea, vomiting, stomatitis, alopecia, leukopenia (10–14 days after the beginning of treatment), hemorrhagic cystitis (up to 40% of patients), increased risk of malignancy (lymphoma, leukemia, bladder carcinoma, and squamous cell carcinoma) [19], and increased risk of infections [62, 67].

39.2.5 Micophenolate Mofetil

Micophenolate mofetil (MM), a medicine acting as an inhibitor of lymphocyte proliferation, has also been used for treatment of DM [72, 73] and inclusion body myositis [74].

Regimen. Micophenolat mofetil should be used at a total dose of 35–45 mg/kg/day, given in divided doses twice daily. The usual dosage of MM is 2 g/day. Two to 3 months of therapy are required to judge impact on antibody production in other autoimmune diseases.

Clinical response. Recently, in one open-label study, four patients with classic DM who failed to respond to conventional therapy with corticosteroids, hydroxylchloroquine and/or methotrexate were treated effectively with micophenolate mofetil [72]. A mean duration of treatment was 13 months and micophenolate mofetil was highly effective in controlling cutaneous disease activity. MM has also been suggested to have steroid-sparing value for cutaneous manifestations of DM. In another open-label study, micophenolate mofetil was used alone or with IVIG in four patients with DM. Three of them improved, and one patient with paraneoplastic DM did not respond [73].

39

Adverse reactions. The main side-effects are gastrointestinal problems (nausea, diarrhea), lymphopenia, and bone marrow suppression.

39.2.6 Chlorambucil

Chlorambucil, another of the challenging agents, has been advocated for resistant disease with modest success [75, 76].

Regimen. Chlorambucil is used in DM patients at 4 mg/kg/day orally, in combination with prednisone or alone.

Clinical response. Five patients with recalcitrant DM were treated with oral chlorambucil, 4 mg/day, after discontinuation of other immunosuppressive drugs — azathioprine or methotrexate [76]. Three patients were treated with chlorambucil and prednisone and two with chlorambucil alone. In all patients, beneficial effects were noted within 4–6 weeks. The treatment with chlorambucil was discontinued after 13–30 months in four patients, and their disease remained in remission. A combination of prednisone, methotrexate, and chlorambucil has also been used with success in cases of severe PM/DM which were not responding to the usual medications [70, 71].

Adverse reactions. Infectious complications and oncogenic potential limit the use of this drug. Leukopenia was reported in two of five patients treated with chlorambucil [76].

39.2.7 Mercaptopurine

Haas [77] described five adults with PM who received 50–150 mg/day of 6-mercaptopurine. Four of five patients improved. Bone-marrow toxicity can ensue [78].

39.2.8 Fludarabine

In one open-label study, 16 patients with recalcitrant IIMs (9 with DM and 7 with PM) were treated with fludarabine 20 mg/m^2 for 3 days/month for 6 months. At the end of treatment, four patients were improved, seven cases were unchanged, and five patients failed to respond [79].

39.2.9 Aminoquinolone Antimalarials

Studies differ with regard to the efficacy of aminoquinolone antimalarials as a steroid-sparing agent in the treatment of the myositis and weakness [19]. Several authors have noted a beneficial response of hydroxychloroquine in the cutaneous eruption of DM [80–83] as well as accompanying myositis [82]. Hydroxychloroquine is deposited in skin as well as in muscles [82]. Although no controlled studies exist, aminoquinolone antimalarials seem to have little effect on adult DM, while in juvenile DM a series of nine patients responded inadequately to prednisone, but improved in both muscle strength and cutaneous eruptions after addition of hydroxychloroquine [82]. Aminoquinolone antimalarials can stabilize lysosome membranes and inhibit activation of complement [80] and impair chemotaxis of formed elements [81].

Regimen. Oral hydroxychloroquine (<6.5 mg/kg/day, or 200 mg twice a day for adults and 2–5 mg/kg/day in children) can aid in control of skin disease in some patients [80, 82]. The addition of quinacrine 100–200 mg/day can be of benefit in some patients [84], while others respond to a switch from hydroxychloroquine to chloroquine (<3.5 mg/kg/day or 250 mg/day) [85].

Clinical response. Hydroxychloroquine is used as an adjunctive treatment, and has been consistently reported to reduce the erythema of DM recalcitrant to steroids and other treatment modalities [80, 82, 83, 86]. Cutaneous manifestations, especially the periorbital and facial heliotope rash and periungual telangiectases, can respond to hyroxychloroquine alone or in combination with systemic corticosteroid or immunosuppressive therapy [80]. Improvement of arthralgias and reduction in the dose of prednisone has also been reported [80]. Partial improvement is more common than complete control [85]. Some patients who do not respond to hydroxychloroquine may have benefit from chloroquine either alone or in combination with quinacrine. Efficacy of antimalarials in combination has been reported in one retrospective series of 17 cases with predominantly cutaneous symptoms of DM [87]. Seven of 17 patients experienced at least near clearance of cutaneous symptoms. Three of them responded well to antimalarial monotherapy, while four of these patients required combination therapy (hydroxychloroquine sulfate–quinacrine hydrochloride or chloroquine phosphate–quinacrine). The median time required to reach the response was 3 months (range from 2 to 14 months) [87]. Six patients did not respond significantly to any type of therapy, including nonantimalarials. The fact that the improvement by hydroxychloroquine is generally in cutaneous rather than muscle symptoms [80, 88, 89] suggests the photoprotective function of this drug, rather than that the immunomodulatory role is important [83].

Adverse reactions. The risk of retinopathy associated with antimalarial therapy requires periodic ophthalmic monitoring at every 6 months. Both hydroxychloquine and chloroquine can cause a reversible myopathy that is almost indistinguishable from IIM on EMG, but can be differentiated by muscle biopsy [90, 91]. Reversible agranulocytosis or neutropenia due to chloroquine have been reported, including in DM patients [92]. Hydroxychloroquine therapy aggravated rash has been reported in a patient with juvenile DM [93]. In one retrospective study, 31% of 39 DM patients developed adverse cutaneous reaction to hydroxychloroquine, and two patients to chloroquine [94].

References

1. Dalakas MC. Polymyositis, dermatomyositis and inclusion body myositis. *N Engl J Med* 1991; 325: 1487–1498.

39

2. Michito H, Sonoko N. Interstitial lung disease in polymyositis and dermatomyositis. *Curr Opin Rheumatol* 2000; 12: 501–508.
3. Villalba L, Adams EM. Update on therapy for refractory dermatomyositis and polymyositis. *Curr Opin Rheumatol* 1996; 8: 544–551.
4. Callen JP. Dermatomyositis. *Lancet* 2000; 355: 53–57.
5. Bohan A, Peter JB, Bowman RL, et al. A computer-assisted analysis of 153 patients with polymyositis and dermatomyositis. *Medicine* 1977; 56: 255–286.
6. Fischer TJ, Rachelefsky GS, Klein RB, et al. Childhood dermatomyositis and polymyositis. *Am J Dis Child* 1979; 133: 386–389.
7. Miller LS, Sisson BA, Tucker LB, et al. Methotrexate treatment of recalcitrant childhood dermatomyositis. *Arthritis Rheum* 1992; 35: 1143–1149.
8. Kaye SA, Isenbery DA. Treatment of polymyositis and dermatomyositis. *Br J Hosp Med* 1994; 52: 463–468.
9. Zieglschmid-Adams ME, Pandya AG, Cohen SB, et al. Treatment of dermatomyositis with methotrexate: presentation of ten cases and the review of the literature. *J Am Acad Dermatol* 1995; 32: 754–757.
10. Kasteler JS, Callen JP. Low-dose methotrexate administered weekly is an effective corticosteroid-sparing agent for the treatment of the cutaneous manifestations of dermatomyositis. *J Am Acad Dermatol* 1997; 36: 67–71.
11. Sokoloff MC, Goldberg LS, Pearson CM. Treatment of corticosteroid-resistant polymyositis with methotrexate. *Lancet* 1971; 1: 14–16.
12. Malaviya AN, Many A, Schwartz RS. Treatment of dermatomyositis with methotrexate. *Lancet* 1968; 2: 485–488.
13. Jacobs JC. Methotrexate and azathioprine treatment of childhood dermatomyositis. *Pediatrics* 1977; 59: 212–218.
14. Metzger Al, Bohan A, Goldberg LS, et al. Polymyositis and dermatomyositis: combined methotrexate and corticosteroid therapy. *Ann Intern Med* 1974; 81: 182–189.
15. Scott DW, Newman ED. Low dose oral methotrexate therapy in polymyositis/dermatomyositis. *Arthritis Rheum* 1993; 36: R9.
16. Oddis CV, Medsger TA. Current management of polymyositis and dermatomyositis. *Drugs* 1989; 37: 382–390.
17. Villalba L, Hicks JE, Adams EM, et al. Treatment of refractory myositis: a randomized crossover study of two new cytotoxic regimens. *Arthritis Rheum* 1998; 41(3): 392–399.
18. Zieglschmid-Adams ME, Pandya A, Cohen SB, et al. The value of methotrexate in dermatomyositis. *J Am Acad Dermatol* 1998; 38(1): 130–132.
19. Kovacs SO, Kovacs SC. Dermatomyositis. *J Am Acad Dermatol* 1998; 39: 899–920.
20. Singsen BH, Goldbach-Mansky R. Methotrexate in the treatment of juvenile rheumatoid arthritis and other pediatric rheumatoid and nonrheumatoid disorders. *Rheum Dis Clin North Am* 1997; 23: 754–757.
21. Joffe MM, Love LA, Leff RL, et al. Drug therapy of the idiopathic inflammatory myopathies: predictors of response to prednisone, azathioprine and methotrexate and a comparison of their efficacy. *Am J Med* 1993; 94: 379–387.
22. Jang K-A, Choi JH, Moon KC, et al. Methotrexate nodulosis. *J Dermatol* 1999; 26: 460–464.
23. Sterba G, Rodriguez C, Sifontes S, et al. Macrophage activation syndrome due to methotrexate in a 12-year-old boy with dermatomyositis. *J Rheumatol.* 2004; 31: 1014–1015.
24. Ravelli A, Caria MC, Buratti S, et al. Methotrexate as a possible trigger of macrophage activation syndrome in systemic juvenile idiopathic arthritis [case report]. *J Rheumatol* 2001; 28: 865–867.
25. Ravelli A. Macrophage activation syndrome. *Curr Opin Rheumatol* 2002; 14: 548–552.

26. Kobayashi I, Yamada M, Kawamura N, et al. Platelet-specific hemophagocytosis in a patient with juvenile dermatomyositis. *Acta Paediatr* 2000; 89: 617–619.
27. Kamel OW, van de Rijn M, Weiss LM, et al. Reversible lymphomas associated with Epstein–Barr virus occurring during methotrexate therapy for rheumatoid arthritis and dermatomyositis. *N Engl J Med* 1993; 328: 1317–1321.
28. Bittar B, Rose CD. Early development of Hodgkin's lymphoma in association with the use of methotrexate for the treatment of dermatomyositis. *Ann Rheum Dis* 1995; 54: 607–608.
29. Chai C, White WL, Shea CR, Prieto VG. Epstein–Barr virus-associated lymphoproliferative disorders primarily involving the skin. *J Cutan Pathol* 1999; 26: 242–247.
30. McFarlin DE, Griggs RC. Treatment of inflammatory myopathies with azathioprine. *Trans Am Neurol Assoc* 1968; 93: 244–246.
31. Bunch TW, Worthington JW, Combs JJ, et al. Azathioprine with prednisone for polymyositis: a controlled clinical trial. *Ann Intern Med* 1980; 92: 365–369.
32. Bunch TW. Prednisone and azathioprine for polymyositis. *Arthritis Rheum* 1981; 24: 45–48.
33. Clements PJ, Davis J. Cytotoxic drugs: their clinical application to the rheumatic diseases. *Semin Arthritis Rheum* 1986; 15: 231–254.
34. Anstey A, Lennard L, Mayou SC, et al. Pancytopenia related to azathioprine — an enzyme deficiency caused by a common genetic polymorphism: a review. *J Roy Soc Med* 1992; 85: 752–756.
35. Schultz E, Gummert J, Armstrong V, et al. Azathioprine pharmacogenetics: the relationship between 6-thioguanine nucleotides and thiopurine methyltransferase in patients after heart and kidney transplantation. *Eur J Clin Chem Clin Biochem* 1996; 34: 199–205.
36. Bunch TW. Polymyositis: clinical trials. *Clin Rheum Dis* 1983; 9: 641–653.
37. Krishnan K, Adams P, Silveira S, et al. Therapy-related acute myeloid leukaemia following immunosuppression with azathioprine for polymyositis. *Clin Lab Haematol* 1994; 16: 285–289.
38. Arnold JA, Ranson SA, Abdalla SH. Azathioprine-associated acute myeloid leukaemia with trilineage dysplasia and complex karyotype: a case report and review of the literature. *Clin Lab Haem* 1999; 21: 289–292.
39. Zabel P, Leimenstoll G, Gross WL. Cyclosporine for acute dermatomyositis. *Lancet* 1984; 1: 343.
40. Ejstrup L. Severe dermatomyositis treated with cyclosporine A. *Ann Rheum Dis* 1986; 45: 612–613.
41. Girardin E, Dayer JM, Paunier L. Cyclosporine for juvenile dermatomyositis. *J Pediatr* 1988; 112: 165–166.
42. Casato M, Bonomo L, Caccavo D, et al. Clinical effects of cyclosporine in dermatomyositis. *Clin Exp Dermatol* 1990; 15: 121–123.
43. Dantzing P. Juvenile dermatomyositis treated with cyclosporine. *J Am Acad Dermatol* 1990; 22: 310–311.
44. Kavanagh GM, Ross JS, Black MM. Dermatomyositis treated with cyclosporine. *J R Soc Med* 1991; 84: 306.
45. Dalakas MC. Current treatment of the inflammatory myopathies. *Curr Opin Rheumatol* 1994; 6: 595–601.
46. Jones EW, Snaith ML, Isenberg DA. Cyclosporine treatment for intractable polymyositis. *Arthritis Rheum* 1987; 30: 959–960.
47. Levi S, Hodgson HJ. Cyclosporine for dermatomyositis? *Ann Rheum Dis* 1989; 48: 85–86.
48. Danko K, Szegedi G. Cyclosporin A treatment of dermatomyositis. *Arthritis Rheum* 1991; 34: 933–934.
49. Heckmatt J, Hasson N, Saunders C, et al. Cyclosporin in juvenile dermatomyositis. *Lancet* 1989; 1(8646): 1063–1066.
50. Gruhn WB, Diaz-Buxo JA. Cyclosporine treatment of steroid-resistant interstitial pneumonitis associated with dermatomyositis/polymyositis. *J Rheumatol* 1987; 14: 1045–1047.

39

51. Maeda K, Kimura R, Komuta K, et al. Cyclosporine treatment for polymyositis/dermatomyositis: is it possible to rescue the deteriorating cases with interstitial pneumonitis? *Scand J Rheumatol* 1997; 26: 24–29.
52. Nawata Y, Kurasawa K, Takabayashi K, et al. Corticosteroid resistant interstitial pneumonitis in dermatomyositis/polymyositis. Prediction and treatment with cyclosporine. *J Rheumatol* 1999; 26: 1527–1533.
53. Pistoia V, Buoncompagni A, Scribanis R, et al. Cyclosporine A in the treatment of juvenile arthritis and childhood polymyositis/dermatomyositis: results of a preliminary study. *Clin Exp Rheumatol* 1993; 11: 203–206.
54. van der Meer S, Imhof JW, Borleffs JC. Severe dermatomyositis treated with cyclosporin A. *Ann Rheum Dis* 1986; 45: 612–613.
55. Saadeh C, Bridges W, Burwick F. Dermatomyositis: remission induced with combined oral cyclosporine and high-dose intravenous immune globulin. *South Med J* 1995; 88: 866–870.
56. Qushmaq KA, Chalmers A, Esdaile JM. Cyclosporin A in the treatment of refractory adult polymyositis/dermatomyositis: population based experience in 6 patients and literature review. *J Rheumatol* 2000; 27: 2855–2859.
57. Vencovsky J, Jarosova K, Machacek S, et al. Cyclosporine A versus methotrexate in the treatment of polymyositis and dermatomyositis. *Scand J Rheumatol* 2000; 29: 95–102.
58. Grau JM, Herrero C, Casademont J, et al. Cyclosporine A as first choice therapy for dermatomyositis. *J Rheumatol* 1994; 21: 381–382.
59. Sanchez Román J, Castello Palma MJ, Ocaña Medina C, et al. Efficacia de la ciclosporina en el tratamiento de las miositis. *Rev Clin Esp* 1995; 195: 449–454.
60. Danieli MG, Malcangi G, Palmieri C, et al. Cyclosporin A and intravenous immunoglobulin treatment in polymyositis/dermatomyositis. *Ann Rheum Dis* 2002; 61: 37–41.
61. Kaşifoğlu T, Korkmaz C, Özkan R. Cytomegalovirus-induced interstitial pneumonitis in a patient with dermatomyositis. *Clin Rheumatol* 2006; 25(5): 731–733.
62. Fries JF, Sharp GC, McDevitt HO, et al. Cyclophosphamide therapy in systemic lupus erythematosus and polymyositis. *Arthritis Rheum* 1973; 16: 154–162.
63. Cronin ME, Miller FW, Hicks JE, et al. The failure of intravenous cyclophosphamide therapy in refractory idiopathic inflammatory myopathies. *J Rheumatol* 1989; 16: 1225–1228.
64. al-Janadi M, Smith CD, Karsh J. Cyclophosphamide treatment of interstitial pulmonary fibrosis in polymyositis/dermatomyositis. *J Rheumatol* 1989; 16(12): 1592–1596.
65. Bombardieri S, Hughes GR, Neri R, et al. Cyclophosphamide in severe polymyositis. *Lancet* 1989; 1: 1138–1139.
66. Kono DH, Klashman DJ, Gilbert RC. Successful IV pulse cyclophosphamide in refractory PM in 3 patients with SLE. *J Rheumatol* 1990; 17: 982–983.
67. Niakan E, Pitner SE, Whitaker JN, et al. Immunosuppressive agents in corticosteroid-refractory childhood dermatomyositis. *Neurology* 1980; 30: 286–291.
68. Marie I, Hatron PY, Hachulla E, et al. Pulmonary involvement in polymyositis and dermatomyositis. *J Rheumatol* 1998; 25: 1336–1343.
69. Leroy JP, Drosos AA, Yiannopoulos D, et al. Intravenous pulse cyclophosphamide therapy in myositis and Sjögren's syndrome. *Arthritis Rheum* 1990; 33: 1579–1581.
70. Wallace DJ, Letzger AL, White KK. Combination immunosuppressive treatment of steroid-resistant dermatomyositis/polymyositis. *Arthritis Rheum* 1985; 28: 590–592.
71. Tiliakos NA. Low-dose cytotoxic combination treatment in intractable dermatomyositis [abstract]. *Arthritis Rheum* 1987; 30: S14.
72. Gelber AC, Nousari HC, Wigley FM. Mycophenolate mofetil in the treatment of severe skin manifestations of dermatomyositis: a series of 4 cases. *J Rheumatol* 2000; 27: 1542–1545.

73. Tausche AK, Meurer M. Mycophenolate mofetil for dermatomyositis. *Dermatology* 2001; 202(4): 341–343.
74. Mowzoon N, Sussman A, Bradley WG. Mycophenolate (CellCept) treatment of myasthenia gravis, chronic inflammatory polyneuropathy and inclusion body myositis. *J Neurol Sci* 2001; 185: 119–122.
75. Tymms KE, Webb J. Dermatomyositis and other connective tissue diseases: a review of 105 cases. *J Rheumatol* 1985; 12: 1140–1148.
76. Sinoway PA, Callen JP. Chloambucil. An effective corticosteroid-sparing agent for patients with recalcitrant dermatomyositis. *Arthritis Rheum* 1993; 36: 319–324.
77. Haas DC. Treatment of polymyositis with immunosuppressive drugs. *Neurology* 1973; 23: 55–62.
78. Rapini RP. Cytotoxic drugs in the treatment of skin diseases. *Int J Dermatol* 1991; 30: 313–322.
79. Adams EM, Pucino F, Yarboro C, et al. A pilot study: use of fludarabine for refractory dermatomyositis and polymyositis, and examination of endpoint measures. *J Rheumatol* 1999; 26: 352–360.
80. Woo TY, Callen JP, Voorhees JJ, et al. Cutaneous lesions of dermatomyositis are improved by hydroxychloroquine. *J Am Acad Dermatol* 1984; 10: 592–600.
81. James WD, Dawson N, Rodman OG. Treatment of dermatomyositis with hydoxychloroquine. *J Rheumatol* 1985; 12: 1214–1216.
82. Olson NY, Lindsley CB. Adjunctive use of hydroxychloroquine in childhood dermatomyositis. *J Rheumatol* 1989; 16: 1545–1547.
83. Cox NH. Amyopathic dermatomyositis, photosensitivity and hydroxychloroquine. *Br J Dermatol* 1995; 132: 1016–1017.
84. Ghate J, Katsambas A, Augerinou G, et al. Review article: a therapeutic update on dermatomyositis/polymyositis. *Int J Dermatol* 2000; 39(2): 81–87.
85. Drake L, Dinehart SM, Farmer ER, et al. Guidelines of care for dermatomyositis. *J Am Acad Dermatol* 1996; 34: 824–829.
86. Bridges BF. The rashes of dermatomyositis in a black patient. *Am J Med* 1991; 91: 661–662.
87. Ang GC, Werth VP. Combination antimalarials in the treatment of cutaneous dermatomyositis: a retrospective study. *Arch Dermatol* 2005; 141: 855–859.
88. Gertner E, Urowitz MB. Discordance of skin and muscle involvement in dermatomyositis. *Int J Dermatol* 1985; 24: 518–519.
89. Euwer RL, Sontheimer RD. Amyopathic dermatomyositis (dermatomyositis sine myositis). *J Am Acad Dermatol* 1991; 24: 959–966.
90. Chapman RS, Ewen WB. Chloroquine-induced myopathy. *Br J Dermatol* 1969; 81: 217–219.
91. Robinson LA. AAEM case report #22: polymyositis. *Muscle Nerve* 1991; 14: 310–315.
92. Don PC, Kahn TA, Bickers DR. Chloroquine-induced neutropenia in a patient with dermatomyositis. *J Am Acad Dermatol* 1987; 16: 629–630.
93. Bloom BJ, Tucker LB, Klein-Gitelman M, et al. Worsening of the rash of juvenile dermatomyositis with hydroxychloroquine therapy. *J Rheumatol* 1994; 21: 2171–2172.
94. Pelle MT, Callen JP. Adverse cutaneous reactions to hydroxychloroquine are more common in patients with dermatomyositis than in patients with cutaneous lupus erythematosus. *Arch Dermatol* 2002; 138(9): 1231–1233.

39

39.3 Immunobiologic (Immunomodulating) Therapy

39.3.1 Intravenous Immunoglobulins

High-dose intravenous immunoglobulins (IVIG) were initially used for refractory PM/DM unresponsive to conventional therapy in the end of the 1980s [1, 2]. A 15-year-old girl with PM who failed to respond from treatment with prednisolone, pulse methylprednisolone, methotrexate, and cyclophosphamide was reported [1]. She received 1 g/kg/day of IVIG for 2 consecutive days/month and experienced an increase in muscular strength, a decrease in serum CK levels and improved cardiopulmonary function. A similar case in a 6-month-old child was reported 2 years later [2]. Several clinical observations and one placebo-controlled study [3] indicate that IVIG are an effective immunomodulating therapy for patients with DM. Cherin et al. [4] were the first to propose IVIG as first-line and monotherapy for IIMs. A good and excellent clinical response from this treatment was reported to range from 30% to 71% of patients [4–6]. However, the exact pathophysiologic mechanisms of IVIG action remain unclear. The possible mechanisms of action of high-dose IVIG are multiple and not fully characterized. The effector mechanisms may differ between diseases, and even between subgroups of patients within a similar disease group [7].

Proposed hypotheses for mechanisms of action of IVIG include [7]: (i) Fc receptor blockade on phagocytic cells and cytotoxic cells mediating antibody-dependent cytotoxicity [8], (ii) anti-idiotypic antibodies blocking endogenous immunoglobulins directed against muscle fibers, (iii) inactivation of lymphocyte activation and their effector functions including cytokine production [9], (iv) blocking of complement activation or effector functions [8], (v) increased catabolism of IgG mediated by FcRn blockade, resulting in the passive loss of pathogenic autoantibodies [10], and (vi) attenuation of immune aggregate-mediated complement activation by enhancing physiologic cleavage of C3b in C3bn-IgG complexes [11] (Table 39.2).

Data from in vivo experiments suggest that intravenous immunoglobulin helps to restore the balance between T helper cells type 1 (Th1) and Th2 cells in autoimmune diseases in which the population of selfreactive Th1 or Th2 clones is expanding [12]. A reduction of TGFβ levels in the muscles [9] and of soluble IL-2 receptor levels in the serum have been demonstrated after IVIG treatment [13].

Regimen. The actual dosage of IVIG is 2 g/kg body weight (120 ml/h) on 2 consecutive days (1 g/kg/day for 2 days), or 0.4 g/kg/day for 5 days at 1-month intervals [3, 4]. The first regiment (used in controlled trial) is preferred. There are no standard treatment protocols for the total number of treatment cycles [13]. In children, doses of 1–2 g/kg/day body weight twice monthly for 9 months have also proved to be efficaceous [5, 14]. DM patients with minimal muscular involvement and pronounced cutaneous lesions responded well to low-dose (0.1 g/kg/day given on 5 consecutive days weekly in two courses) IVIG therapy [15, 16].

Clinical response. In the first double-blind, placebo-controlled, randomized crossover trial, Dalakas et al. [3] found significant but transient results in patients with DM treated with IVIG. The patients treated with IVIG showed a significant improvement in muscle strength scores ($p < 0.018$), and neuromuscular symptoms ($p < 0.035$) in contrast to

Table 39.2 Immunoregulatory effects of immunoglobulin (Adapted from [12])

Effect over	Mechanism
Fc receptors	1. Blockade of Fc receptors on macrophages and effector cells
	2. Induction of antibody-dependent cellular cytotoxicity
	3. Induction of inhibitory Fcg receptor IIB
Inflammation	1. Attenuation of complement-mediated damage
	2. Decrease in immune-complex-mediated inflammation
	3. Induction of anti-inflammatory cytokines
	4. Inhibition of activation of endothelial cells
	5. Neutralization of microbial toxins
	6. Reduction in corticosteroid requirements
B cells and antibodies	1. Control of emergent bone marrow B-cell repertoires
	2. Negative signaling through Fcg receptors
	3. Selective down-regulation and up-regulation of antibody production
	4. Neutralization of circulating autoantibodies by anti-idiotypes
T cells	1. Regulation of the production of helper-T-cell cytokines
	2. Neutralization of T-cell superantigens
Cell growth	1. Inhibition of lymphocyte proliferation
	2. Regulation of apoptosis

patients assigned to placebo. Serum CK levels, elevated up to tenfold before IVIG treatment, fell by 50% after the first infusion and decreased further or normalized by the second infusion. Although the improvement in strength is usually short-lived, not lasting more than 4–8 weeks, a number of patients experienced long-lasting remissions. Most of them, however, require IVIG every 4–8 weeks to maintain the beneficial results [3]. The efficacy of IVIG was demonstrated in 20 patients by Cherin et al. [4] and in groups of patients studied by Saadeh et al. [17], and Mastaglia et al. [18]. In a prospective study, this successful trend was confirmed by long-term follow-up analysis in 70% of 35 patients with chronic refractory PM [19]. In the same group, however, 11 patients with IIMs (PM or DM) did not find a clear benefit for IVIG as first-line treatment [4]. The benefit of IVIG has also been documented in more than 30 patients treated in several institutions [20]. In several patients the prednisone dose can be lowered; however, later others may require the addition of another immunosuppressant.

In patients who showed major improvement, repeat open muscle biopsies showed a marked improvement in muscle histology such as an increase in the muscle fiber diameter, increased number and decreased size on capillaries, and a decrease or normalisation of the mean ratio of muscle fiber to capillaries [3]. The main immunological markers were down-regulation of MHCI and ICAM-I expression on the surface of muscle fibers and endomysial blood vessels, and reduction of the TGF-β expression on the connective tissue, along with reduction of TGF-β mRNA [3]. IVIG intercepted the formation and intramuscular deposition of the MAC, the lytic component of the complement pathway [8]. C3bNEO, an neoantigen, which is immune-complex-specific, and MAC were no longer detected in the endomysial capillaries [8, 21]. It was concluded that IVIG inhibits the incorporation of C3 into the C5 convertase assembly, thereby preventing the formation of C3bNEO and intercepting the formation and deposition of MAC on the endomysial capillaries [21]. In one series, a steroid, cyclosporine A and IVIG regimen in DM/PM patients gave the best and statistically significant results as compared with a steroid and cyclosporine A based treatment [22]. Nonresponders to IVIG treatment are patients with severe skin and muscle disease, concomitant with MSAs or malignancy [13].

Some case reports have confirmed life-threatening gastrointestinal complications of DM such as hemorrhage, ulcerations, duodenal perforation, or paralytic ileus, all of which have been reported to be refractory to corticosteroids but were responsive to IVIG therapy [23–26].

Adverse reactions. The realistic use of IVIG in DM patients is limited by the high cost of the medication and has been recommended only for "off label" use in cases with recalcitrant DM cases who have failed on standard immunosuppressive regimens [27, 28]. Side-effects such as fever, headache, nausea, vomiting, and systolic hypertension during infusion were observed [4, 13, 28] in 10% of cases [29]. Serious reactions are rare: anaphylaxis (mainly in IgA-deficient patients who are hypersensitive against IgA antibodies), lymphocytic meningitis, acute renal insufficiency from tubular precipitation of saccharose, and potential risk from transmission of infectious agents, as human immunoglobulins are a part of many donors' plasma [29].

39.3.2 Anticytokines

Based on experimental evidence indicating an important role for TNF-α in the pathogenesis of DM, anticytokines have been used in DM patients, in both the muscular and cutaneous manifestations of the disease [30]. The usefulness of anti-TNF therapy in certain individuals with juvenile DM has also been reported [31]. Several drugs have been used experimentally: infliximab, etanercept, tacrolimus, thalidomide, etc. No randomized clinical trials with these agents have been conducted yet, and the impetus for their use arises from either small case series or the accumulated clinical experience gathered in large clinics [32].

39.3.2.1 Infliximab

Infliximab (Remicade®) is a chimeric human TNF-α monoclonal antibody, derived from mice, that specifically binds to TNF-α, blocking its biologic activity, and has been established in the treatment of rheumatoid arthritis. There is preliminary evidence to support its use in several other inflammatory diseases, and a few patients with juvenile and "classic" DM have been published in literature [33–35].

Regimen. Infliximab is administered in DM patients via intravenous infusion in doses 3 mg/kg or 5 mg/kg given at 0, 2, and 6 weeks, and then every 8 weeks thereafter. Infliximab therapy is instituted, initially, at 200 mg (3.3 mg/kg).

Clinical response. Two patients with PM and DM receiving intravenous infusion of infliximab have been reported [33]. The myopathy responded well, but efficacy with regard to cutaneous lesions in DM is unclear. Three similar cases with refractory juvenile DM were managed successfully with infliximab [36]. Recently five children with juvenile DM and calcinosis showed marked improvement after starting treatment with infliximab [35].

Adverse reactions. Infusion reactions (chills, headache, flushing, nausea, dyspnea), infectious complications (cholecystitis, pyelonephritis, and sepsis), oncogenic potential (non-Hodgkin's lymphoma) and elevated transaminases have been reported [37]. Over time, neutralizing antibodies to drug develop and make treatment less effective. There are concerns regarding the potential development of malignancy following TNF-α blockade. A 48-year-old woman with refractory DM, who became persistently unwell following treatment with infliximab (5 mg/kg), developed non-Hodgkin's lymphoma [37]. Two days after the third infusion of infliximab, the previously normal CRP and ESR were elevated to 120 mg/l and 68 mm/h.

39.3.2.2 Etanercept

Etanercept (Enbrel®) is a recombinant TNF-α receptor fusion protein, which binds to TNF-α and forms a complex, so the cytokine is no longer available to perform its biologic activity. This TNF-α antagonist was administered to ameliorate the symptoms of acute and chronic dermatoses [38, 39].

Regimen. Etanercept is administered subcutaneously in doses 25 mg twice weekly for 12 weeks.

Clinical response. Four cases of severe DM, refractory to conventional therapy with steroids and other immunosuppressive agents, were treated successfully with TNF-α inhibitor etanercept [40]. No data of efficacy upon cutaneous manifestations were noted. Treatment with etanercept in DM patients successfully improved the clinical symptoms and quality of life in patients from two other studies[38, 39].

Adverse reactions. Side-effects with a low incidence from etanercept include aplastic anemia, reactivation of latent tuberculosis, demyelinating diseases and different types of antibodies (neutralizing, ANA, ss-DNA) in some patients.

39.3.2.3 Tacrolimus

Tacrolimus (Protopic®) is a immunosuppressive macrolide, acting as an inhibitor of calcineurin and thus inhibiting both T-lymphocyte signal transduction and IL-2 transcription [42]. It is a new, promising, effective, well-tolerated therapy for managing refractory ILD and myositis as part of the antisynthetase syndrome [43, 44].

Regimen. Tacrolimus is administered in oral applications of 3 mg/day.

Clinical response. Tacrolimus up to a dose of 2 mg b.i.d. was initiated in a 48-year-old woman with refractory DM, but this was withdrawn when the patient developed nausea and a sensory axonal neuropathy [37]. Two cases of progressive ILD associated with PM and DM, refractory to treatment with corticosteroids pulse, cyclosporine, and intermittent pulse cyclophosphamide, have been successfully treated with tacrolimus. Tacrolimus showed high effectiveness in achieving clinical, laboratory, and radiographic improvement in both patients [45]. Another 31-year-old patient with therapeutically resistant DM achieved significant improvement after initiation of tacrulimus treatment [46]. In a study by Martín Nalda et al., a significant improvement in both muscular straight and cutaneous lesions was observed in all six patients with juvenile DM treated with tacrolimus to the end of the follow-up period [47].

Topical 0.1% tacrolimus cream adjunct to sunscreens and weekly pulse of superpotent topical corticosteroids has been reported highly effective in cutaneous lesion management in DM [48].

39.3.2.4 Eculizumab

A small clinical trial of a recombinant monoclonal antibody to the fifth component of complement eculizumab (Alexion®) resulted in an improvement of both the cutaneous and the muscular manifestations of DM [49].

39.3.2.5 Rituximab

Rituximab is a chimeric monoclonal antibody against CD 20, used for treatment of B-cell lymphomas. A recent study reports results of rituximab treatment in three patients with long-standing PM or DM poorly responsive to prednisone combined with several immunosuppressants [50].

Rituximab was given intravenously in a dose of 1.0 g on days 0 and 14 [50]. Short-term beneficial effects were observed in all reported cases as muscle strength improved in all of them. Average daily prednisone and methotrexate dose significantly decreased [50].

39.3.3 Thalidomide

Thalidomide, a TNF-α production inhibitor, has been observed anecdotally to be in value for treatment of cutaneous lesions in DM [41].

39.3.4 Dapsone

A successful treatment of both the cutaneous and muscular manifestations of DM by dapsone has been observed [51, 52]. Dapsone (4,4′-diaminodiphenylsulfone) is a sulfone chemotherapeutic used for the treatment of leprosy and dermatitis herpetiformis; however, it also has anti-inflammatory actions, primarily by inhibiting the functions of polymorphonuclear leukocytes and complement activation via the alternative pathway [53].

Regimen. A quantitative glucose-6 phosphate dehydrogenase (G-6-PD) should be normal prior to starting dapsone 25 mg twice daily along with cimetidine 400 mg twice daily [52]. Dapsone dose may increase to 100 mg daily in 2 weeks, without any side effects.

Clinical response. Konohana and Kawashima [51] reported dapsone to be a successful treatment of both the cutaneous and muscular manifestations of DM. Recently, two patients who failed to respond to combined treatment with prednisone, hydroxychloroquine, quinacrine, and mycofenolat mofetil, but showed rapid improvement from dapsone addition, were published [52].

Adverse reactions. Side-effects from dapsone therapy are generally minor and dose-dependent, including morbilliform or urticarial eruptions, gastrointestinal intolerance, hemolysis, and methemoglobinemia (may be minimized with concomitant administration of cimetidine). Severe toxic idiosyncratic reactions are rare, but cases of LE, aplastic anemia, exfoliative dermatitis, peripheral neuropathy, Stevens–Johnson syndrome, and allergic hypersensitivity syndrome have been reported.

39.4 Combination of Regimes

The following sequential, step-by-step, empirical escalating approach has been successful in DM patients [54]. Step 1 is prednisone. Step 2 is azathioprine or methotrexate (the choice depends on personal experience). In aggressive cases, steps 1 and 2 may be combined from the outset. Step 3 is intravenous immunoglobulin (this may be used as step 2). Step 4 is cyclosporin, mycophenolate mofetil, chlorambucil, or cyclophosphamide, used individually or in various combinations with steps 1–3 [55], as dictated by disease severity, coexisting disorders, or the patient's age. Several reports have supported the use of combination therapy. Twelve children with severe juvenile DM (mainly with dysphagia and severe cutaneous vasculitis) were treated with intravenous methylprednisolone (30 mg/kg/dose) and methotrexate [56]. The six patients who were treated early with intravenous methylprednisolone and methotrexate showed a significant clinical improvement, and none developed calcinosis. In contrast, two of six patients who were treated late with methotrexate developed calcinosis [56]. Superiority of a specific combination remains unproven [55].

References

1. Raifman CM, Schaffer FM, Wachsmuth SE. Reversal of chronic polymyositis following intravenous immune serum globin therapy. *JAMA* 1987; 258: 513–515.
2. Gelfand EW. The use of intravenous immune globulin in collagen vascular disorders: a potentially new modality of therapy. *J Allergy Clin Immunol* 1989; 84(4 Pt 2): 613–615.
3. Dalakas MC, Illa I, Dambrosia JM, et al. A controlled trial of high-dose intravenous immunoglobulin infusions as treatment for dermatomyositis. *N Engl J Med* 1993; 329: 1993–2000.
4. Cherin P, Herson S, Wechsler B, et al. Efficacy of intravenous gammaglobulin therapy in chronic refractory polymyositis and dermatomyositis: an open study with 20 adult patients. *Am J Med* 1991; 91: 162–168.

39

5. Lang BA, Laxer RM, Murphy G, et al. Treatment of dermatomyositis with intravenous gammaglobulin. *Am J Med* 1991; 91: 169–172.
6. Dalakas MC. Intravenous immunoglobulin for dermatomyositis. *N Engl J Med* 1994; 330: 1392–1393.
7. Patel SY, Kumararatne DS. From black magic to science: understanding the rationale for the use of intravenous immunoglobulin to treat inflammatory myopathies. *Clin Exp Immunol* 2001; 124: 169–171.
8. Basta M, Dalakas MC. High-dose intravenous immunoglobulin exerts its beneficial effect in patients with dermatomyositis by blocking endomysial deposition of activated complement fragments. *J Clin Invest* 1994; 94: 1729–1735.
9. Amemiya K, Semino-Mora C, Granger RP, et al. Downregulation of TGF-β1 mRNA and protein in the muscles of patients with inflammatory myopathies after treatment with high-dose intravenous immunoglobulin. *Clin Immunol* 2000; 94: 99–104.
10. Yu Z, Lennon VA. Mechanism of intravenous human globin therapy in antibody-mediated autoimmune disease. *N Engl J Med* 1999; 340: 227–228.
11. Lutz HU, Stammler P, Jelezarova E, et al. High doses of immunoglobulin G attenuate immune aggregate-mediated complement activation by enhancing physiologic cleavage of C3b in C3bn-IgG complexes. *Blood* 1996; 88: 184–193.
12. Kazatchkine MD, Kaveri SV. Immunomodulation of autoimmune and inflammatory disease with intravenous immunoglobulin. *N Engl J Med* 2001; 345: 747–755.
13. Götterfied I, Seeber A, Anegg B, et al. High dose intravenous immunoglobulin (IVIG) in dermatomyositis: clinical responses and effect on sIL-2R levels. *Eur J Dermatol* 2000; 10: 29–35.
14. Sansome A, Dubowitz V. Intravenous immunoglobulin in juvenile dermatomyositis — four year review of nine cases. *Arch Dis Child* 1995; 72(1): 25–28.
15. Morita R, Nakano K, Hirano Y, et al. Dramatic effects of high-dose intravenous gammaglobulin in each patient with intractable dermatomyositis and polymyositis. *No To Hattatsu* 1989; 21(6): 523–528 [Japanese].
16. Sadayama T, Miyagawa S, Shirai T. Low-dose intravenous immunoglobulin therapy for intactable dermatomyositis skin lesions. *J Dermatol* 1999; 26: 457–459.
17. Saadeh C, Bridges W, Burwick F. Dermatomyositis: remission induced with combined oral cyclosporine and high-dose intravenous immune globulin. *South Med J* 1995; 88(8): 866–870.
18. Mastaglia FL, Phillips BA, Zilko PJ. Immunoglobulin therapy in inflammatory myopathies. *J Neurol Neurosurg Psychiatry* 1998; 65: 107–110.
19. Cherin P, Pelletier S, Teixeira A, et al. Results and long-term follow-up of intravenous immunoglobulin infusions in chronic refractory polymyositis: an open study with 35 adult patients. *Arthritis Rheum* 2002; 46(2): 467–474.
20. Dalakas MC. High-dose intravenous immunoglobulin in inflammatory myopathies: experience based on controlled clinical trials. *Neurol Sci* 2003; 24: S256–S259.
21. Dalakas MC. Intravenous immunoglobulin in the treatment of autoimmune neuromuscular diseases: present status and practical therapeutic guidelines. *Muscle Nerve* 1999; 22: 1479–1497.
22. Danieli MG, Malcangi G, Palmieri C, et al. Cyclosporin A and intravenous immunoglobulin treatment in polymyositis/dermatomyositis. *Ann Rheum Dis* 2002; 61: 37–41.
23. Eshraghi N, Farahmand M, Maerz LL, et al. Adult-onset dermatomyositis, with severe gastrointestinal manifestations: case report and review of the literature. *Surgery* 1998; 123: 356–358.
24. Rigby SP, Schott JM, Bliss P, et al. Dilated stomach and weak muscles. *Lancet* 2000; 356: 1898.
25. Marie I, Levesque H, Cailleux N, et al. Intravenous immunoglobulin for treatment of gastrointestinal haemorrhage in dermatomyositis. *Ann Rheum Dis* 2001; 60: 723–724.
26. Fukunaga E, Kunishigea M, Mitsuia T, et al. Severe dermatomyositis with rhabdomyolysis and paralytic ileus: a case successfully treated with plasmapheresis and intravenous immunoglobulin. *EFNS Eur J Neurol* 2002; 9: 687–702.

27. Ratko TA, Burnett DA, Foulke GE, et al. Recommendations for off-label use of intravenously administered immunoglobulin preparations. *JAMA* 1995; 273: 457–492.
28. Jolles S, Hughes J, Whittacker S. Dermatological uses of high-dose intravenous immunoglobulin. *Arch Dermatol* 1998; 134: 80–86.
29. Roujeau JC. Dermatomyositis. In: *Therapeutique Dermatologique*, Dubertret L (ed.), Medecine-Sciences, Flammarion, Paris, 2001; 178–182.
30. Hengstman GJ, van den Hoogen FH, Barrera P, et al. Successful treatment of dermatomyositis and polymyositis with anti-tumor-necrosis-factor-alpha: preliminary observations. *Eur Neurol* 2003; 50: 10–15.
31. Maillard SM, Wilkinson N, Davidson JE, Murray KJ. The treatment of persistent severe idiopathic inflammatory myositis with anti TNF therapy. *Ann Rheum Dis* 2002; 61: S143.
32. Mastaglia FL, Garlepp MJ, Phillips BA, et al. Inflammatory myopathies: clinical, diagnostic and therapeutic aspects. *Muscle Nerve* 2003; 27(4): 407–425.
33. Hengstman G, van den Hoogen F, van Engelen B, et al. Anti-TNF-α blockade with infliximab (Remicade) in polymyositis and dermatomyositis [abstract]. *Arthritis Rheum* 2000; 43: S193.
34. Musial J, Undas A, Celinska-Lowenhoff M. Polymyositis associated with infliximab treatment for rheumatoid arthritis. *Rheumatology* 2003; 42: 1566–1568.
35. Riley P, McCann LJ, Maillard SM, et al. Effectiveness of infliximab in the treatment of refractory juvenile dermatomyositis with calcinosis. *Rheumatology* 2008; 47(6): 877–880.
36. Nzeusseu A, Durez P, Houssiau F, et al. Successful use of infliximab in a case of refractory juvenile dermatomyositis. *Arthritis Rheum* 2001; 44: S90.
37. Roddy E, Couriney PA, Morris A. Non-Hodgkin's lymphoma in a patient with refractory dermatomyositis which had been treated with infliximab [letter]. *Rheumatology* 2002; 41: 1194–1195.
38. Norman R, Greenber RG, Jackson JM. Case report of etanercept in inflammatory dermatoses. *J Am Acad Dermatol* 2006; 54(Suppl 2): S139–142.
39. Hall HA, Zimmermann B. Evolution of dermatomyositis during therapy with a tumor necrosis factor alpha inhibitor. *Arthritis Rheum* 2006; 55(6): 982–984.
40. Saadeh CK. Etanercept is effective in the treatment of polymyositis/dermatomyositis which is refractory to conventional therapy including steroids and other disease modifying agents [abstract]. *Arthritis Rheum* 2000; 43: S193.
41. Sontheimer RD. Skin manifestations of systemic autoimmune connective tissue disease: diagnostics and therapeutics. *Best Pract Res Clin Rheumatol* 2004; 18 (3): 429–462.
42. Liu J, Farmer JD Jr, Lane WS, et al. Calcineurin is a common target of cyclophilin–cyclosporin A and FKBP-FK506 complexes. *Cell* 1991; 66(4): 807–815.
43. Oddis CV. Current approach to the treatment of polymyositis and dermatomyositis. *Curr Opin Rheumatol* 2000; 12(6): 492–497.
44. Wilkes MR, Sereika SM, Fertig N, et al. Treatment of antisynthetase-associated interstitial lung disease with tacrolimus. *Arthritis Rheum* 2005; 52(8): 2439–2446.
45. Ochi S, Nanki T, Takada K, et al. Favorable outcomes with tacrolimus in two patients with refractory interstitial lung disease associated with polymyositis/dermatomyositis. *Clin Exp Rheumatol* 2005; 23: 707–710.
46. Mitsui T, Kuroda Y, Kunishige M, et al. Successful treatment with tacrolimus in a case of refractory dermatomyositis. *Intern Med* 2005; 44(11): 1197–1199.
47. Martín Nalda A, Modesto Caballero C, Arnal Guimeral C, et al. Efficacy of tacrolimus (FK-506) in the treatment of recalcitrant juvenile dermatomyositis: study of 6 cases. *Med Clin (Barc)* 2006; 127(18): 697–701.
48. Jorizzo JL. Dermatomyositis: practical aspects. *Arch Dermatol* 2002; 138: 114–116.
49. Kaplan M. Eculizumab (Alexion). *Curr Opin Invest Drugs* 2002; 3: 1017–1023.

39

50. Noss EH, Hausner-Sypek DL, Weinblatt ME. Rituximab as therapy for refractory polymyositis and dermatomyositis. *J Rheumatol* 2006; 33(5): 1021–1026.
51. Konohana A, Kawashima J. Successful treatment of dermatomyositis with dapsone. *Clin Exp Dermatol* 1994; 19(4): 367.
52. Cohen JB. Cutaneous involvement of dermatomyositis can respond to dapsone therapy. *Int J Dermatol* 2002; 41: 182–184.
53. Coleman MD. Dapsone: modes of action, toxicity, and possible strategies for increasing patient tolerance. *Br J Dermatol* 1993; 129: 507–513.
54. Dalakas MC, Hohfeld R. Polymyositis and dermatomyositis. *Lancet* 2003; 362: 971–982.
55. Choy EH, Isenberg DA. Treatment of dermatomyositis and polymyositis. *Rheumatology (Oxford)* 2002; 41(1): 7–13.
56. Al-Mayouf S, Al-Mazyed A, Bahabri S. Efficacy of early treatment of severe juvenile dermatomyositis with intravenous methylprednisolone and methotrexate. *Clin Rheumatol* 2000; 19: 138–141.

40 Treatment of Cutaneous Manifestations and Complications of Dermatomyositis

40.1 Therapy of Cutaneous Manifestations

Generally there is a lack of correlation between the degree and severity of the muscle disease and the skin disease [1]. Systemic corticosteroids in doses of 60–80 mg/day of prednisone are frequently required to control cutaneous involvement [2]. Some use moderate doses of prednisone (40–60 mg/day) for patients with amyopathic DM [3]. The cutaneous manifestations of DM are recalcitrant to therapy in many patients. Parenteral steroids and/or immunosuppressive agents in sufficient quantities to suppress the muscle disease are ineffective in the treatment of the skin disease, and topical potent corticosteroids are seldom of benefit. Topical steroids likewise can be of help, but have also been reported to fail [4]. Topical potent fluorinated steroids are only marginally effective in suppressing the inflammatory condition.

Severe involvement of the skin associated with superficial, painful erosions, or epidermal necrosis, although unusual, may occur in the axillary region and on the sides of the neck. In these patients, pulse corticosteroid therapy with dose of 1.0 g methylprednisolone for 3–5 consecutive days is effective. Among cutaneous features of DM, Gottron's papules, vasculitis, and mechanic's hands disappeared after the first pulse, while periungual erythema and poikiloderma were remarkably persistent, even at the 3-month treatment [5]. Cyclosporin A and mycophenolate appear to be reasonable alternatives in the treatment of the cutaneous features of DM, especially in severe, recalcitrant disease [6, 7]. In recalcitrant cases of cutaneous DM, low-dose methotrexate (2.5–30 mg/week) can be effective [8]. Four out of 13 patients experienced complete clearing, and all patients showed moderate improvement [8]. Patients may respond to combination of antimalarials and methotrexate. A study showed that 15 of 35 patients had resistant cutaneous lesions despite treatment with oral corticosteroids, antimalarials, and methotrexate [9]. Other immunosuppressive agents have not been systemically studied; however, it is suggested that mycophenolate mofetil might be beneficial [10]. Intravenous immunoglobulin administered monthly can result in clearing of cutaneous lesions [11].

Commonly overlooked is the fact that the cutaneous manifestations of DM are photosensitive. Aminoquinoline antimalarials have beneficial effect upon the photosensitive dermatitis of DM, and can be helpful in treating DM skin disease [4]. However, DM skin disease is relatively resistant to antimalarial therapy. Partial improvement in up to 80% is more common than complete control [12]. Patients who do not respond well to hydroxychloroquine can be treated with 250–500mg daily chloroquine phosphate [10] or quinacrine 100mg/day, twice daily [10, 13]. The patients with DM have an increased risk of drug eruptions from antimalarial agents. The patients should be advised to avoid sun exposure. Emollients and photoprotection are essential. It is a rule in practice to recommend the use of broad-spectrum sunscreens with a skin protection factor of more than 25. Patients should be instructed in the use of protective clothing, and practice sun-avoidance behavior.

Dapsone has been found to be a successful treatment alternative of both the cutaneous and muscular manifestations of DM [14, 15]. Pentoxiphylline, an anticoagulant and viscosity-lowering agent, has also been reported to induce rapid response to DM eruption and reduction of CK level in a 60-year-old woman [16].

The generalized pruritus associated with DM is very distressing to some patients. The use of topical anti-pruritic lotions should also be a part of the regimen. Bland emollients can be used to combat the skin dryness that is a complicating factor of the pruritus/burning sensations often experienced by adults with active DM skin disease [17]. Unfortunately, topical emollient formulations containing mild-potency steroids, pramoxine, menthol, phenol and/or camphor phenol or diphenhydramine or doxepin can provide only short-term relief [18]. Various antihistamines appear to offer only limited control of this very annoying symptom. Systemic antipruritic therapy can serve as an adjunct. While nonsedating antihistamines such as cetirizine, loratadine, and fexofenadine are preferred during the day, potent, long-acting, sedating hydroxyzine, doxepin, or tricyclic antidepressant doxepine given at bedtime can ameliorate pruritus and excoriations experienced during the evening [12, 19].

Very potent topical corticosteroids such as clobetasol propionate are helpful but rarely curative [2]. The cutaneous eruption can be intensively pruritic, producing marked secondary lichenoid change superimposed on the poikiloderma lesions, scalp, and over the knuckles. Foam-based preparations containing clobetasol can be especially useful for the pruritus/burning of the scalp. Topical formulations of tacrolimus can provide some benefit for the cutaneous inflammation of DM, especially on the face and around the eyes. High efficacy in cutaneous lesion treatment has been reported from a new topical 0.1% tacrolimus adjunct to sunscreens and weekly pulse superpotent local clobetasol propionate [20, 21]. Formulations containing 0.3% tacrolimus could provide greater value to DM skin disease patients, as has been reported for refractory cutaneous LE patients [22].

Calcium channel blockers are helpful in treating associated Raynauds's phenomenon in DM patients [23]. Nifedipine, 10–20mg t.i.d is generally the drug of choice, but may aggravate lower esophageal discomfort, making diltiazem and prazosin an alternative [23].

40.2 Treatment of Pulmonary Disease

Pulmonary involvement appears responsive to corticosteroid therapy [24]. Treatment usually includes prednisone in 40–60mg/day dosages for initial control, followed by lower-dose prednisone plus an immunosuppressive agent such as azathioprine or methotrexate for disease suppression [25]. However, some DM patients with ILD show steroid resistance [26]. In addition, acute respiratory failure as a complication of methotrexate therapy can be avoided by immediate initiation of high-dose steroids after discontinuing methotrexate. Hydroxychloroquine has also been proposed as a steroid-sparing agent in periods of remission [25]. Colchicine has been used as a potentially antifibrotic drug; however, it has not been proven to be effective in treating the interstitial pneumofibrosis [27]. Intravenous immunoglobulins did not alter the outcome [25]. Others have reported success in treating Jo-1 positive ILD with a combination of low-dose prednisone, cyclosporine, and azathioprine [28], in a regimen similar to those currently used for prevention of organ transplantation rejection. Recently, it has been reported that i.v. pulse cyclophosphamide is efficaceous in patients with ILD and PM or DM [29].

Patients with a variant of ILD, called rapid progressive ILD, have a rapidly aggravating clinical course, and are mostly unresponsive to corticosteroid therapy [30–32]. The prognosis is very poor unless aggressive immunosuppressive agents such as cyclophosphamide are started early enough to prevent irreversible pulmonary damage [33]. Two cases with PM/DM associated with progressive ILD, refractory to conventional therapy with high-dose corticosteroids, cyclosporine, and intermittent pulse cyclophosphamide, have been successfully treated with tacrolimus. Tacrolimus was found markedly effective in achieving subjective, laboratory, and radiographic improvement in both patients [34].

40.3 Treatment of Calcinosis

Once established, calcification of soft tissue and muscle in DM patients is problematic and difficult to treat [35, 36]. Some authors believe that calcinosis in juvenile DM could be prevented by aggressive early treatment [36]. Intermittent high-dose intravenous methylprednisolone has been suggested, which may prevent and decrease the severity of calcinosis in juvenile DM [37, 38]; however, randomized controlled trials have not yet corroborated this suggestion [36].

Several remedies, such as aluminum hydroxide [39], warfarin [40, 41], colchicine [42], probenecid [43], and calcium channel blocker diltiazem have been reported to be effective in treating calcinosis.

Bassett et al. [44] first described the use of disodium ethane-1-hydroxy-1,1-diphosphonate (EHDP) administered orally in dose of 10 mg/kg/day in two children with myositis ossificans and severe limitation of motion. Symptoms resolved within a few days, and no calcification ensued. Diphosphonates inhibit calcium deposit [45, 46] and hold in check the absorption of intestinal calcium [45]. Disphosphonates can inhibit macrophage pro-inflammatory production of IL1, IL6, and TNF-α [47].

Aledronate is speculated to exert a two-fold activity in DM patients, by inhibiting bone resorption followed by reducing calcium turnover and inhibiting calcium accretion in existing calcifications. A 6-year-old boy with juvenile DM developed severe and debilitating calcinosis, unresponsive to diltiazem, and probenecid [48]. Alendronate produced dramatic improvement within 1 month, and 1 year later calcinosis had virtually resolved [48].

Warfarin, a different calcium antagonist, has been used to treat and prevent calcification [40, 41, 49]. Patients with calcinosis universalis secondary to DM have elevated tissue levels of, and raised urinary excretion of gamma carboxyglutamic acid [50]. The carboxylation of glutaminate is sensitive to the inhibitory effects of warfarin [51]. Berger and Hadler [40] reported four patients with calcinosis universalis due to DM or SSc, all treated with 1 mg/day of warfarin orally for 18 months. A decrease in lesion size in three of them and inhibition of further lesion development was observed. Recently, warfarin has been reported to reduce the amount of subcutaneous calcinosis and to improve mobility in a 27-year-old male with DM, calcinosis universalis, and very high serum vitamin K levels [52].

Treatment with aluminum hydroxide gel has been successful and safe [35]. Aluminum hydroxide is presumed to prevent the absorption of ingested phosphate by binding it in the gut and results in the reduction of calcium phosphate product in plasma [53]. Nassim and Connolly (1970) described a child with calcinosis universalis who was given oral aluminum hydroxide in divided doses of 2.4 g/day for about 6 months, resulting in "considerable clearing" [54]. Eighteen months later, the contractures were improved and only solitary lesions remained. Wang et al. [55] reported a remarkable response to aluminum hydroxide in a juvenile DM patient with cutaneous calcinosis. Aluminum hydroxide is widely used to treat calcinosis because of a lack of adverse effects [39, 53].

Chelation therapy has shown some modest success using D-penicillamine [43, 56, 57]. D-penicillamine may be effective by increasing renal phosphate clearance [58]. However, the efficacy of ethylene diamine tetraacetic acid (EDTA) in doses of 50 mg/kg intravenously in 3–5 day courses over 3 weeks has been disappointing [59].

Colchicine 0.6 mg once or twice daily has been effective in decreasing the inflammation and healing of chronic ulcers, but not affected the size of calcified plaques in two adolescents with DM [60].

Palmieri et al. [61] suggest that the benzothiazepine calcium channel blocker, diltiazem, which inhibits mitochondrial sodium–calcium exchange, may have a beneficial therapeutic effect in treating calcinosis. Neither verapamil nor the nifedipine type calcium channel blockers have this inhibiting effect on mitochondrial sodium–calcium exchange. Diltiazem, reducing the influx of calcium ions into the cells, corrects cellular calcium disorder to a certain extent. An 8-year-old girl with juvenile DM and dystrophic calcinosis was treated with oral diltiazem (5 mg/kg/day) and oral pamidronate in addition to calcium and vitamin D supplementation for 3 years [62]. Twenty-one months after the initiation of the treatment, the clinical and radiological examination revealed dramatic regression of the calcinosis. More recently, a few case reports of calcinosis successfully treated with diltiazem in "classic" DM in adults [63] and juvenile DM have been published [64]. Some believe that diltiazem alone or in combination with other drugs could be a useful therapy in patients with juvenile DM and pronounced calcification. Moreover, a high dosage of 360 mg/day diltiazem significantly reduced the mineral content of calcified tissues in a wheelchair-bound patient with adult DM [63].

Evidence-based data show that aggressive initial immunosuppression therapy can prevent or ameliorate the process of calcium deposition [65]. Early initiation of aggressive treatment with intravenous methylprednisone and methotrexate in 12 children with juvenile-onset DM prevented the development of calcinosis in those who initiate the treatment within 6 weeks of diagnosis [66].

Recently, peripheral blood stem cell autograft resulted in total disappearance of calcinosis and remission of disease activity in a bedridden teenage girl with DM, arthritis, myalgia, skin ulcers, and diffuse calcinosis [67].

A surgical approach to the management of large calcium deposits in DM patients is also appropriate [68]. Successful surgical removal of soft-tissue sacral calcifications in DM has been described [69]. Surgical excision or drainage of calcinosis is possible if dangerous ulceration or infection occurs or if the calcinosis is in hazardous locations, but is rarely curative. Surgical excision is a successful option for a limited involvement.

Low-calcium or high-phosphate diets have previously been advocated in calcinosis and juvenile DM [68]. Aggressive physiotherapy is as useful as any medications for severe calcinosis, at least in preventing functional complications. Occasionally, subcutaneous calcinosis may resolve spontaneously in some patients [68].

40.4 Treatment of Dermatomyositis in Pregnant Women

Pregnant women with DM/PM should be monitored as to the usual clinical and laboratory parameters [70]. Prednisone is the treatment of choice, and should be given in the same doses as for nonpregnant patients. Aggressive use of this drug may minimize the potential for fetal wastage [71]. If steroids are ineffective, more potent immunosuppressants should be used [35].

40.5 Treatment of Paraneoplastic Dermatomyositis

Malignancy-associated DM/PM often portends a difficult and recalcitrant course [2]. An improvement in myopathy may be seen after cancer therapy [72], but a paradoxal worsening has also been reported [2]. The disease may become quiescent and even go into remission, only to flare with appearance of metastases [72]. Other patients may experience no change in their disease activity, regardless of the treatment or tumor behavior. It seems to be difficult to predict the response of a DM when associated with a malignancy. Patients with malignant tumors that developed simultaneously with DM have required more aggressive treatment [73]. After adequate surgery or radiotherapy of tumor, the skin and muscle symptoms respond better to immunosuppressive therapy [73].

References

1. Gertner E, Urowitz MB. Discordance of skin and muscle involvement in dermatomyositis. *Int J Dermatol* 1985; 24: 518–519.
2. Tuffanelli DL, Lavole PE. Prognosis and therapy of polymyositis/dermatomyositis. *Clin Dermatol* 1988; 6: 93–104.

3. Euwer RL, Sontheimer RD. Amyopathic dermatomyositis (dermatomyositis sine myositis). Presentation of six new cases and review of the literature. *J Am Acad Dermatol* 1991; 24: 959–966.
4. Woo TY, Callen JP, Voorhees JJ, et al. Cutaneous lesions of dermatomyositis are improved by hydroxychloroquine. *J Am Acad Dermatol* 1984; 10: 592–600.
5. Bolosiu HD, Man L, Rednie S. The effect of methylprednisolone pulse therapy in polymyositis/dermatomyositis. *Adv Exp Med Biol* 1999; 455: 349–357.
6. Gelber AC, Nousari HC, Wigley FM. Mycophenolate mofetil in the treatment of severe skin manifestations of dermatomyositis: a series of 4 cases. *J Rheumatol* 2000; 27: 1542–1545.
7. Danieli MG, Malcangi G, Palmieri C, et al. Cyclosporin A and intravenous immunoglobulin treatment in polymyositis/dermatomyositis. *Ann Rheum Dis* 2002; 61: 37–41.
8. Kasteler JS, Callen JP. Low-dose methotrexate administered weekly is an effective corticosteroid-sparing agent for the treatment of the cutaneous manifestations of dermatomyositis. *J Am Acad Dermatol* 1997; 36: 67–71.
9. Dawkins MA, Jorizzo JL, Walkler FO, et al. Dermatomyositis: a dermatology-based case series. *J Am Acad Dermatol* 1998; 38: 397–404.
10. Callen JP. New and emerging therapies for collagen-vascular diseases. *Dermatol Clin* 2000; 18: 139–146.
11. Dalakas MC, Illa I, Dambrosia JM, et al. A controlled trial of high dose intravenous immunoglobulin infusions as treatment for dermatomyositis. *N Engl J Med* 1993; 329: 1993–2000.
12. Trüeb RM. Dermatomyositis. *Dermatol Ther* 2001; 14: 70–80.
13. Ghate J, Katsambas A, Augerinou G, Jorizzo JL. A therapeutic update on dermatomyositis/polymyositis. *Int J Dermatol* 2000; 39: 81–87.
14. Cohen JB. Cutaneous involvement of dermatomyositis can respond to dapsone therapy. *Int J Dermatol* 2002; 41: 182–184.
15. Konohana A, Kawishima J. Successful treatment of dermatomyositis with dapsone. *Clin Exp Dermatol* 1994; 69: 367.
16. Person JR. Dermatomyositis responding to pentoxiphylline [Letter]. *Br J Dermatol* 1995; 134: 593.
17. Sontheimer RD, Geers DL. Skin disease in dermatomyositis — what patients and their families often want to know. *Dermatology Online J* 2002; 20: 387–408.
18. Sontheimer RD. Skin manifestations of systemic autoimmune connective tissue disease: diagnostics and therapeutics. *Best Pract Res Clin Rheumatol* 2004; 18 (3): 429–462.
19. Koler RA, Montemarano A. Dermatomyositis. *Am Fam Physician* 2001; 64(9): 1565–1572.
20. Jorizzo JL. Dermatomyositis: practical aspects. *Archiv Dermatol* 2002; 138: 114–116.
21. Jordan JR, Paruthi S, Pichardo RO, et al. Spontaneously remitting dermatomyositis. *JEADV* 2004; 18: 495–498.
22. Walker SL, Kirby B, Chalmers RJG. The effect of topical tacrolimus on severe recalcitrant chronic discoid lupus erythematosus. *Br J Dermatol* 2002; 147: 405–406.
23. Oddis CV, Medsger TA. Current management of polymyositis and dermatomyositis. *Drugs* 1989; 37: 382–390.
24. Dickey BF, Meyers AR. Pulmonary disease in polymyositis and dermatomyositis. *Sem Arthritis Rheum* 1984; 14: 60–76.
25. Douglas WW, Tazelaar HD, Hartman TE, et al. Polymyositis/dermatomyositis associated interstitial lung disease. *Am J Respir Crit Care Med* 2001; 164: 1182–1185.
26. Takada T, Suzuki E, Nakano M, et al. Clinical features of polymyositis/dermatomyositis with steroid-resistant interstitial lung disease. *Intern Med* 1998; 37: 669–673.
27. Douglas WW, Ryu JH, Schroeder DR. Idiopathic pulmonary fibrosis: impact of oxygen and colchicine, prednisone or no therapy on survival. *Am J Respir Crit Care Med* 2000; 161: 1172–1178.

28. Sauty A, Rochat T, Schoch OD, et al. Pulmonary fibrosis with predominant CD8 lymphocytic alveolitis and anti-Jo-1 antibodies. *Eur Respir J* 1997; 10: 2907–2912.
29. Meyer O, Hayem G, Palazzo E, et al. Interstitial lung disease due to polymyositis or dermatomyositis: effect of a 6-month course of i.v. pulse cyclophosphamide. *Clin Exp Rheumatol* 2005; 23: 724.
30. Nawata Y, Kurasawa K, Takabayashi K, et al. Corticosteroid resistant interstitial pneumonitis in dermatomyositis polymyositis; prediction and treatment with cyclosporine. *J Rheumatol* 1999; 26: 1527–1533.
31. Ito M, Kaise S, Suzuki S, et al. Clinico-laboratory characteristics of patients with dermatomyositis accompanied by rapidly progressive interstitial lung disease. *Clin Rheumatol* 1999; 18: 462–467.
32. Hirakata M, Nagai S. Interstitial lung disease in polymyositis and dermatomyositis. *Curr Opin Rheumatol* 2000; 12: 501–508.
33. Yoshida T, Koga H, Saitoh F, et al. Pulse intravenous cyclophosphamide treatment for steroid-resistant interstitial pneumonitis associated with polymyositis. *Intern Med* 1999; 38: 733–738.
34. Ochi S, Nanki T, Takada K, et al. Favorable outcomes with tacrolimus in two patients with refractory interstitial lung disease associated with polymyositis/dermatomyositis. *Clin Exp Rheumatol* 2005; 23: 707–710.
35. Boyd AS, Neldner KH. Therapeutic options in dermatomyositis/polymyositis. *Int J Dermatol* 1994; 33: 240–250.
36. Callen JP. Dermatomyositis. *Lancet* 2000; 355: 53–57.
37. Callen JP, Pachman LM, Hayford J, et al. Intermittent high dose intravenous methylprednisolone (IV pulse) prevents calcinosis and shortens disease course in juvenile dermatomyositis (JDMS) [abstract]. *Arthritis Rheum* 1994; 37: R10.
38. Klein-Gitleman MS, Waters T, Pachman LM. The economic impact of intermittent high-dose intravenous versus oral corticosteroid treatment of juvenile dermatomyositis. *Arthritis Care Res* 2000; 13: 360–368.
39. Nakagawa T, Takaiwa T. Calcinosis cutis in juvenile dermatomyositis responsive to aluminium hydroxide treatment. *J Dermatol* 1993; 20: 558–560.
40. Berger RG, Hadler NM. Treatment of calcinosis universalis secondary to dermatomyositis or sceroderma with low dose warfarin [abstract]. *Arthritis Rheum* 1983; 26: S11.
41. Berger RG, Featherstone GL, Raasch RH, et al. Treatment of calcinosis universalis with low-dose warfarin. *Am J Med* 1987; 83: 72–76.
42. Kotliar SN, Roth SI. Cutaneous mineralization and ossification. In: *Dermatology in General Medicine*, Fitzpatrick TB, Eisen AZ, Wolff K, Freedberg IM, Austen KF (eds), 4th ed, McGraw–Hill, New York, 1993; 1940–1948.
43. Eddy MC, Leelawattana R, McAlister WH, et al. Calcinosis universalis complicating juvenile dermatomyositis: resolution during probenecid therapy. *J Clin Endocrinol Metab* 1997; 82: 3536–3542.
44. Bassett CAL, Donath A, Macagno F, et al. Diphosphonates in the treatment of myositis ossificans. *Lancet* 1969; 2(7625): 845.
45. Cram RL, Barmada R, Geho WB, et al. Diphosphonates in the treatment of calcinosis universalis. *N Engl J Med* 1971; 285: 1012–1013.
46. Russel RG, Smith R. Diphosphonates: experimental and clinic aspects. *J Bone Joint Surg Br* 1973; 55: 66–86.
47. Mukamel M, Horev G, Mimouni M. New insight into calcinosis of juvenile dermatomyositis: a study of composition and treatment. *J Pediatrics* 2001; 138 (5): 763–766.
48. Ambler GR, Chaitow J, Rogers M, et al. Rapid improvement of calcinosis in juvenile dermatomyositis with alendronate therapy. *J Rheumatol* 2005; 32: 1837–1839.
49. Lassoued K, Saiag P, Anglade MC, et al. Failure of warfarin in treatment of calcinosis universalis. *Am J Med* 1988; 84: 795–796.

40

50. Lian J, Pacman L, Gunberg C, et al. Gamma carboxyglutamate excretion and calcinosis in juvenile dermatomyositis. *Arthritis Rheum* 1982; 25: 1094–1100.
51. Levy R, Lian J. Gamma carboxyglutamate excretion and warfarin therapy. *Clin Pharmacol Ther* 1979; 25: 562–570.
52. Matsuka Y, Miyajima S, Okada N. A case of calcinosis universalis successfully treated with low-dose warfarin. *J Dermatol* 1998; 25(11): 716–720.
53. Aihara Y, Mori M, Ibe M, et al. A case of juvenile dermatomyositis with calcinosis universalis: remarkable improvement with aluminium hydroxide therapy. *Ryumachi* 1994; 34: 879–884 [Japanese].
54. Nassim JR, Connolly CK. Treatment of calcinosis universalis with aluminium hydroxide. *Arch Dis Child* 1970; 45: 118–121.
55. Wang WJ, Lo WL, Wong CK, et al. Calcinosis cutis in juvenile dermatomyositis: remarkable response to aluminium hydroxide therapy. *Arch Dermatol* 1988; 124: 1721–1722.
56. Dent CE, Stamp TC. Treatment of calcinosis circumscripta with probenecid. *Br J Med* 1972; 1: 216–218.
57. Skuterud E, Sydnes OA, Haavik TK. Calcinosis in dermatomyositis treated with probenecid. *Scand J Rheumatol* 1981; 10: 92–94.
58. Harel L, Harel G, Korenreich L, et al. Treatment of calcinosis in juvenile dermatomyositis with probenecid: The role of phosphorus metabolism in the development of calcification. *J Rheumatol* 2001; 28(5): 1129–1132.
59. Herd JK, Vaughan JH. Calcinosis universalis complicating dermatomyositis. Its treatment with Na2EDTA. *Arthritis Rheum* 1964; 7: 259–271.
60. Taborn J, Bole GG, Thompson GR. Colchicine suppression of local and systemic inflammation due to calcinosis universalis in chronic dermatomyositis. *Ann Intern Med* 1978; 89: 648–649.
61. Palmieri GM, Sebes JI, Aelion JA, et al. Treatment of calcinosis with diltiazem. *Arthritis Rheum* 1995; 38: 1646–1654.
62. Oliveri MB, Palermo R, Mautalen C, et al. Regression of calcinosis during diltiazem treatment in juvenile dermatomyositis. *J Rheumatol* 1996; 23: 2152–2155.
63. Vienen C, Patel S, Bruckner FE. Regression of calcinosis associated with adult dermatomyositis following diltiazem therapy. *Rheumatology* 2000; 39: 333–334.
64. Ichiki Y, Akiyama T, Shimozawa N, et al. An extremely severe case of cutaneous calcinosis with juvenile dermatomyositis, and successful treatment with diltiazem. *Br J Dermatol* 2001; 144: 894–897.
65. Halbert AR. Juvenile dermatomyositis. *Austral J Dermatol* 1996; 37: 106–108.
66. Fisler RE, Liang MG, Fuhlbrigge RC, et al. Aggressive management of juvenile dermatomyositis results in improved outcome and decreased incidence of calcinosis. *J Am Acad Dermatol* 2002; 47(4): 505–511.
67. Elhasid R, Rowe JM, Berkowitz D, et al. Disappearance of diffuse calcinosis following autologous stem cell transplantation in a child with autoimmune disease. *Bone Marrow Transplant* 2004; 33(12): 1257–1259.
68. Sewell JR, Liyanage B, Ansell BM. Calcinosis in juvenile dermatomyositis. *Skeletal Radiol* 1978; 3: 137–143.
69. Carlson M, Lindesth RE, DeRosa GP. Surgical removal of soft tissue calcifications in dermatomyositis. *Arch Surg* 1975; 110: 755–756.
70. Mintz G. Dermatomyositis. *Rheum Dis Clin North Am* 1989; 15: 375–382.
71. King CR, Chow S. Dermatomyositis and pregnancy. *Obstet Gynecol* 1985; 66: 589–592.
72. Burnes BE. Dermatomyositis and malignancy. *Ann Intern Med* 1976; 84: 68–76.
73. Andras C, Ponyi A, Constantin T, et al. Association of myositis with tumors. *Hungarian Oncol* 2002; 46: 253–259.

41 Non-pharmacological Treatment of Dermatomyositis, Physical Therapies and Rehabilitation of Dermatomyositis

Nonpharmacological management includes physical methods for treatment as well as physiotherapy that should be considered as components of the overall management of patients with DM [1]. Plasmapheresis, extracorporal photochemotherapy, and total body irradiation are adjunctive methods of treatment in therapy-resistant cases of DM and PM. Early physiotherapy from the illness onset is beneficial in preventing development of soft-tissue contractures and severe muscle wasting. Physical therapy preserves muscle function and activity, and is an important adjuvant in the treatment and rehabilitation of these patients [2].

41.1 Plasmapheresis (Plasma Exchange)

Removal of circulating immunoglobulins in adults and children with DM/PM has been reported to be effective [3–5]. The benefit of plasmapheresis is still uncertain, and the results of various studies are contradictory. In 1981, Dau [3] was the first to report the efficacy of plasmapheresis associated with immunosuppressive drugs (cyclophosphamid, chlorambucil, and/or prednisone) in corticosteroid-resistant patients with PM/DM. A double-blind, placebo-controlled trial failed to demonstrate the efficacy of plasma exchange and leukopheresis in chronic refractory PM/DM [6].

Plasmapheresis reduces the amount of circulating antibodies and cytokines [7]. A study of plasmapheresis posttreatment muscle biopsies demonstrated a diminished degree of atrophy and improvement in pathologic findings [8].

Regimen. Plasma exchange involves the removal of a patient's plasma and giving fresh frozen replacement [9]. Treatment is usually once or twice a week. Immunoglobulins can be given at the end of a session. Concomitant medications, such as prednisone and immunosuppressive agents continue.

Clinical response. The largest study included 35 patients with IIMs (11 with DM and 15 with PM), who were steroid- or immunosuppressant drug therapy-resistant [3].

L.A. Dourmishev and A.L. Dourmishev, *Dermatomyositis: Advances in Recognition, Understanding and Management,* © Springer-Verlag Berlin Heidelberg 2009

41

Plasmapheresis were administered once per week for 10 weeks and then at gradually increasing intervals. At the end, 30 of 35 patients improved clinically and according to laboratory findings. Moderate to major improvement of muscle weakness has also been reported in juvenile DM [4], and in a case report of adult DM [10]. Paraneoplastic DM also responded to plasmapheresis treatment [11]. Successful treatment of severe DM with rhabdomyolysis and paralytic ileus with plasmapheresis and IVIG have been reported [12].

Plasma exchange therapy was initiated in a 15-year-old girl with childhood-onset DM, in whom previous therapy with coricosteroids and immunosuppressors had failed [13]. Treatment with prednisone and cyclophosphamide were continued. The patient was remarkably improved after her 22nd exchange. Two large European studies showed 63% [14] and 71% response rate of plasma exchange therapy [15]. An improvement in two-thirds of 21 patients with DM, most of whom had juvenile DM, has been reported [15]. Plasma exchange therapy appears to work better in acute disease [14].

Adverse reactions. Seven patients developed herpes zoster during plasmapheresis [3].

41.2 Extracorporeal Photochemotherapy

Regimen. The extracorporeal photochemotherapy procedure used in the study by Salvaneschi et al. consisted of three steps: (i) peripheral blood mononuclear cells were collected by the cytopheresis of two total blood volumes, (ii) 8-methoxypsoralen (200 ng/mL) was added to the collection bag, followed by ultraviolet A radiation (2 J/cm^2 of white cell-surface area), and (iii) the 8-methoxypsoralen photoactivated cells were returned to the patient by intravenous transfusion within 30 min of collection [16].

Clinical response. Extracorporeal photochemotherapy has also been proposed as adjunctive therapy in juvenile DM [17] and in "classic" DM in adults [16].

Adverse reactions. Reported side-effects associated with extracorporeal photochemotherapy include chills, headache, and post-transfusion fever (<38°C) [16].

41.3 Total-Body Irradiation

Ionizing radiation has a limited place in the treatment of DM/PM [9]. This treatment is used for patients with very severe and progressed disease. Whole-body radiation has been used as a last-chance effort in severely recalcitrant IIM; however, no controlled studies have been performed so far, and most of the information of this mode of treatment has been culled from case reports [7].

Regimen. Usually 15 rad is given twice weekly over a 5-week period for a total of 150 rad. Repeat courses can be given successfully [18].

Clinical response. Dramatic improvements have been reported in patients with PM [19, 20], and DM [21]. A 40-year-old woman with PM, in whom therapy with prednisone, methotrexate, azathioprine, and cyclophosphamide had failed, was moribund [19]. Improvement of treatment with total body irradiation was noted during the second week. Similar cases in adult PM have also been reported [18, 22]. Two patients with severe DM refractory to immunosuppressive therapy and treated with total body irradiation responded promptly and remained in partial remission 42 and 18 months respectively after completion of treatment [21]. However, some studies have shown failure, and the conclusion of specialists is that this treatment is not uniformly curative [23].

Adverse reactions. Total-body irradiation is better tolerated than total nodal irradiation, since nausea and malaise are not seen [19, 21, 22]. The side-effects include pancytopenia, lymphopenia (for several years after treatment), increased risk of malignancy (lymphoma), and death [19, 23].

41.4 Thymectomy

In a small number of patients with IIM (PM and DM), surgical thymectomy has been performed [24, 25]. A patient with DM, who was refractory to corticosteroids and plasmapheresis, started improving in muscle strength 1 month after thymectomy and continued his medication for 2 years [25].

41.5 Transplantation of Autologous Stem Cells

Autologous stem cell transplant, reported to be potentially effective in a number of children with autoimmune disorders, could be considered for very severe, resistant, or life-threatening cases with DM [26]. Disappearance of diffuse calcinosis following autologous stem cell transplantation in a child with DM has been reported [27].

41.6 Physical Therapies and Rehabilitation of Dermatomyositis

Many adjunctive therapies have been used in patients with DM. An important but controversial treatment of IIMs is physical exercise. Because of a fear for causing disease flare-ups, patients with myositis have been recommended to avoid active exercise. Bed rest is recommended, particularly during the acute stage of disease and may result in decreased CK levels [28]. Although it has been reported that reduction in muscle strength is a symptom that mostly impairs quality of life [29], some debate of the appropriateness of therapeutic exercises during the acute stage exists because of a fear of aggravating the inflammatory process [30]. Active exercise should be avoided during the acute phase of muscle inflammation, however, passive range of motion should start early in the disease and can prevent development of soft-tissue contractures, since no data exist to support the contention that every exercise will exacerbate the inflammatory response [31].

Although reestablishment of muscle strength through a physical therapy program is the proposed long-term intervention for DM [32], the progressive nature of the disease suggests that the patient's current physical status (deterioration or recovery) should dictate the balance between physical therapy intervention and rest. In addition, since CK is an indicator of the acuity of the disease [33], CK levels should be used as a guide to the intensity of a physical therapy program. After CK have normalized, gradually introduced and advanced active exercises help to restore the muscle strength lost from disease activity, immobility, and muscle atrophy. A patient's body temperature also should be monitored because a fever may be indicative of an exacerbation [34]. Preliminary MRI studies suggest some changes in inflammatory edema in active myositis (and normal healthy children) after exercise but this is relatively minimal and rapidly reversible [35–37].

Involvement of the multidisciplinary team is essential for the optimal care of all patients with DM. Consultation with a physiotherapist is recommended to prevent contractures, particularly in severely affected children. Mild weight-bearing exercises are encouraged [2]. Physiotherapy treatment from the beginning of illness is beneficial to prevent development of soft-tissue contractures and severe muscle wasting. As soon as a general improvement in clinical state is achieved, a more intensive graded program should begin. Such a program includes passive stretching and range of motion exercises, and hydrotherapy, building up to resisted exercises, gait correction, and stamina work.

A physical training program should be recommended for patients with chronic DM as an adjunct to drug therapy. Training must be carried out under medical supervision and must be adjusted to fit the needs of patients. Studies have supported the hypothesis that exercise is beneficial in the treatment of patients with inflammatory diseases of muscle. Escalante et al. [38] investigated the effects of six exercise sessions (three resistive and three nonresistive) in one patient, using CK levels as the indicator of disease acuity. The patient did not exhibit an increase in muscle strength; however, the patient's performance of daily living activities improved. During the study, however, CK increased, and the authors speculated that the increased CK was related to attempts to taper the dose of prednisone. Heikkila et al. [32] also demonstrated that short-term (3-week) intensive therapeutic exercise programs designed by a physical therapist resulted in improvements in function in 22 patients diagnosed with myositis (four of them with DM). During the study, CK serum levels were monitored and remained stable, indicating that the therapeutic exercise did not result in an increase of muscle inflammation. The benefit of physical training of 14 patients with IIMs (DM/PM) was investigated in a prospective randomized controlled study [39]. Disease duration was more than 6 months, and the drug therapy was stable for at least 3 months before the initiation of the training program. The training consisted of bicycle-based exercise and step aerobics, and took place over 6 weeks. No rise in inflammatory activity was observed; moreover, a significant improvement in muscle strength, oxygen uptake, and well-being were found in DM/PM patients as a result of physical training. Results demonstrated an improvement in both muscle strength and oxygen uptake compared with a control group, with no rise in inflammatory activity as indicated by CK levels. In a follow-up study, Wiesinger et al. [40] investigated the effects of the same exercise program carried out over a 6-month period with eight patients (six with DM and two with PM). The findings were similar to those of the first study, in which both isometric muscle strength and maximum oxygen uptake increased, with no change in serum CK levels. The patients' performance of daily living activities also improved. It has been found [41–43] a sustained increase in inorganic phosphate (Pi) in muscles of DM patients. After an exercise regimen phosphate bound to organic creatine (PCr). The Pi/PCr ratio in muscles reflects an inverse measure of energy reserve: the lower the ratio, the more energy is available for muscle contraction. During exercise, the Pi/PCr ratio increased in patients with DM and controls and rapidly returned to baseline in controls, but both Pi and PCr remained above baseline in DM patients as result of irregular Pi/PCr ratios [44]. Pi/PCr ratio increase in patients with DM is a sensitive indicator of disturbed energy metabolism. In addition to presenting higher Pi/PCr ratios than controls, DM patients also revealed prolonged recovery time for Pi and PCr before and after exercise [43]. The slow postexercise recovery was found to be associated with defects in aerobic metabolism secondary to impaired blood supply, but not primarily to abnormalities of mitochondria [43].

Although these studies give us insight about the effects of exercise when treating patients with inflammatory muscle disease in general, they are of limited usefulness in understanding the specific response of individuals with DM.

Respiratory muscle exercises and chest physiotherapy are valuable for myositis patients with generalized weakness, who are at risk of aspiration and infection.

Occupational therapists have a role in initial functional assessment. They may help with task-modification, school/classroom, and home assessment for those patients with ongoing disabilities. Apart from caring for the acutely unwell child, specialist nursing input provides for family education support for parental provision of medical care in home.

Clinical psychologists have a role to play in providing counseling to families with a child with a chronic illness such as juvenile DM, with potential major morbidity and occasional mortality. They have a particular role together with the specialist nurse in helping adolescents deal with body-image issues, educational vocational and lifestyle choices, and independence from their family group over time [45].

Physical therapy diagnoses are focused on classifying dysfunction rather than the disease itself and, therefore, are different from a medical diagnosis [34].

41.7 Diet

Many patients with DM are in negative nitrogen balance due to their wasting disease [9, 46]. A patient's diet should consist of high-calorie, rich in protein products with supplementation if necessary [47]. Vitamins should also be given [46]. Total parenteral nutrition should be administered if the patient is unable to swallow, or if dysphagia or another gastrointestinal complaint are present [47]. Low-calcium or high-phosphate diets have been previously advocated in calcinosis and juvenile DM [48]. Attention to general nutrition and prophylactic therapy for calcium/vitamin D should also be considered.

An association between DM and celiac disease in children has been documented [49–51]. Celiac disease was found to be more prevalent in patients with inflammatory myopathies than in the general population [51]. HLA-DQ2 and HLA-DQ8 allele carriers, who are known to be found more frequently among patients with IIMs, could explain the high prevalence of antigliadin antibodies in this population [51]. Song et al. [50] have suggested that patients with newly diagnosed dermatomyositis be investigated for concomitant celiac disease, even if they have no gastrointestinal symptoms. Moreover, in some patients a strict gluten-free diet may resolve both nutritional deficiencies and DM [50].

41.8 Prevention

The etiology of DM is unknown. No preventive measures have been identified. The cutaneous manifestation of disease can be induced by sunlight. Patients should avoid unnecessary sun exposure.

References

1. Mehta DP, Wortmann RL. Management guidelines for idiopathic inflammatory myopathies. *J Musculoskeletal Med* 1994; 11(9): 38–43.
2. Oddis CV, Medsger TA. Current management of polymyositis and dermatomyositis. *Drugs* 1989; 37: 382–390.
3. Dau PC. Plasmapheresis in idiopathic inflammatory myopathy. Experience with 35 patients. *Arch Neurol* 1981; 38: 544–552.
4. Dau PC, Bennington JL. Plasmapheresis in childhood dermatomyositis. *J Pediatr* 1981; 98: 237–240.
5. Anderson L, Ziter FA. Plasmapheresis via central catheter in dermatomyositis: a new method for selected pediatric patients. *J Pediatr* 1981; 98: 240–241.
6. Miller FW, Leitman SF, Cronin ME, et al. Controlled trial of plasma exchange and leukopheresis in polymyositis and dermatomyositis. *N Engl J Med* 1992; 326: 1380–1384.
7. Kovacs SO, Kovacs SC. Dermatomyositis. *J Am Acad Dermatol* 1998; 39: 899–920.
8. Bennington JL, Dau PC. Patients with polymyositis and dermatomyositis who undergo plasmapheresis therapy. *Arch Neurol* 1981; 38: 553–560.
9. Boyd AS, Neldner KH. Therapeutic options in dermatomyositis/polymyositis. *Int J Dermatol* 1994; 33: 240–250.
10. Heriksson KG, Sandstedt P. Polymyositis: treatment and prognosis. *Acta Neurol* 1982; 65: 280–300.
11. Macpherson A, Berth Jones J, Graham-Brown R. Carcinoma associated dermatomyositis responding to plasmapheresis. *Clin Exp Dermatol* 1989; 14: 304–305.

12. Fukunaga E, Kunishigea M, Mitsuia T, et al. Severe dermatomyositis with rhabdomyolysis and paralytic ileus: a case successfully treated with plasmapheresis and intravenous immunoglobulin. *EFNS Eur J Neurol* 2002; 9: 687–702.
13. Brewer EJ, Gianini EH, Rossen RD, et al. Plasma exchange therapy of a childhood onset dermatomyositis patient. *Arthritis Rheum* 1980; 23: 509–513.
14. Herson S, Lok C, Roujeau JC, et al. Plasma exchange in dermatomyositis and polymyositis. Retrospective study of 38 cases of plasma exchange. *Ann Med Interne (Paris)* 1989; 140(6): 453–455 [French].
15. Lok C, Herson S, Roujeau JC, et al. Echanges plasmatiques au cours des dermatomyositis. *Ann Dermatol Venereol* 1989; 116: 219–224.
16. Salvaneschi L, Perotti C, Torretta L. Adverse effects associated with extracorporeal photochemotherapy. *Transfusion* 2000; 40: 121.
17. De Wilde A, Dispalatro FX, Geller A, et al. Extracorporeal photochemotherapy as adjunctive treatment in juvenile dermatomyositis: a case report. *Arch Dermatol* 1992; 128: 1656–1657.
18. Morgan SH, Bernstein RM, Coppen J, et al. Total body irradiation and the course of polymyositis. *Arthritis Rheum* 1985; 28: 831–835.
19. Engel WK, Lichter AS, Galdi AP. Polymyositis: remarkable response to total body irradiation. *Lancet* 1981; 1: 658.
20. Hubbard WH. Remission from polymyositis after total body irradiation. *BMJ* 1982; 284: 1915–1916.
21. Kelly JJ, Madoc-Jone H, Adelman LS, et al. Response to total body irradiation in dermatomyositis. *Muscle Nerve* 1988; 11: 120–123.
22. Schalon F, Thomas PK, Senanayke LF. Remission from polymyositis after total body irradiation [letter]. *Br Med J* 1982; i: 658.
23. Cherin W, Herson S, Coutellier A, et al. Failure of total body irradiation in polymyositis: report of three cases. *Br J Rheumatol* 1992; 31: 282–283.
24. Lane R, Hudgson P. Thymectomy for polymyositis. *Lancet* 1984; 1: 626.
25. Cumming W. Thymectomy for refractory dermatomyositis. *Muscle Nerve* 1989; 12: 424–425.
26. Samarsinghe SR, Cleary G, Veys P, et al. Autologous stem cell transplantation for juvenile dermatomyositis. *Arch Dis Child* 2002; 86: S48–49.
27. Elhasid R, Rowe JM, Berkowitz D, et al. Disappearance of diffuse calcinosis following autologous stem cell transplantation in a child with autoimmune disease. *Bone Marrow Transplant* 2004; 33(12): 1257–1259.
28. Bohan A, Peter JB, Bowman RL, et al. A computer-assisted analysis of 153 patients with polymyositis and dermatomyositis. *Medicine* 1977; 56: 255–286.
29. Stoll T, Bruhlmann P, Stucki G, et al. Muscle strength assessment in polymyositis and dermatomyositis evaluation of the reliability and clinical course of a new, quantitative, easily applicable method. *J Rheumatol* 1995; 22: 473–477.
30. Brown CB, Marshall SF. Connective tissue disease update: focus on dermatomyositis. *Consultant* 1999; 28: 67–75.
31. Alexanderson H, Stenstrom CH, Lundberg I. Safety of a home exercise regimen programme in patient with polymyositis and dermatomyositis: a pilot study. *Rheumatology* 1999; 38: 608–611.
32. Heikkila S, Viitanen JV, Kautiainen H, et al. Rehabilitation in myositis. *Physiotherapy* 2001; 87: 301–309.
33. Rendt K. Inflammatory myopathies: narrowing the differential diagnosis. *Clev Clin J Med* 2001; 68: 505–519.
34. Cleland JA, Venzke JW. Dermatomyositis: evolution of a diagnosis. *Phys Ther* 2003; 83: 932–945.
35. Summers RM, Brune AM, Choyke PL, et al. Juvenile idiopathic inflammatory myopathy: exercise-induced changes in muscle at short inversion time inversion-recovery MR, imaging. *Radiology* 1998; 209: 191–196.

36. Maillard SM, Jones R, Owens C, et al. The effects of exercise on the MRI parameters of inflammation of thigh muscle in children with juvenile dermatomyositis. *Ann Rheum Dis* 2002; 61: S144.
37. Maillard SM, Jones R, Owens CM, et al. Quantitative assessments of the effects of a single exercise session on muscles in juvenile dermatomyositis. *Arthritis Rheum* 2005; 53: 558–564.
38. Escalante A, Miller L, Beardmore TD. Resistive exercise in the rehabilitation of polymyositis/dermatomyositis. *J Rheumatol* 1993; 20: 1340–1344.
39. Wiesinger GF, Quittan M, Aringer M, et al. Improvement of physical fitness and muscle strength in polymyositis/dermatomyositis patients by a training programme. *Br J Rheumatol* 1998; 37(2): 196–200.
40. Wiesinger GF, Quittan M, Graninger M, et al. Benefit of 6 months long-term physical training in polymyositis/dermatomyositis patients. *Br J Rheumatol* 1998; 37(12): 1338–1342.
41. Chung YL, Smith EC, Williams SC, et al. In vivo proton magnetic resonance spectroscopy in polymyositis and dermatomyositis: a preliminary study. *Eur J Med Res* 1997; 28: 183–187.
42. Park JH, Nierman KJ, Ryder NM, et al. Muscle abnormalities in juvenile dermatomyositis patients: P-31 magnetic resonance spectroscopy studies. *Arthritis Rheum* 2000; 13: 2359–2367.
43. Cea G, Bendahan D, Manners D, et al. Reduced oxidative phosphorylation and proton efflux suggest reduced capillary blood supply in skeletal muscle of patients with dermatomyositis and polymyositis: a quantitative (31)P-magnetic resonance spectroscopy and MRI study. *Brain* 2002; 125: 1635–1645.
44. Pfleiderer B, Lange J, Loske KD, et al. Metabolic disturbances during short exercises in dermatomyositis revealed by real-time functional ^{31}P magnetic resonance spectroscopy. *Rheumatology* 2004; 43: 696–703.
45. Uziel Y, Nemet D, Maimon E, et al. Juvenile dermatomyositis: medical and psychosocial team approach. *Clin Exp Rheumatol* 2002; 20(2): 256.
46. Tuffanelli D, Lavole PE. Prognosis and therapy of polymyositis/dermatomyositis. *Clin Dermatol* 1988; 6: 93–104.
47. Winkelmann RK. Dermatomyositis in childhood. *Clin Rheum Dis* 1982; 8: 353–368.
48. Sewell JR, Liyanage B, Ansell BM. Calcinosis in juvenile dermatomyositis. *Skeletal Radiol* 1978; 3: 137–143.
49. Marie I, Lecomte F, Hachulla E, et al. An uncommon association: celiac disease and dermatomyositis in adults. *Clin Exp Rheumatol* 2001; 19(2): 201–203.
50. Song MS, Farber D, Bitton A, et al. Dermatomyositis associated with celiac disease: response to a gluten-free diet. *Can J Gastroenterol* 2006; 20(6): 433–435.
51. Selva-O'Callaghan A, Casellas F, de Torres I, et al. Celiac disease and antibodies associated with celiac disease in patients with inflammatory myopathy. *Muscle Nerve* 2007; 35(1): 49–54.

Management and Control

Evolution and Prognosis of Dermatomyositis

42

The initial cases of DM in German literature were fatal [1–3], but recoveries were soon observed [4, 5]. In the precorticosteroid era, the largest review, of 153 cases with adequate follow-up, determined a mortality rate of 61% [6]. Most surviving patients had permanent sequelae (e.g., muscle atrophy, joint contractures, and calcinosis). Later, in more studies of noncorticosteroid-treated patients, the mortality rate improved to 37%, and 33% of patients had good recoveries [7–9]. However, the prognosis of DM was significantly worse in older patients.

In contrast, case reports of "spontaneous" recoveries are documented in classic DM [4–6] and amyopathic DM [10].

Relapses tended to occur within the first 2 years after the initiation of treatment, and during the tapering phase of treatment [11]. Patients with PM and CTD-associated myositis had a higher relapse rate than that for "classic" DM and paraneoplastic DM patients. Relapses were defined as a sustained elevation in serum CK levels in absence of an alternative etiology. Advanced age and increased duration of symptoms prior to treatment initiation had nonsignificant associations with an increased risk of relapse [11].

42.1 Prognosis

Classic factors that affect prognosis of DM include:

(i) Age of patient
(ii) Male sex
(iii) African-American race
(iv) Severity of myositis
(v) Presence of complications (dysphagia, dysphonia, pulmonary, and cardiac involvement)
(vi) Associated malignancy
(vii) Presence of anti-Jo-1 or anti-SRP autoantibodies

L.A. Dourmishev and A.L. Dourmishev, *Dermatomyositis: Advances in Recognition, Understanding and Management,* © Springer-Verlag Berlin Heidelberg 2009

(viii) Delayed or inadequate treatment or resistance to applied therapy [12–16]

The prognosis in the patient with amyopathic DM is good if there is an absence of malignancy or pulmonal involvement.

In juvenile DM, systemic vasculitis and vascular occlusion were important factors for prognosis. Fatal cases of childhood DM in which systemic vasculitis and vascular occlusion were evident have been reported [17, 18].

Morbidity and mortality in DM and PM remain a significant problem. Several studies have attempted to identify independent risk factors predicting a poor outcome. In some analyses of populations reflecting inflammatory myositis, poor prognostic factors included recalcitrant disease, delay in diagnosis and therapy, advanced age, malignancy, fever, asthenia–anorexia, pulmonary interstitial fibrosis, dysphagia, and leukocytosis [14, 19]. ILD has also been regarded as a major cause of death, in addition to malignancy, cardiac complications, and iatrogenic complications [20, 21]. ILD, cardiac complications, including cor pulmonale, esophageal involvement, or calcinosis have tended to occur in patients with noncancer-associated DM/PM [22].

Available data on survival of patients with IIMs, based on studies with sufficient numbers of patients, from the USA, France, UK, Israel, and Hungary [12, 14, 16, 23–26] are presented in Table 42.1. All of these long-term large series had different inclusion criteria, especially concerning the studied subgroups of IIMs, particularly of cancer-associated myositis patients. In one long-term follow-up study, 46 patients with IIMs (23 with adult-onset PM, 14 "classic" DM in adults, one with childhood-onset DM and eight with overlap syndrome) were reported [26]. During the disease course, seven patients (15.2%) went into full remission, eight (17.4%) had monophasic illness, nine (19.6%) had a relapsing-remitting course, 16 (34.8%) had chronic progressive illness, and six (13.04%) died. Patients with myositis displayed significantly poorer health than the general population. Those with

Table 42.1 Long-term survival data for patients with PM/DM

Author	Period	No of Patients	Survival (%) 1 Year	5 Years	>5 Years
Medsger et al. (1971) USA [23]	1947–1968	124	72	65	53 (7 years)
Benbassat et al. (1985) Israel [12]	1956–1976	92	72	52	–
Hochberg et al. (1986) USA [24]	1970–1981	76	94.5	80.4	72.8 (8 years)
Maugars et al. (1996) France [14]	1973–1984	69	82.6	66.7	55.4 (9 years)
Marie et al. (2001) France [25]	1983–1998	77	83	77	61 (15 years)
Sultan et al. (2002) England [26]	1978–1999	46	–	95	83.8 (10 years)
Danko et al. (2004) Hungary [16]	1976–2002	162	95	92	89 (10 years)

chronic progressive illness had significantly greater bodily pain than those with a relapsing–remitting illness. The 5-year survival rate was 95% and 10-year survival rate was 83.8%.

Survival rates for PM/DM are higher than those reported before the corticosteroid era. Many factors have contributed to this, such as the earlier use of immunosuppressive agents during the course of disease and better general medical care. The differences may also be due to changes in the case mix, therapy, and comorbidity. Long-term prognosis cannot be determined during a follow-up period of less than 5 years, as many cases are still active at this time and the prognosis can improve over time.

Improved survival of patients with IIM in the past years could be due to the following factors [16]:

(i) Early diagnosis and recognition of milder forms of the disease due to use of new diagnostic tools and serologic testing
(ii) Early use of more appropriate and more aggressive immunosuppressive and supportive therapy
(iii) Regular follow-up in departments specialized in the diagnosis and treatment of the disease
(iv) Better general medical care
(v) Better understanding of the natural history of the disease

Prior to the corticosteroid era, juvenile DM had a high mortality rate (>30%), and left 50% of those who survived with serious permanent impairments. After the introduction of corticosteroids, mortality rapidly dropped, to less than 10%, and is currently reported to be less than 2–3% [27]. Since most of the children with this illness survive now, the greater is the interest in long-term outcomes. However, for the present relatively little is known in long-term outcomes about morbidity, mortality, physical function, quality of life, pain, educational and vocational achievement, patient satisfaction, and ongoing disease activity.

References

1. Hepp P. Über Pseudo-trichinose, eine besondere Form von acuter parenchymatose Polymyositis. *Berl Klin Wochenschr* 1887; 24: 297, 332.
2. Unverricht H. Über eine eigenthümliche Form von akuter Muskelentzündung mit einem der Trichinose ähnelnden Krankheitsbilde. *Müncher Med Wochenschr* 1887; 34: 488–492.
3. Wagner E. Fall einer seltnen Muskelkrankheit. *Dtsch Arch Heilk* 1863; 4: 282–283.
4. Lewy B. Zur Lehre von der primären acuten Polymyositis. *Berlin Klin Wochenschr* 1893; 30: 475–477.
5. Unverricht H. Dermatomyositis acuta. *Dtsch Med Wochenschr* 1891; 17: 41–44.
6. Schuermann H. Zur Klinik und Pathogenese der Dermatomyositis (Polymyositis). *Arch Dermat Syph (Wien)* 1939; 178: 414–468.
7. Wedgwood RJ, Cook CD, Cohen J. Dermatomyositis. Report of 26 cases in children with a discussion of endocrine therapy in 13. *Pediatrics* 1953; 12: 447–466.
8. Everett MA, Curtis AC. Dermatomyositis. A review of nineteen cases in adolescents and children. *Arch Intern Med* 1957; 100: 70–76.

9. Winkelmann RK, Mulder DW, Lambert EH, et al. Course of dermatomyositis–polymyositis: comparison of untreated and cortisone-treated patients. *Mayo Clin Proc* 1968; 43: 545–556.
10. Jordan JR, Paruthi S, Pichardo RO, et al. Spontaneously remitting dermatomyositis. *JEADV* 2004; 18: 495–498.
11. Agarwal SK, Monach PA, Docken WP, et al. Characterization of relapses in adult idiopathic inflammatory myopathies. *Clin Rheumatol* 2006; 25(4): 476–481.
12. Benbassat J, Geffel D, Larholt K, et al. Prognostic factors in polymyositis/dermatomyositis: a computer-assisted analysis of 92 cases. *Arthritis Rheum* 1985; 28: 249–255.
13. Love LA, Leff RL, Fraser DD, et al. A new approach to the classification of idiopathic inflammatory myopathy: myositis-specific autoantibodies define useful homogeneous patient groups. *Medicine* 1991; 70: 360–374.
14. Maugars YM, Berthelot JMM, Abbas AA, et al. Long term prognosis of 69 patients with dermatomyositis or polymyositis 1996. *Clin Exp Rheumatol* 1996; 14: 263–274.
15. Marie I, Hatron P-Y, Levesque H, et al. Influence of age on characteristics of polymyositis and dermatomyositis in adults. *Medicine* 1999; 78: 139–147.
16. Danko K, Ponyi A, Constantin T, et al. Long-term survival of patients with idiopathic inflammatory myopathies according to clinical features. A longitudinal study of 162 cases. *Medicine* 2004; 83: 35–42.
17. Falcini F, Trapani S, Ermini M, et al. Systemic vasculitis in juvenile dermatomyositis: a fatal case. *Clin Exp Rheumatol* 1995; 13: 531–532.
18. Takeda T, Fujisaku A, Jodo S, et al. Fatal vascular occlusion in juvenile dermatomyositis. *Ann Rheum Dis* 1998; 57: 172–176.
19. Mautner GH, Grossman ME, Silvers DN, et al. Epidermal necrosis as a predictive sign of malignancy in adult dermatomyositis. *Cutis* 1998; 61: 190–194.
20. Basset-Seguin N, Roujeau JC, Gherardi R, et al. Prognostic factors and predictive signs of malignancy in adult dermatomyositis. A study of 32 cases. *Arch Dermatol* 1990; 126: 633–637.
21. Xue L, Chen X, Chen S. Prognostic factors of dermatomyositis: analysis of 119 cases. *Chin J Intern Med* 1997; 36: 32–35.
22. Chen YJ, Wu CY, Shen JL. Predicting factors of malignancy in dermatomyositis and polymyositis: a case-control study. *Br J Dermatol* 2001; 144: 825–831.
23. Medsger TA, Robinson H, Masi AT. Factors affecting survivorship in polymyositis. A lifetable study of 124 patients. *Arthritis Rheum* 1971; 14: 249–258.
24. Hochberg MC, Feldman D, Stevens MB. Adult onset polymyositis–dermatomyositis: an analysis of clinical and laboratory factors and survival in 76 patients with a review of the literature. *Semin Arthritis Rheum* 1986; 15: 168–191.
25. Marie I, Hachulla E, Hatron P-Y, et al. Polymyositis and dermatomyositis: short term and long term outcome, and predictive factors of prognosis. *J Rheumatol* 2001; 28: 2230–2237.
26. Sultan SM, Ioannou Y, Moss K, et al. Outcome in patients with idiopathic inflammatory myositis: morbidity and mortality. *Rheumatology* 2002; 41: 22–26.
27. Huber A, Feldman BM. Long-term outcomes in juvenile dermatomyositis: how did we get here and where are we going? *Curr Rheumatol Rep* 2005; 7: 441–446.

Index

MIX
Papier aus verantwortungsvollen Quellen
Paper from responsible sources
FSC® C105338

If you have any concerns about our products,
you can contact us on
ProductSafety@springernature.com

In case Publisher is established outside the EU,
the EU authorized representative is:
Springer Nature Customer Service Center GmbH
Europaplatz 3, 69115 Heidelberg, Germany

Printed by Libri Plureos GmbH
in Hamburg, Germany